The
Dark Art
of Blood
Cultures

The *Dark Art* of Blood Cultures

EDITED BY

Wm. Michael Dunne, Jr.
bioMérieux, Inc.
Durham, North Carolina
Washington University School of Medicine in St. Louis
St. Louis, Missouri
Duke University School of Medicine
Durham, North Carolina

and

Carey-Ann D. Burnham
Washington University School of Medicine in St. Louis
St. Louis, Missouri

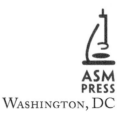

ASM
PRESS
WASHINGTON, DC

Disclaimer: To the best of the publisher's knowledge, this publication provides information concerning the subject matter covered that is accurate as of the date of publication. The publisher is not providing legal, medical, or other professional services. Any reference herein to any specific commercial products, procedures, or services by trade name, trademark, manufacturer, or otherwise does not constitute or imply endorsement, recommendation, or favored status by the American Society for Microbiology (ASM). The views and opinions of the author(s) expressed in this publication do not necessarily state or reflect those of ASM, and they shall not be used to advertise or endorse any product.

Library of Congress Cataloging-in-Publication Data

Names: Dunne, W. Michael, editor. | Burnham, Carey-Ann D., editor.
Title: The dark art of blood cultures / edited by William Michael Dunne, Jr., bioMerieux, Inc. Durham, North Carolina, and Carey-Ann Burnham, Washington University School of Medicine in St. Louis, St. Louis, Missouri.
Description: Washington, DC : ASM Press, [2018] | Includes index.
Identifiers: LCCN 2017032783 (print) | LCCN 2017034981 (ebook) |
ISBN 9781555819828 (ebook) | ISBN 9781555819811 (pbk.)
Subjects: LCSH: Blood–Cultures and culture media. | Septicemia–Microbiology.
| Diagnostic microbiology.
Classification: LCC QR66 (ebook) | LCC QR66 .D37 2018 (print) | DDC 579–dc23
LC record available at https://lccn.loc.gov/2017032783

10   9   8   7   6   5   4   3   2   1

Address editorial correspondence to
ASM Press, 1752 N St., N.W.,
Washington, DC 20036-2904, USA

Send orders to ASM Press, P.O. Box 605, Herndon, VA 20172, USA
Phone: 800-546-2416; 703-661-1593
Fax: 703-661-1501
E-mail: books@asmusa.org
Online: http://www.asmscience.org

Cover Image: An ill man who is being bled by his doctor. Coloured etching by J. Sneyd, 1804, after J. Gillray. 1804. Courtesy of Wellcome Library, London https://wellcomeimages.org/indexplus/image/V0011195.html. Copyrighted work available under Creative Commons Attribution only licence CC BY 4.0 http://creativecommons.org/licenses/by/4.0/.

To Linda and Ryley for keeping us sane.

Editors' Disclaimer

While references are used extensively to support observations, published data, clinical trials, and laboratory comparisons of blood culture systems, culture media, protocols and procedures, etc., it is inevitable that personal opinions and small biases might have unintentionally snuck in to the final copy. The editors were very attuned and sensitive to this possibility and made every attempt to avoid blatant conflicts of interest without interrupting the independence of the authors. All of the individuals and commercial entities that have contributed to the advancement of the science of blood cultures have had a significant influence on the field and we thank them all.

Contents

Contributors

Neil W. Anderson
Washington University School of Medicine
Saint Louis, Missouri

Robyn Atkinson-Dunn
Utah Public Health Laboratory
Taylorsville, Utah

Eileen M. Burd
Department of Pathology and Laboratory
  Medicine
Department of Medicine
Division of Infectious Diseases
Emory Antibiotic Resistance Center
Emory University School of Medicine
Atlanta, Georgia

Carey-Ann D. Burnham
Washington University School of Medicine
St. Louis, Missouri

Robin R. Chamberland
Saint Louis University School of Medicine
Saint Louis, Missouri

Carl O. Deetz
Analytical Pathology Services
Saint Louis, Missouri

Christopher Doern
Department of Pathology
Virginia Commonwealth University
  Health System
Richmond, Virginia

Wm. Michael Dunne, Jr.
bioMérieux, Inc.
Durham, North Carolina
Washington University School of Medicine
St. Louis, Missouri
Duke University School of Medicine
Durham, North Carolina

Matthew L. Faron
Medical College of Wisconsin
Milwaukee, Wisconsin

Bradley Ford
Department of Pathology
University of Iowa Carver College of
  Medicine
Iowa City, Iowa

Mark D. Gonzalez
Department of Pathology and Laboratory
  Medicine
Children's Healthcare of Atlanta
Atlanta, Georgia

Robert C. Jerris
Department of Pathology and Laboratory
  Medicine
Children's Healthcare of Atlanta
Atlanta, Georgia

George Kallstrom
Department of Pathology and Laboratory
  Medicine
Summa Health System

Akron, Ohio
Department of Pathology
Northeast Ohio Medical University
    (NEOMED)
Rootstown, Ohio

William Lainhart
Washington University School of Medicine
St. Louis, Missouri

Nathan A. Ledeboer
Medical College of Wisconsin
Milwaukee, Wisconsin

Robert S. Liao
PeaceHealth Laboratories
Springfield, Oregon

Erin McElvania TeKippe
University of Texas Southwestern and
    Children's Health
Dallas, Texas

Allison R. McMullen
Medical College of Georgia at Augusta
    University
Augusta, Georgia

Morgan A. Pence
Cook Children's Medical Center
Fort Worth, Texas

Paula Revell
Departments of Pathology and
    Pediatrics
Baylor College of Medicine
Houston, Texas

Barbara Robinson-Dunn
Beaumont Health System
Royal Oak, Michigan

Robert J. Tibbetts
Henry Ford Health System
Detroit, Michigan

Lars F. Westblade
Department of Pathology and Laboratory
    Medicine
Department of Medicine
Division of Infectious Diseases
Weill Cornell Medicine
New York, New York

Craig B. Wilen
Washington University School of
    Medicine
St. Louis, Missouri

Melanie L. Yarbrough
Washington University School of
    Medicine
Saint Louis, Missouri

Preface

Many years ago, we began kicking around the possibility of devoting an entire text to the subject of blood culture technology and the continuing evolution that has occurred over the past decades (and centuries if you start with historical perspective). As with any idea, there is often an energy of activation to get the project underway but once that occurred, we were able to gain the support of those involved.

This project was a team effort, and each of the chapters was authored and/or coauthored by the fellows of the Medical and Public Health Microbiology training program established at Washington University School of Medicine and Barnes-Jewish Hospital in 2001. We are equally proud of each of the fellows, and any proceeds generated from this publication will be funneled back into the training program to help keep it alive. We are also thankful for those contributors who worked with former or current fellows to generate some of the chapters presented in the text. The title and cover we selected for this book underscores the slightly warped sense of humor we have integrated into the training program over the years, and even today, there are a number of inside jokes shared by this family as it continues to grow. In that vein (there's the first pun), a good microbiologist who recovers *Eikenella corrodens* from a blood culture will always ask about bite marks. It is our hope that this compendium of all things blood culture will also continue to expand with future editions and will always include graduates of the Washington University program both before and after they leave to direct clinical microbiology laboratories of their own. We might have not provided a complete evaluation of all the technologies that have come and gone over the years, but we'll stick with it (second pun).

WM. MICHAEL DUNNE, JR.
CAREY-ANN D. BURNHAM

About the Editors

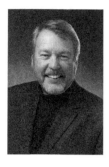

Wm. Michael Dunne, Jr., PhD, is currently a senior research fellow for bioMérieux, Inc. in Durham, North Carolina. Prior to joining bioMérieux, he was Medical Director of the Diagnostic Microbiology Laboratory at Barnes-Jewish Hospital and Professor of Pathology and Immunology, Molecular Microbiology, Pediatrics, and Medicine at Washington University School of Medicine in St. Louis from 2000–2011 and remains on the faculty there. During that time, he established an internationally-recognized training program in medical and public health microbiology, which is still active under the direction of Carey-Ann Burnham. He has previously served as Medical Director of Microbiology Laboratories at Henry Ford Hospital (Detroit, Michigan), Texas Children's Hospital (Baylor College of Medicine, Houston, Texas) and Children's Hospital of Wisconsin (Medical College of Wisconsin, Milwaukee, Wisconsin, where he had received his PhD in 1982). Dr. Dunne is a Diplomate of the American Board of Medical Microbiology and a Fellow of the American Academy of Microbiology, the Infectious Diseases Society of America, the Pediatric Infectious Diseases Society, and the Canadian College of Microbiology. He served as a senior editor of the *Journal of Clinical Microbiology* for ten years and remains on the editorial board. He is also an Adjunct Professor of Pediatrics at Duke University School of Medicine, Durham, North Carolina. He has authored or coauthored over 170 peer-reviewed publications and 10 chapters, in addition to this book.

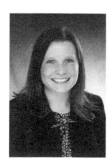

Carey-Ann D. Burnham, PhD, completed her PhD in Medical Sciences at the University of Alberta in Edmonton, Alberta, Canada and her postdoctoral training in Medical and Public Health Microbiology at Washington University under the direction of Wm. Michael Dunne, Jr. Currently, Burnham is an Associate Professor of Pathology & Immunology, Molecular Microbiology, and Pediatrics at Washington University in St. Louis School of Medicine. Burnham has a keen interest in education and is the Program Director for the Medical and

Public Health Microbiology Fellowship at Washington University, the co-editor of Medical Microbiology Question of the Day, and the section editor of "The Brief Case" for the *Journal of Clinical Microbiology*. Burnham's research program focuses on development of diagnostic assays for infectious diseases and the transmission and epidemiology of antimicrobial resistance in bacteria. Burnham has authored or coauthored more than 100 peer-reviewed publications in addition to numerous invited articles and book chapters.

The Dark Art of Blood Cultures
Edited by Wm. Michael Dunne, Jr. and Carey-Ann D. Burnham
© 2018 American Society for Microbiology, Washington, DC
doi:10.1128/9781555819811.ch1

Historical Perspectives on the Art and Science of Blood Culture

Wm. Michael Dunne, Jr.[1,2,3]

From an historic point of view, one can divide the evolution of blood culture technology into four distinct "archeological" periods that I refer to (tongue in cheek) as the "Manualithic" (pre-1970), the "Bactecene" (1970 to 1990), the "Continuous Monitorassic" (1990 to 2000), and the "Ampliaissance" (post-2000) ages (Fig. 1). Each of these denotes a quantum shift in the use of technology to increase the sensitivity and decrease the time-to-detection of microorganisms in blood. While the rate of improvement in both speed and sensitivity has clearly reached steady state over recent years, and the ultimate goal of directly detecting microorganisms causing bacteremia/fungemia/sepsis from blood has not yet been achieved, progress is most definitely moving forward and the tools being developed for that purpose are impressive. However, before we find out how far we have come, it is best to review where the concept of finding microorganisms in blood began, and some historians would conclude that it started with Athanasius Kircher (Fig. 2).

Kircher was an ordained Jesuit priest whose life nearly spanned the entire 17th century (1602 to 1680). He is referred to as a polymath/savant and his life story reads more like Indiana Jones and the Arc of the Covenant (1). Kircher was a scholar and true renaissance man who became well versed in linguistics, astronomy, magnetism, volcanology, archeology, and acoustics, just to name a few of his scientific hobbies. When the bubonic plague struck Rome in full force in 1656, Kircher extended his credentials to include

[1]bioMérieux, Inc., Durham, NC 27712
[2]Washington University School of Medicine, St. Louis, MO 63110
[3]Duke University School of Medicine, Durham, NC 27703

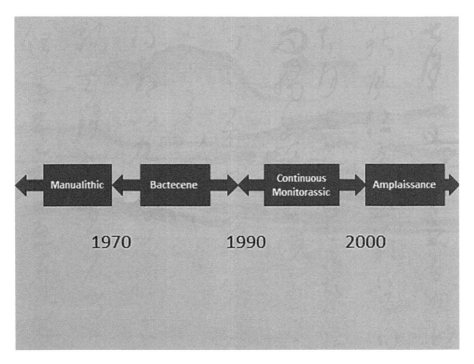

Figure 1 The archeological periods of blood culture evolution.

ad hoc pathologist and infectious diseases researcher (1, 2). Using a primitive microscope, he described observing tiny worms or *vermes* (*contagia animate*) in the "verminous blood of fever patients" and became the first to develop a germ theory of disease, which was published 2 years later (*Scrutinium physico-medicum contagiosæ luis*. Romæ: Typis Mascardi, 1658; references 2, 3). In this treatise, he describes the disease thusly: "*Pestis est flagellum and sagitta Dei ob peccata hominibus immissa*," which loosely translates into "plague is the whip and arrows of an angry God used to punish sinful humans." From a purely microbiological standpoint, two words in this description jump out: pestis and flagellum. Of course, the former became the species name for the causative agent of bubonic plague. However, the latter was inaccurate, because *Yersinia pestis* is nonmotile and lacks flagella. He further stated that "vinegar, milk, and the blood of those sick with fever are full of worms invisible, however, to the unaided eye. That the matter is not otherwise than I have said, the putrid blood of those afflicted by fevers has fully convinced me; I have found it, an hour or so after letting, so crowded with worms as to well high dumbfound me; and I had even been persuaded forthwith that man

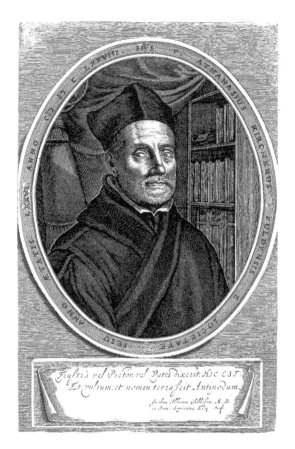

Figure 2 Cornelis Bloemaert II, *Portrait of Athanasius Kircher*, 1664/1678. Kircher was a Jesuit priest who launched the notion that certain diseases were caused by microscopic organisms carried in the blood and published his germ theory of disease in 1658 amid the plague epidemic in Rome. The quotation loosely translates to "Plague is the whip and arrows of an angry God used to punish humans." Note the Latin words *pestis* and *flagellum* in the quotation that had unintended contemporary application in current bacteriology. Reprinted from reference 1, with permission.

both alive and dead swarms with numberless but yet invisible worms; and that this may be the meaning of the words of Job: 'I have said to corruption, thou art my father; to the worms, my mother and my sister.'" As fate would have it, the microscope Father Kircher used likely lacked the resolution to visualize *Y. pestis*. What he actually observed remains a mystery, but it was probably clumps of red blood cells (3, 4). However, his speculation that bubonic plague was indeed blood borne and caused by a microorganism was entirely spot on, albeit perhaps a lucky guess (2, 4). He also opined that infectious diseases were not transmitted through the air but rather by person-to-person contact or via another living thing. Kircher also unintentionally invented infection prevention by offering ways of avoiding disease through piety, repentance, and acts of mercy which did not preclude leaving the city, having adequate ventilation, or using odorous substances (2, 4). In fact, it was not until nearly 25 years later that Antonie van Leeuwenhoek had developed a microscope with sufficient resolution (most likely in combination with some form of dark-field illumination) to observe a microorganism the size of *Y. pestis* (5, 6). So in a sense, Father Kircher was the father of the concept of blood-borne disease.

In a continuation of the theory that blood harbors agents of infection, Professor Jean Antoine Villemin (Fig. 3), a French physician, reported to the Académie de Médecine in 1868 that the injection of blood, sputum, or granulomatous material from animals or humans with tuberculosis into the veins of laboratory animals (rabbits, dogs, cows, etc.) generated lesions in the lungs, bone, and viscera of these animals that were indistinguishable from those produced by active infection (7). Furthermore, Dr. Villemin stressed that the lesions thusly generated via venous inoculation were quite distinct from embolic lesions generated by the inoculation of inert materials such as dust or even pus from other infectious processes. In the strictest sense, Villemin had just described a "biological blood culture," i.e., the use of laboratory animals to recover agents of blood-borne infection.

At the turn of the 20th century, just prior to the outbreak of World War I, the process of culturing blood from septic patients was already a complex

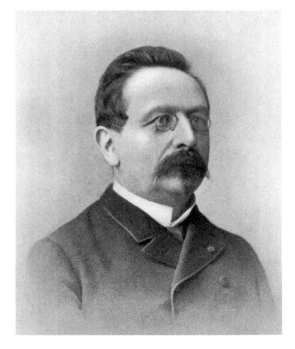

Figure 3 Dr. Jean Antoine Villemin, a French physician, reported to the Académie de Médecine in 1868 that the injection of blood, sputum, or granulomatous material from animals or humans with tuberculosis into the veins of laboratory animals (rabbits, dogs, cows, etc.) generated lesions in the lungs, bone, and viscera of these animals that were indistinguishable from those produced by active infection.

affair beginning with preparation of the skin surface prior to drawing a sample (8). It was recommended that preparation for a blood draw should take place at least an hour prior to collection by using green soap, alcohol, and bichloride of mercury in succession to cleanse the skin as one would do to prepare for surgery. Blood should be collected using a sterilized syringe (30 min of boiling or hot-air chamber) using a linen bandage as a tourniquet. Approximately 10 ml was the target collection volume, and this could be mixed with sterile 2% ammonium oxalate to prevent clotting so that "transfers can be made more leisurely to culture media." In cases where transportation to the laboratory might be delayed, cultures could be prepared at bedside (point-of-care system?). Recommended media combinations consisted of glucose-meat-infusion agar and broth; the former to be melted and combined with blood (0.25 to 1.0 ml) to prepare pour plates. Three flasks containing between 100 and 150 ml of broth were to be inoculated with "varying" volumes of blood, but one flask should be at high dilution. It was further suggested to add powdered calcium carbonate to one flask to ensure a neutral pH, thus supporting the growth of either pneumococci or streptococci that are "sensitive to acid" (do not tell oral streptococci this!) and to "develop and retain their vitality." It was recognized at this point in time that contaminants posed a challenge to interpretation, but one could look at the frequency of isolation (one flask or one plate only) or location (near the edges or on the surface of the pour plate) as an indication of contamination. It was also considered a good idea to regard all staphylococci recovered from blood with suspicion. *Staphylococcus albus* (now *S. epidermidis*/coagulase-negative *Staphylococcus* spp.) should most often be deemed a skin contaminant, whereas the isolation of *Staphylococcus pyogenes aureus* from a single blood culture should be substantiated with a second (8). Patients with suspected typhoid fever prompted an entirely different blood culture strategy that was based on clinical investigations of Coleman and Buxton, Conradi, Schottmueller, and Castellani, as discussed in reference 9. For this method, flasks containing 20 ml of a mixture of ox bile, glycerin, and pepton (peptone) were inoculated with 3 ml of blood and incubated for 18 to 24 h. At that time, samples were subcultured to lactose-litmus agar, and isolated colonies were identified using agglutination or additional biochemical tests. This protocol produced a positivity rate of 89% during the first week of illness, 73% during the second, 60% during the third, 38% during the fourth, and 26% thereafter. In the eighth edition of the *Manual of Bacteriology*, Muir and Ritchie promote two approaches for the culture of blood depending on the organism(s) being sought (10). For enteric bacilli, it was recommended to mix 5 ml of blood with 10 ml of sterilized ox bile or 50 ml of a 0.5% solution of bile salts in a 1% solution of sodium citrate and incubate the mixture. When examining for other organisms such as streptococci, however, it was suggested that 5 to 10 ml of blood be added to a large volume of liquid medium (e.g., 100 ml)—an interesting observation considering that the recommended blood-to-broth ratio in the absence of neutralizing resins remains the same even today. They also mention the use of trypsin added to broth to neutralize the antibacterial properties of blood and to prevent clotting (Douglas and Colebrook cited in the chapter but no reference provided). The trypsin/broth blood culture medium could be made ahead of time and stored in the ice chest for several weeks.

At the onset of World War I, Mildred Clough, a physician/microbiologist at Johns Hopkins University, first reported on the use of a lysis-centrifugation procedure for the recovery of *Mycobacterium tuberculosis* from the blood of patients with miliary tuberculosis (11). Ten milliliters of blood was lysed with distilled water and the lysate was "centrifugulized" for 1.5 h at high speed. The sediment was then washed over the surface of blood agar slants and incubated. It was noted that colonies of *M. tuberculosis* could sometimes be visualized within 7 to 10 days, which, even by today's standards, would be considered rapid.

One of the more important developments in modern blood culture technology occurred during the 1930s and 1940s and concerned the recognition of "Liquoid" (Hoffman-LaRoche; sodium polyanethol sulfonate) as a potent anticoagulant, anticomplement, and antiphagocytic agent. This substance was found to be useful as a blood transport medium (thus avoiding complicated bedside inoculation of media), an additive to liquid blood culture media, and indeed a self-contained culture medium that could be subcultured periodically during incubation to solid, agar-based media (12). Initially used at a concentration of 0.16%, later experiments suggested that concentrations higher than 0.05% could inhibit the growth of certain organisms (13). Liquoid essentially replaced saponin and trypsin as a blood culture anticoagulant over the next few decades, although the most effective final concentration and its use for the recovery of anaerobes remained an issue of some debate (12).

At about this same time, an interesting protocol for the recovery of streptococci was reported (14). This method (credited to Cecil without reference) called for the collection of 20 ml of blood in two tubes that were allowed to clot overnight in the icebox. The clots were then disrupted with a glass rod and placed in 50 ml of beef heart infusion broth and incubated at

37°C for a month. Subcultures were made every fifth day to blood agar and broth. The authors noted that the risk for contamination was high.

By the end of World War II, blood culture techniques would be fairly recognizable by clinical microbiologists today with a few exceptions. Blood samples were to be collected when patients exhibited temperature spikes, although the logistics of doing so would make timing a nightmare (15). Several (number not stated) specimens should be collected at hourly intervals to increase the likelihood of obtaining a positive result. Special consideration should be given to the choice of vein for collection. Drawing from a vein draining an infected area should be used whenever feasible. Blood collection from the femoral artery was believed to be better than venous blood for culture, although this too was disputed. If blood cultures proved negative, one could try sternal marrow as an alternative. It was recognized that pneumonia and meningitis were associated with bacteremia in about 50% of cases and duplicate bottles should be obtained in cases of subacute bacterial endocarditis, puerperal sepsis, and subacute focal infections, one bottle each being incubated aerobically and anaerobically. The latter was always to be included for patients with postsurgical infections using thioglycollate broth. Once collected, blood cultures should be examined once daily for 3 weeks. If *Brucella* spp., *Neisseria gonorrhoeae*, or *Neisseria meningitidis* infection was suspected, the atmosphere of the bottles should include 10% CO_2.

To avoid contamination, the following process was suggested. Blood should not be collected within 8 h of any intravenous injection. All electric fans should be turned off and windows and doors closed. The best vein for the infectious process at hand should be selected and a sterile towel placed under the collection site. Wash the site with soap or tincture of green soap in a circular motion. Remove the soap with a sterile gauze. Apply tincture of iodine or merthiolate over the area and cover with a sterile gauze until dry. Wash this off with 95% alcohol and allow to dry under a sterile gauze or towel. At bedside, withdraw about 15 ml of blood and inoculate a bottle containing 150 ml of dextrose beef infusion hormone broth with 5 ml of the total volume collected. Place another 5 ml in a citrated tube and mix to prevent clotting. In the laboratory, prepare two pour plates with 1 and 2 ml of citrated blood mixed with melted beef infusion agar cooled to 45°C and poured into sterile petri plates. Allow to harden, and label the volume of blood in each (these will be used to estimate the level of bacteremia). Place another 2 ml of blood into 25 ml of thioglycollate glucose broth for anaerobes. Prepare a Spray dish. (Note: a Spray dish is like a pineapple upside-down cake. It is a pour plate with the agar-blood mix in the top of the petri dish, which is then covered by the bottom of the dish and inverted.) A mixture of sodium bicarbonate, sulfuric acid, and water is added to the bottom to generate CO_2 for cases of suspected *Brucella* spp., *N. gonorrhoeae*, or *N. meningitidis* infection. The plate is then sealed with paraffin and incubated. All cultures are incubated at 37°C for 24 h, examined, and an initial report generated based on Gram stains of the broth cultures which are subsequently subcultured to blood agar slates. This process is repeated every 2 to 3 days for 10 to 21 days until being reported as negative.

Scott's method simplified things a bit (16). It used 2-oz.-square, clear glass bottles with a screw-cap top and a rubber septum underneath. The aerobic bottle consisted of 15 ml of melted Trypticase soy agar dispensed into the bottle, which was turned on its side and cooled. Then, 10 ml of Trypticase soy broth was added to the bottle to create a modified Castaneda bottle (Fig. 4). Various iterations of this type of a system would be seen in later years, e.g., the Septi-Chek system from Becton Dickinson (Sparks, MD). The anaerobic bottle consisted of 25 ml of thioglycollate broth that had been autoclaved and stoppered to remove O_2. The aerobic/anaerobic bottles were inoculated with 5 and 2 ml of blood, respectively (the difference

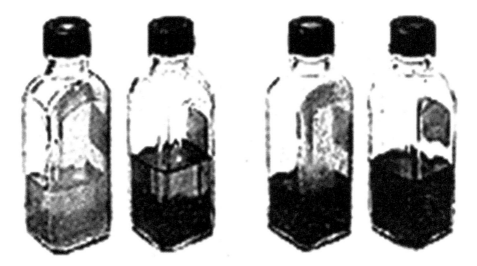

Figure 4 The advent of the modern blood culture set of E. G. Scott (16) consisting of a thioglycollate anaerobic bottle and a broth/agar slant combination bottle for aerobes fashioned after the *Brucella* bottle designed by Castaneda (17). The bottle set on the left demonstrates no growth in either bottle, while the set on the right shows growth in both. Reproduced from reference 15, with permission.

in volume was not elucidated). *p*-Aminobenzoic acid (PABA) and penicillinase could be added if the patient was receiving sulfonamides or penicillin, respectively (first antimicrobial removal system?). The bottles were again incubated at 37°C and examined at 24 h and every 2 days thereafter. The agar side of the aerobic bottle could be "washed" with the blood/broth mixture if no growth was observed and the atmosphere of the bottle could be recharged by venting in the presence of 10% CO_2. Most isolates were recovered in 24 to 72 h unless antibiotics were on board. This method was also amenable for bedside inoculation.

If the blood sample clotted, serum was removed and the clot was placed in the barrel of a 10- to 20-ml syringe. The plunger was replaced, and the clot was forced through the tip of the syringe into a 100-ml bottle containing 50 ml of 0.12% beef infusion agar (semisolid).

Recognized contaminants of the day included diphtheroids (19% of the total) and skin cocci (*S. albus*, 24% of the total). Scott reported an overall contamination rate of 4.7% using his system, which included diphtheroids, *S. albus* (*S. epidermidis* and coagulase-negative staphylococci), *Escherichia coli*, and *Proteus* spp. One has to wonder about the latter two being designated contaminants.

Other standard blood culture media of the mid-20th century included hormone broth with 0.2% glucose, peptone colloid medium, tryptose phosphate broth, and Kracke's blood culture media designed to fix complement (15).

In all fairness, the first description of a biphasic liquid-solid medium interface was made by Castaneda in 1947 (17), and specifically designed for the recovery of *Brucella* species from blood. But, with time, it gained a more general appeal for the recovery of most organisms, including fungi and intracellular organisms causing bacteremia. Unfortunately, the popularity of biphasic blood culture bottles was offset by the complexity of producing them.

Advances in blood culture technology progressed at a glacier pace over the next decade, but two notable events paved the way for more significant developments down the road. The first of these seems like a non sequitur, but bear with me, because the connection will be made later. Levin et al., in a 1962 *Science* article, described a system developed by the National Aeronautics and Space Administration (NASA) by which microbial life in Martian soil could be detected using radiospirometry (18). The system was to be loaded on board a small probe called "Gulliver," which was intended to be delivered to the surface of Mars. Once there, the probe would launch two cylindrical projectiles attached by 23 feet of wire onto the surface and reel the projectiles back into the probe, collecting soil samples in the cylinders in the process (Fig. 5). The contents would then be emptied into a microbial growth chamber containing a defined broth medium supplemented with glucose-^{14}C (uniformly labeled) and formate-^{14}C. If microorganisms were present in the sample and they utilized glucose or formate as a carbon source for growth, detectable levels of ^{14}CO$_2$ would be generated and detected (after precipitation as barium carbonate) by a solid-state beta detector coated with barium hydroxide and situated directly above the growth chamber. Field tests on terra firma showed that the system worked with a wide variety of aerobic, microaerophilic, and anaerobic microorganisms. The system was also equipped with a nonlabeled CO$_2$-generating system that permitted flushing of the growth chamber prior to inoculation to eliminate any labeled gas that was generated during the long trip to Mars. This same approach would appear later as a microbial growth detection system specifically applied to the detection of microorganisms in blood cultures.

Similar to the Gulliver story, the second involved the development of a "rapid" blood culture method and modeled the way for future advancements years later. Winn et al. (19) described a novel membrane filtration blood culture technique that was more extensively evaluated later by Finegold et al. in 1969 (20). Although quite labor intensive, the method demonstrated the value of separating microorganisms from whole blood via dextran sedimentation of erythrocytes followed by differential capture of bacteria and yeasts on a filter and direct plating on solid media. The process allowed for removal of antimicrobial substances, promoted more rapid growth, provided discrete colonies for quantitation and rapid identification, and, hence, better discrimination between potential contaminants and significant isolates. It also allowed for the recognition of multiorganism bacteremia. Despite being more rapid than standard broth cultures (average time-to-detection 28 h versus 61 h for broth), the latter proved to be more sensitive for overall detection of microorganisms in blood.

In a hallmark proof-of-principle publication in 1969, Deland and Wagner (21) connected the dots between radiospirometric detection of bacteria on Mars and automated blood culture technology. Using a rudimentary closed-circuit system composed of a culture flask, circulating pump, and an analog ionization chamber connected via Tygon tubing to a readout meter and recorder, they were able to demonstrate active bacterial metabolism in liquid medium through the release of radiolabeled CO$_2$ (Fig. 6). The culture medium consisted of 20 ml of glucose-free thioglycollate broth supple-

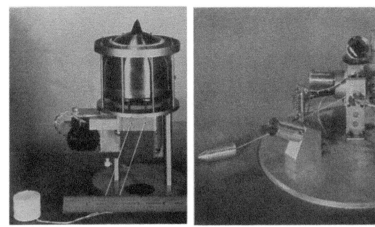

Fig. 6 (left). The first model of Gulliver, designed to probe for microbial life on Mars. Fig. 7 (right). The most recent model of Gulliver. This view shows the projectiles used to carry the soil-sample retrieval lines, the reel-in motor (at left), the broth chamber (at right and center), and the end of the solid detector, resting on the top of the culture chamber. The instrument shown has been used for field testing.

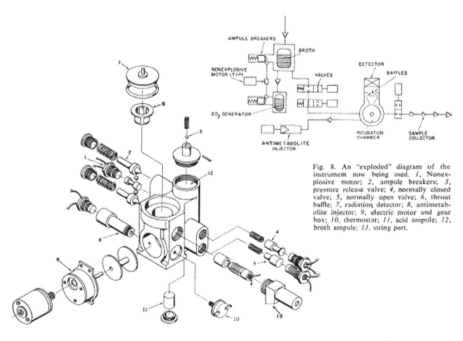

Fig. 8. An "exploded" diagram of the instrument now being used. *1*, Nonexplosive motor; *2*, ampule breakers; *3*, pressure release valve; *4*, normally closed valve; *5*, normally open valve; *6*, throat baffle; *7*, radiation detector; *8*, antimetabolite injector; *9*, electric motor and gear box; *10*, thermostat; *11*, acid ampule; *12*, broth ampule; *13*, string port.

Figure 5 Working models (above) and mechanical and schematic views of the Gulliver system, a radiospirometry system designed to collect soil samples on Mars, inoculate broth containing ^{14}C-labeled carbon substrates, and detect the evolution of $^{14}CO_2$ in an ionization chamber. Reproduced from reference 18, with permission.

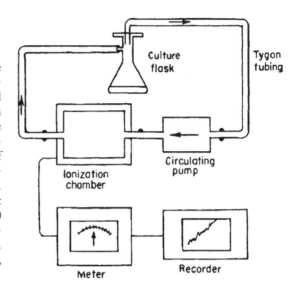

Figure 6 Schematic of the original microbial growth detection system designed by DeLand and Wagner. Culture medium containing ^{14}C-labeled glucose was inoculated with microorganisms, and the production of ^{14}CO$_2$ was measured in an ionization chamber and recorded. In initial trials, the instrument detected the growth of 100 strains from 15 species of clinically important microorganisms. Reproduced from reference 21, with permission.

mented with 0.5 µCi of ^{14}C-D-glucose (36 µg glucose) at a pH of 7.0. To this, approximately 10 CFU of bacteria representing 15 species and 100 strains initially recovered from human infection were inoculated, and all produced detectable levels of ^{14}CO$_2$ during the course of growth. They speculated that a similar system could be used for the routine diagnosis of bacteremia from broth cultures of blood and that the same technology could be applied to determine the susceptibility of bacteria to antimicrobial agents. Two years later, DeBlanc et al. (which included DeLand and Wagner) published the results of the first clinical trial of the Johnston Laboratories Bactec bacterial growth detector (22). Although similar in principle to their 1969 publication, this iteration processed 25 blood culture samples in one run. Patient blood samples (2 ml) were placed in a Bactec culture vial containing 30 ml of glucose-free Trypticase soy broth (TSB) supplemented with 0.5 µCi of ^{14}C-glucose (uniformly labeled) and a magnetic stir bar. The sample bottles were incubated offline at 37°C and analyzed for released, labeled CO$_2$ hourly for the first 2 days and once again after 12 days of incubation. To accomplish this, bottles were loaded on a 25-sample circular tray and placed in the instrument which maintained constant temperature at 37°C. The tray revolved around a sampling station that would first irradiate the rubber septum of the bottle with UV light for 70 s. A two-needle set would then penetrate the septum where 200 ml of unlabeled, filtered air was pumped into the headspace through one needle. The displaced air escaped through the other needle into an ionization chamber for measurement of free $^{14}CO_2$. The measurement cycle took 30 min (72 s/bottle) after which the bottles were returned to the incubator. For comparison in this study, a conventional culture set consisting of 8 ml of blood in 70 ml of TSB and 2 ml of blood in 20 ml of thioglycollate medium incubated for 12 days and inspected visually was used as the reference method. They evaluated 2,967 cultures from 1,280 patients, and in 125 cultures from 50 patients, at least one of the conventional bottles was positive for bacterial growth. The Bactec growth detector identified 111 positive cultures from 48 patients. Neither method detected all patients with bacteremia. The routine method identified 87% of all bacteremic patients while the radiometric method identified 85%. More importantly, however, 70% of the positive cultures identified by both systems were detected first by the radiometric method, and 65% of these signaled positive on the first day of incubation. This initial design, which was marketed as the Bactec 225 radiometric microbial growth detection system, was followed by a model with increased specimen-processing capabilities (Bactec 460); designs that utilized infrared growth detection with various sample capacities and levels of automation (Bactec NR-660, -730, and -860); and, finally, the 9000 series (9050, 9120, and 9240) and the FX, all of which utilized fluorescent CO_2 sensors for growth detection (23–29). Along with instrument evolution, a plethora of media types compatible with each of the systems were developed along the way. A more detailed history of the Bactec system is reviewed by Chamberland in chapter 4.

One blood culture technology advance that could certainly fall in the category of groundbreaking was reported by Gordon Dorn and colleagues in 1976 in a series of two back-to-back publications (30, 31). In these reports, they described the use of a centrifugation technique in which microorganisms are extracted from lysed, whole-blood samples into a density cushion (sucrose gel or Ficoll) contained within a vacutainer-like collection tube (Fig. 7). The sedimented material containing microbial cells was then removed from the tube using a syringe and plated directly to solid agar medium. The method was evaluated for recovery of microorganisms from 1,000 patient samples from which there were 176 positive cultures. The lysis-centrifugation method generated more positive recoveries (73%) than standard broth or pour plate used for comparison. Furthermore, they observed better recovery of *Pseudomonas*, Gram-positive cocci, and fungi (primarily yeast) and in a shorter time-to-detection. This innovative technology eventually became known as the Isolator blood culture system and was initially marketed by E. I. du Pont de Nemours & Co., Wilmington,

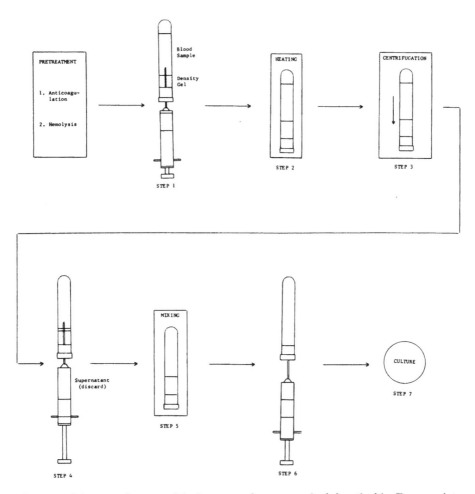

Figure 7 Schematic diagram of the lysis centrifugation method described by Dorn et al. in 1976. The system consisted of a vacutainer tube that allowed for the separation of microorganisms from lysed, anticoagulated whole blood into a density gel that was removed and plated directly to solid media. The system led to the commercialization of the product known as the Isolator (DuPont, then Wampole). Reproduced from references 30 and 31, with permission.

DE, and later by Wampole Laboratories, Cranbury, NJ, and is reviewed in much greater detail by McElvania TeKippe and Pence in chapter 3.

Another milestone in blood culture technology was reported by Wallis et al. in 1980 (32). Along with his colleagues at Baylor College of Medicine in Houston, this publication was the first to describe the Antimicrobial Removal Device (ARD) system. The ARD consisted of a 60-ml rubber septum-capped vial containing 10 g of a cationic resin (C249-Ionac, Birmingham, NJ) and 15 g of a polymeric adsorbent resin (Amberlite XAD_4, Rohm & Haas, Philadelphia, PA) in 5 ml of normal saline. To use the device, 5 to 10 ml of whole blood was injected into the ARD bottle, which was then rotated at 84 rpm for 15 min. Afterward, the treated blood was removed and transferred to a standard blood culture bottle. A small study comparing one 5-ml processed blood sample with two unprocessed blood samples inoculated to standard blood culture bottles was conducted involving 51 patients who had been or were being treated with antimicrobial therapy. The three blood culture bottles were subcultured at selected intervals and the plates examined for bacterial growth. Thirty-one of the 51 patients were determined to be bacteremic and the ARD-processed blood generated earlier growth on subculture for 21 of the matched cultures. Four of the cultures were positive only for ARD-processed specimens versus one for the unprocessed samples. As most readers will recognize, the ARD technology was eventually simplified by Becton Dickinson (Cockeysville, MD) and later bioMérieux, Inc. (Durham, NC) by placing the antimicrobial removal materials directly into blood culture bottles (see chapters 4 and 5).

Two other major events in blood culture history deserve mention but will be explored in greater detail in separate chapters that follow. The first is the initial published clinical evaluation of the Organon Teknika Corp. (OT, Durham, NC) BacT/Alert colorimetric microbial detection system in 1990 (33). This system actually preceded the introduction of the Becton Dickinson Bactec 9000 series by several years and could be considered the first "continuously monitored," fully automated blood culture system to be cleared for routine use in the clinical microbiology laboratory (Fig. 8). The system was based on colorimetric detection of pH changes secondary to microbial growth, metabolism, and the concomitant evolution of CO_2 by a sensor located at the bottom of the blood culture bottle. The second was heralded by a report of a multicenter evaluation of the Difco (Detroit, MI) ESP blood culture system in 1994 (34). This system was unique in its method of microbial growth detection in that it monitored changes in the pressure of the bottle headspace secondary to microbial metabolism via an electronic pressure sensor connected to the septum of the bottle through a sterile vent. Together, the BacT/Alert, Bactec 9000 series, and ESP ushered in the "Continuous Monitorassic" period of blood culture evolution.

Similar to the automobile industry, the side of the road of blood culture history is littered with Packards, Hudsons, Plymouths, DeSotos, Oldsmobiles, and Pontiacs. If the bioMérieux VITAL, Diagnostic Pasteur

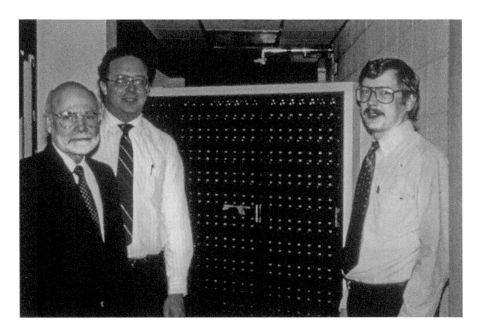

Figure 8 Original prototype of the Organon Teknika BacT/Alert continuously monitored blood culture system. From left: James Turner, James DiGuiseppi, and Therman Thorpe, developers of the BacT/Alert system. Courtesy of bioMérieux, Inc., Durham, NC.

Bio Argos, Difco Sentinel, and ESP and Unipath Ltd. o.a.s.i.s. systems ring a familiar bell, the readers are dating themselves. These systems worked on a variety of principles for the detection of growth, including headspace pressure changes (ESP and o.a.s.i.s.), fluorescent dye redox indicator (VITAL), and electrical impedance (Sentinel). Some of these systems worked quite well compared with the standards of the day, but, alas, market pressures and/or corporate acquisitions led to their transformation into contemporary systems (ESP to VersaTREK; Roche Septi-Chek to BBL Septi-Chek) or ultimate demise (35–40).

Clearly, there have been many additional improvements in contemporary blood culture technology since 1994. Many of these concern the speed at which an identification of bacteremia is made—either directly from patient blood or indirectly from a positive blood culture—and utilized molecular-based assays or high-resolution spectrometry. Rather than highlight all these advancements from the early 1990s to the present time, separate chapters have been created in this book specifically for that purpose, and in much greater detail, so I hope the reader will use this historic perspective as a starting point to explore the fascinating art of blood culture.

References

1. **Findlen P.** 2004. Introduction: the last man who knew everything...or did he? Antanasius Kircher, S.J. (1602-80) and his world, p 1–48. *In* Findlen P (ed), *Athanasius Kircher. The Last Man Who Knew Everything.* Routledge, London, NY.

2. **Baldwin M.** 2004. Reverie in time of plague. Athanasius Kircher and the plague epidemic of 1656, p 1–48. *In* Findlen P (ed), *Athanasius Kircher. The Last Man Who Knew Everything.* Routledge, London, NY.

3. **Torrey HB.** 1938. Anthanasius Kircher and the progress of medicine. *Osiris* 5:246–275.

4. **Wilson C.** 1951. Anamalcula and the theory of animate contagion, p 140–175. *In* Wilson C (ed), *The Invisible World: Early Modern Philosophy and the Invention of the Microscope.* Princeton University Press, Princeton NJ. [Third printing, 1997.]

5. **Wilson C.** 1951. Instruments and applications, p 70–102. *In* Wilson C (ed), *The Invisible World: Early Modern Philosophy and the Invention of the Microscope.* Princeton University Press, Princeton NJ. [Third printing, 1997.]

6. **Frischknecht F, Renaud O, Shorte SL.** 2006. Imaging today's infectious animalcules. *Curr Opin Microbiol* 9:297–306.

7. **Villemin JA.** 2015. On the virulence and specificity of tuberculosis. *Int J Tuberc Lung Dis* 19:256–266.

8. **Hiss PH, Zinsser H.** 1911. The bacteriological examination of materials from patients, p 178–180. *In* Hiss PH, Zinsser H (ed), *A Text-Book of Bacteriology: A Practice Treatise for Students and Practitioners of Medicine.* D Appleton and Co, New York, NY.

9. **Hiss PH, Zinsser H.** 1911. Bacilli of the colon-typhoid-dysentery group: the bacillus of typhoid fever, p 399–427. *In* Hiss PH, Zinsser H (ed), *A Text-Book of Bacteriology: A Practice Treatise for Students and Practitioners of Medicine.* D Appleton and Co, New York, NY.

10. **Muir R, Ritchie J.** 1927. Methods of examining the properties of serum – preparation of vaccines – inoculation of animals – methods of obtaining pathological materials for examination, p 122–149. *In* Muir R, Ritchie J (ed), *Manual of Bacteriology*, 8th ed. Humphrey Milford Oxford University Press, London, UK.

11. **Clough MC.** 1917. The cultivation of tubercle bacilli from the circulating blood in military tuberculosis. *Am Rev Tuberc* 1:598–621.

12. **Stuart RD.** 1948. The value of Liquoid for blood culture. *J Clin Pathol* 1:311–314.

13. **Von Haebler T, Miles AA.** 1938. The action of sodium polyanethol sulphonate ("liquoid") on blood cultures. *J Pathol Bacteriol* 48:245–252.

14. **Stitt ER, Clough PW, Clough MC.** 1938. Blood cultures, p 702–705. *In* Stitt ER, Clough PW, Clough MC (ed), *9th edition of Practical Bacteriology, Haematology and Parasitology.* P. Blakiston's Son and Co, Inc, Philadelphia, PA.

15. **McBurney R.** 1952. Bacteriological examination of blood and feces, p 559–592. *In* Miller SE (ed), *A Textbook of Clinical Pathology.* The Williams & Wilkins Co, Baltimore, MD.

16. **Scott EG.** 1951. A practical blood culture procedure. *Am J Clin Pathol* 21:290–294.

17. **Castaneda MR.** 1947. A practical method for routine blood cultures in brucellosis. *Proc Soc Exp Biol Med* 64:114–115.

18. **Levin GV, Heim AH, Clendenning JR, Thompson MF.** 1962. "Gulliver"–a quest for life on Mars: radioisotopes are used in a miniature instrument designed to detect life during early probes of the planet. *Science* 138:114–121.

19. Winn WR, White ML, Carter WT, Miller AB, Finegold SM. 1966. Rapid diagnosis of bacteremia with quantitative differential-membrane filtration culture. *JAMA* **197**:539–548.
20. Finegold SM, White ML, Ziment I, Winn WR. 1969. Rapid diagnosis of bacteremia. *Appl Microbiol* **18**:458–463.
21. DeLand FH, Wagner HN Jr. 1969. Early detection of bacterial growth, with carbon-14-labeled glucose. *Radiology* **92**:154–155.
22. DeBlanc HJ Jr, DeLand F, Wagner HN Jr. 1971. Automated radiometric detection of bacteria in 2,967 blood cultures. *Appl Microbiol* **22**:846–849.
23. Gröschel D, Hopfer RL, French JE. 1979. Blood cultures with the BACTEC 225 radiometric microbial growth detection system. *Zentralbl Bakteriol [Orig A]* **244**:316–323.
24. Phillips LE, Martin RR, Gentry LO, Rogers TE. 1979. Assay of serum tobramycin levels with the Bactec 460. *Antimicrob Agents Chemother* **16**:463–467.
25. Courcol RJ, Fruchart A, Roussel-Delvallez M, Martin GR. 1986. Routine evaluation of the nonradiometric BACTEC NR 660 system. *J Clin Microbiol* **24**:26–29.
26. Schnur ER, Azimi PH, Belchis DA. 1989. Poor performance of BACTEC NR 730 blood culture system in early detection of *Neisseria meningitidis*. *J Clin Microbiol* **27**:654–656.
27. Nolte FS, Williams JM, Jerris RC, Morello JA, Leitch CD, Matushek S, Schwabe LD, Dorigan F, Kocka FE. 1993. Multicenter clinical evaluation of a continuous monitoring blood culture system using fluorescent-sensor technology (BACTEC 9240). *J Clin Microbiol* **31**:552–557.
28. Arpi M, Bremmelgaard A. 1993. Comparison of detection speed and yield in BACTEC NR-860 and Roche BCB blood culture systems. *APMIS* **101**:545–550.
29. Riedel S, Eisinger SW, Dam L, Stamper PD, Carroll KC. 2011. Comparison of BD Bactec Plus Aerobic/F medium to VersaTREK Redox 1 blood culture medium for detection of *Candida* spp. in seeded blood culture specimens containing therapeutic levels of antifungal agents. *J Clin Microbiol* **49**:1524–1529.
30. Dorn GL, Haynes JR, Burson GG. 1976. Blood culture technique based on centrifugation: developmental phase. *J Clin Microbiol* **3**:251–257.
31. Dorn GL, Burson GG, Haynes JR. 1976. Blood culture technique based on centrifugation: clinical evaluation. *J Clin Microbiol* **3**:258–263.
32. Wallis C, Melnick JL, Wende RD, Riely PE. 1980. Rapid isolation of bacteria from septicemic patients by use of an antimicrobial agent removal device. *J Clin Microbiol* **11**:462–464.
33. Thorpe TC, Wilson ML, Turner JE, DiGuiseppi JL, Willert M, Mirrett S, Reller LB. 1990. BacT/Alert: an automated colorimetric microbial detection system. *J Clin Microbiol* **28**:1608–1612.
34. Morello JA, Leitch C, Nitz S, Dyke JW, Andruszewski M, Maier G, Landau W, Beard MA. 1994. Detection of bacteremia by Difco ESP blood culture system. *J Clin Microbiol* **32**:811–818.
35. Thomson RB Jr, File TM Jr, Tan JS, Evans BL. 1987. Yield, clinical significance, and cost of a combination BACTEC plus Septi-Chek blood culture system. *J Clin Microbiol* **25**:819–823.
36. Trombley C, Anderson JD. 1987. SIGNAL blood culture system for detection of bacteremia in neonates. *J Clin Microbiol* **25**:2098–2101.

37. Stevens M, Patel H, Walters A, Burch K, Jay A, Dowling N, Mitchell CJ, Swann RA, Willis AT, Shanson DC. 1992. Comparison of Sentinel and Bactec blood culture systems. *J Clin Pathol* **45**:815–818.

38. Aubert G, Vautrin AC, Michel VP, Fresard A, Dorche G. 1993. Evaluation of three automated blood culture systems. Bio Argod, Bact T/Alert, bactec NR-860. *Pathol Biol (Paris)* **41**:434–440. (In French.)

39. Stevens CM, Swaine D, Butler C, Carr AH, Weightman A, Catchpole CR, Healing DE, Elliott TS. 1994. Development of o.a.s.i.s., a new automated blood culture system in which detection is based on measurement of bottle headspace pressure changes. *J Clin Microbiol* **32**:1750–1756.

40. Wilson ML, Mirrett S, McDonald LC, Weinstein MP, Fune J, Reller LB. 1999. Controlled clinical comparison of bioMérieux VITAL and BACTEC NR-660 blood culture systems for detection of bacteremia and fungemia in adults. *J Clin Microbiol* **37**:1709–1713.

The Dark Art of Blood Cultures
Edited by Wm. Michael Dunne, Jr. and Carey-Ann D. Burnham
© 2018 American Society for Microbiology, Washington, DC
doi:10.1128/9781555819811.ch2

Conventional Blood Culture Methods

Robyn Atkinson-Dunn[1] and Wm. Michael Dunne, Jr.[2,3,4]

Chapter 1 took us on a time-travel journey spanning the evolution of blood cultures. All the experimentation and discovery since the 17th century have led to a common understanding of which microorganisms cause bloodstream infections and what essential nutrition is required to grow and recover them from blood. Even today, blood culture remains the best option to determine microbial causes of sepsis. Detection of microbial nucleic acids in blood by PCR or sequencing may not represent the presence of viable organisms (see chapter 13 on the blood microbiome). Often, manual culture methods are used as a reference standard for newer iterative protocols like current-generation automated blood culture systems (1). While the routine use of manual blood culture methods in modern diagnostic microbiology laboratories in 2017 is no longer commonplace, the practice remains quite prevalent in the developing world where purchase and maintenance of automated blood culture instruments are both unaffordable and impractical. But in the developed world, manual blood culture protocols often serve as a backup plan if automated systems experience problems. The comedian Mitch Hedberg once said, "An escalator can never break: it can only become stairs." The same holds true for automated blood culture systems. Regardless of how blood cultures are performed, however, the same set of parameters must be attained to ensure optimal microbial recovery. The list of best practice benchmarks includes the following and can also be found in chapter 10:

[1]Utah Public Health Laboratory, Taylorsville, UT 84129
[2]bioMérieux, Inc., Durham, NC 27712
[3]Washington University School of Medicine, St. Louis, MO 63110
[4]Duke University School of Medicine, Durham, NC 27703

Timing of collection. It is commonly believed that microorganisms or associated by-products like lipopolysaccharide gain access to the bloodstream about 1 h before fever (2). Therefore, it has long been believed that blood for culture should be collected adjacent to febrile episodes and prior to the introduction of antimicrobial therapy. However, a multicenter study of 1,436 patients with positive blood cultures concluded that "The likelihood of documenting bloodstream infections was not significantly enhanced by collecting blood specimens for culture at the time that patients experienced temperature spikes." (3)

Blood to broth ratio. This is also a key determinant for increasing the odds of organism recovery (4). This ratio must ensure there is proper balance between nourishment for the pathogens, dilution of inhibitors naturally found in blood, and enough anticoagulant to prevent clotting. The optimal blood:broth ratio ranges from 1:5 to 1:10 depending on the blood culture bottles used, with the former being adapted for bottles containing antimicrobial removal polymeric resins and the latter for larger-volume bottles without added resins (2).

Volume of blood. This needs to be optimized to reduce the likelihood of falsely negative results. In general, it has been determined that 20 to 30 ml/culture for adults with two to three total cultures collected per 24-h period are necessary to achieve successful pathogen isolation (1, 2, 4). This is usually collected over a number of separate draws rather than all at one time. For pediatric patients, maximum volume is a function of patient age and weight (see chapter 8).

Broth composition. The types and combinations of blood culture broth vary by institution or manufacturer, but all agree that the broth must have nutrients for growth of a spectrum of microorganisms, including aerobic, microaerophilic, and anaerobic, with an anticoagulant to prevent clotting. On the aerobic side, bottles containing brain heart infusion (BHI), Trypticase soy, and Columbia broths are quite common, while thiol or thioglycollate broths generally suffice for anaerobes (4). The most common anticoagulant is sodium polyanethol sulfonate (SPS) with a typical concentration of 0.025 to 0.05%.

Length of incubation. For manual blood cultures, this is typically 7 days at 35 to 37°C. Because basic manual blood cultures have no indicator to signal bacterial growth, blind subcultures (i.e., plating blood culture liquid in the absence of visual growth) are sometimes performed at 24 h, 48 h, and 7 days after inoculation (1, 5), although terminal subcultures of bottles without evidence of growth have proven to be of little value (4, 6, 7).

Transportation. Ideally, inoculated blood cultures should be sent to the laboratory within 2 h of collection. In the absence of off-site incubators, cultures can be kept at room temperature for only a few hours but should never be refrigerated or frozen.

Unsatisfactory samples. In general, an unsatisfactory sample is a sample that is hemolyzed (unless hemolysis is caused by organism growth), clotted, or contains an anticoagulant that is not suitable for recovery of potential pathogens (1, 2).

Manual Blood Culture

Most blood culture bottles for manual cultures will not have an indicator of growth other than obvious turbidity or the visual appearance of microcolonies floating in the broth or at the blood/broth interface of stationary bottles. As a result, bottles need to be checked visually for growth at 6 to 12 h after inoculation and then several times daily for 7 days (1, 2, 4, 8). This should be done with care, because blood samples with certain properties (i.e., lipemic) can result in broth turbidity with the potential to mimic bacterial growth. Growth can also be assessed by observing color changes, lysis of red blood cells, or gas production (1). Most often, blood culture bottles are placed in racks and inspected with the assistance of backlighting ("candling" for those familiar with egg inspection). Unlike automated systems where most positives are detected after 3 to 4 days of incubation (9, 10), blood cultures from patients suspected of infection with fastidious or slowly growing organisms like *Brucella* spp. might benefit from additional incubation beyond the recommended 7-day incubation cycle to better visualize growth (1).

As with any other blood culture system, Gram stains are necessary to determine the nature of growth in positive bottles. If Gram stain is performed prior to plating, the results can be used to guide the type of medium that is selected for the subculture process. In addition, the description of the growth in the blood culture bottle can inform the clinician with regard to selection of initial antimicrobial therapy (1). Many times, bottles that appear visually positive, i.e., turbid, will be negative on Gram stain. In this case, it may be helpful to perform an acridine orange stain to visualize organisms using a UV microscope (see chapter 11).

Subculture is necessary to fully characterize organisms growing in culture in terms of identification and antimicrobial susceptibility. Often with manual blood cultures, this occurs via a blind subculture where a small amount of culture liquid is removed from a visually negative aerobic blood culture bottle and struck onto standard media, blood, chocolate, and MacConkey agar. Similarly, anaerobic bottles can be subcultured to suitable anaerobic agar, e.g., CDC blood agar and incubated in the appropriate atmosphere. Plates are usually held at 35°C for at least 24 h. If growth is detected at this stage, normal microbiological identification and susceptibility testing, manual or automated, can be initiated.

When Is Manual or Conventional Blood Culture Still Useful?

Although the majority of clinical laboratories in industrialized countries rely on automated blood culture systems, resources (or the lack thereof) in many parts of the world still dictate the use of manual or conventional blood culture methods, and some areas have to consider whether culture is even relevant. Often laboratories are not even equipped with reliable electrical or water resources to accommodate even the simplest of testing, so hard decisions have to be made. In resource-poor areas, clinical judgment might dictate therapeutic options rather than rely on the collection of routine blood cultures, or perhaps only utilize aerobic blood culture. However, clinics in developing nations might establish more rigorous guidelines and set up both aerobic and anaerobic blood culture bottles (see "Manual Blood Culture Production in Cambodia" below). A study published in 2009 (5) describes the practices of the largest pediatric hospital in Georgia that used conventional blood cultures because of the complete collapse of their health care infrastructure in the early 1990s. They collected two aerobic blood cultures (2 to 3 ml each) for pediatric patients and performed blind subcultures at 24 h, 48 h, and 7 days after blood bottle inoculation. All blood cultures were discarded after 7 days, and often nothing more than a Gram stain was used to identify growth, because more sophisticated systems for pathogen identification were not available.

Commercially Available Manual Blood Culture Media

Although commercially produced conventional blood culture bottles are likely available from regional manufacturers across the globe, a number of companies have stopped producing bottles specifically for manual culture and have shifted to production of bottles for automated systems. Regardless, blood culture bottles intended for continuously monitored systems can always be used for conventional blood cultures if necessary. However, two interesting blood culture systems that are still available commercially for use with conventional blood culture procedures deserve mentioning. The first of these is the Septi-Chek system that was originally developed and marketed by Roche Diagnostics in the early 1980s but is now manufactured by BD Diagnostic Systems (Fig. 1). The system consists of two components. The bottom unit is a broth bottle containing two different volumes of broth for adults or pediatrics with a selection of broth formulations for aerobic, facultative, and anaerobic organisms. One formula (tryptic soy broth) is also available with antimicrobial removal resins. The second part of the system consists of a hollow cylinder containing an agar-coated paddle with choco-

Figure 1 Septi-Chek blood culture system by BBL. This is a two-piece manual culture system designed for culture of blood. The system consists of a broth bottle available in five formulations and two media fill volumes with or without antimicrobial removal resins and an upper slide unit consisting of paddles with solid agar media. Blood is introduced into the broth, and the slide unit is attached to the top. Periodically, the blood/broth mixture is inverted such that it washes over the surface of the agar paddles. It is then incubated in the upright position and the bottles are inspected for growth in the broth and colonies on the agar surface. Image used with permission from BD Biosciences.

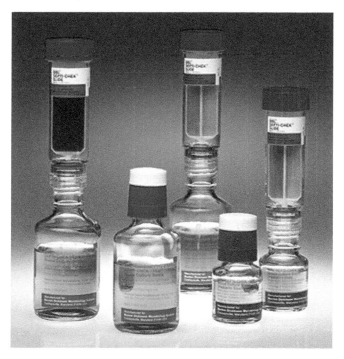

late, MacConkey, and malt agars. After inoculation of the broth with blood, the slide chamber is attached to the top of the bottle. During the course of incubation, bottles are inverted, allowing the broth/blood mixture to wash over the surface of the agar. The system is then incubated in the upright position and monitored for the appearance of turbidity in the broth or isolated colonies on the surface of the agar. The agar allows for more rapid identification and/or susceptibility testing of isolated colonies by avoiding the need for subculture to solid media (4). Of course, this system is simply a technically advanced version of the biphasic culture bottle described by Casteneda in 1947 (11; see also chapter 1).

The second of these is the Oxoid Signal blood culture system. This too is a two-piece system consisting of a single one-size-fits-all multipurpose media bottle and a growth indicator device that connects to the top of the bottle after blood inoculation. The bottle is incubated under standard conditions, and, when growth occurs, a positive buildup of pressure forces a volume of the blood/broth mixture to be displaced into a chamber at the top of the indicator tube (Fig. 2). Like the Septi-Chek, the Signal was developed for use and evaluated during the mid-1980s. While neither of these systems represents new technology, each provides laboratories that cannot acquire automated systems a means to process manual blood cultures in a more expedient way. Even though many of the initial clinical evaluations of these two products were compared with systems that are no longer available,

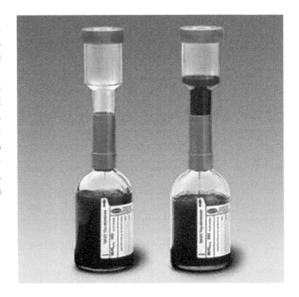

Figure 2 Oxoid Signal blood culture system by Oxoid. Also a two-piece manual blood culture system consisting of a broth-containing bottle and a growth indicator device that is attached to the top of the bottle. Organism growth generates positive pressure in the bottle that displaces a volume of the blood-broth mixture into the detection chamber. Image used with permission from BD Biosciences.

the reports provide some indication of expected performance. A study of Murray et al. in 1988 (12) was a head-to-head comparison of the Oxoid Signal and the Roche Septi-Chek. Using 5,034 equal volume paired cultures, they found that the Septi-Chek recovered significantly more isolates including *Pseudomonas*, *Acinetobacter*, and yeast species, whereas the signal recovered significantly more anaerobes and viridans group streptococci. Both products were equivalent in terms of time to detection (TTD), but the authors observed a 71.7% false positivity rate for the Oxoid Signal, one that likely corresponded to increased workload. In 1990, Daley et al. (13) compared the Signal to the now-defunct Bactec NR-660 using a two-stage approach: simulated blood cultures inoculated with 88 clinically relevant strains of bacteria and yeast (including anaerobes) and a clinical arm comparing 3,321 paired patient blood cultures. Both approaches demonstrated greater isolation rates for the Bactec system, while the Signal showed poor growth detection for yeasts, nonfermentative Gram-negative rods, *Neisseria meningitidis*, *Nocardia* spp., and *Corynebacterium jeikeium*. The two were equivalent for recovery of staphylococci, *Enterobacteriaceae*, streptococci, and anaerobes. TTD was in favor of the Bactec system, but, as noted above, the Oxoid system had a false positivity rate of 58.5% versus 7.7% for Bactec. Rohner and colleagues (14) performed a more recent comparison between the Organon Teknika (now bioMérieux, Inc., Durham, NC) BacT/Alert automated blood culture system and the Oxoid Signal using 5,284 paired sets consisting of aerobic and anaerobic bottles inoculated with 5 ml of blood each for the BacT/Alert and a Signal bottle containing 10 ml of blood. They found that the BacT/Alert was superior to the Signal for recovery of significant microorganisms ($P < 0.0001$) including *Escherichia coli*, Gram-negative rods other than *Pseudomonas* spp. and *Enterobacteriaceae*, and yeast. The BacT/Alert system also detected significantly more septic cases but was higher than the Signal for contaminants and false-positive results (interestingly different from previous reports). Overall, TTD also favored the BacT/Alert system ($P = 0.001$). Moving to the Septi-Chek system, a large number of clinical evaluations appeared after the introduction of this product by Roche in the early 1980s, and most of these come to similar conclusions.

The multicenter trial by Weinstein et al. (15) evaluated the performance of the Septi-Chek against the Bactec system using the Plus 26 aerobic bottle containing antimicrobial removal resins. A total of 5,293 paired aerobic blood cultures were obtained, and the Bactec system surpassed the performance of the Septi-Chek in terms of total recovered organisms, including staphylococci, enterococci, *Enterobacteriaceae*, and TTD (all statistically significantly different). There was no difference observed in recovery for *Pseudomonas aeruginosa*, yeasts and other fungi, other Gram-negative rods, and other Gram-positive organisms. Finally, Welby et al. (16) evaluated the performance of the Bactec and Septi-Chek systems for pediatric patients using the Peds Plus bottles and the Pediatric Septi-Chek bottles; 4,112 paired blood cultures were collected with equal volumes of blood. While no differences were seen in overall recovery of organisms, the Bactec system bested the Septi-Chek in terms of TTD, but the reverse was true when considering time to isolated colonies.

Manual Blood Culture Production in Cambodia

As an example of the use of conventional blood culture in a developing country (in this case, Cambodia), the following description and protocol are provided so that the reader can appreciate the construction of a process suited for a particular geographic region and the attention to detail that is necessary to provide quality diagnostic services. The Diagnostic Microbiology Development Program (DMDP) was founded in 2008 by Drs. James C. McLaughlin and Ellen Jo Baron. The objective was to implement diagnostic microbiology laboratory services in Cambodian government referral hospitals in provinces throughout the country. Because Cambodia is a resource-limited country, it was essential to provide inexpensive blood culture bottles to these government hospitals. In 2013, the DMDP established a Central Media Making Laboratory (CMML) in collaboration with faculty and staff at the Cambodian University of Health Sciences (UHS) and began producing blood culture broth bottles for distribution to the provincial hospitals with diagnostic microbiology laboratories supported by DMDP. In addition to blood culture broth bottles, the CMML is now producing a wide variety of bacteriological media for organism isolation and identification. In 2015, the CMML staff produced and distributed 7,300 blood culture bottles. That volume increased to 12,400 in 2016, and production continues to increase.

The standard operating procedure (SOP), "Preparation of Blood Culture Bottles," has been developed in collaboration with DMDP partners at the Cambodian UHS and the Integrated Quality Laboratory Services (IQLS) based in Lyon, France. Refer to Appendix A below.

A blood collection of 10 ml/bottle into at least two bottles for adult patients and 2 to 5 ml in one bottle for children is suggested. To encourage the medical staff to collect this volume of blood, continuing education efforts are presented on a regular basis to stress the importance of the relationship between volume of blood collected and yield of pathogens. Bottles are weighed in the laboratory before distribution to the wards and again when returned to the laboratory in an effort to monitor the volumes of blood collected in individual bottles. The protocol also emphasizes the importance of collecting blood prior to initiation of antibiotic treatment, but in a resource-poor setting, most patients start treatment recommended by local pharmacists before presenting to hospital. Blood culture bottles are incubated and processed according to the "Standard Operating Procedure: Blood Culture" (see Appendix B).

Conclusion

The development of continuously monitored blood culture systems has led to a high penetrance technology, one that has been implemented throughout the world and dominated by a small number of competitors. While it is likely that improvements in these systems will be continuous, it is unlikely that that any near-term developments will obviate the need for alternative methods of culturing blood, especially those that can be performed anywhere in the world and without special resources. There is always a place for "low-tech" and low-cost methods. We tend to lose sight of this when working in high-complexity clinical laboratories. So there will always be a need for conventional blood culture in the diagnostic clinical microbiology laboratory, especially at those times when an escalator becomes a stair.

Acknowledgments

The authors are indebted to Joanne Letchford, Dr. James McLaughlin, Dr. Ellen Jo Baron, Dr. Chou Monidarin and Dr. Chrea Makteyka (University of Health Sciences), and Dr. Antoine Pierson and Dr. Laura Rumèbe (Integrated Quality Laboratory Services) for providing the bottle preparation and blood culture procedures from their DMDP Cambodia program.

References

1. Baron EJ, Weinstein MP, Dunne WM Jr, Yagupsky P, Welch DF, Wilson DM. 2005. *Cumitech 1C, Blood Cultures IV*. Baron EJ, Coordinating ed. ASM Press, Washington, DC.
2. Wilson ML, Mitchell M, Morris AJ, Murray PR, Reimer LG, Reller LB, Towns M, Weinstein MP, Wellstood SA, Dunne WM Jr, Jerris RC, Welch DF. 2007. *Principles and Procedures for Blood Cultures; Approved Guideline M47-A*. CLSI, Wayne, PA.
3. Riedel S, Bourbeau P, Swartz B, Brecher S, Carroll KC, Stamper PD, Dunne WM, McCardle T, Walk N, Fiebelkorn K, Sewell D, Richter SS, Beekmann S, Doern GV.

2008. Timing of specimen collection for blood cultures from febrile patients with bacteremia. *J Clin Microbiol* **46**:1381–1385.

4. **Dunne WM Jr, LaRocco M.** 2001. Blood culture systems, p 189–209. *In* Cimolai N (ed), *Laboratory Diagnosis of Bacterial Infections.* Marcel-Dekker, New York, NY.

5. **Schaffner J, Chochua S, Kourbatova EV, Barragan M, Wang YF, Blumberg HM, del Rio C, Walker HK, Leonard MK.** 2009. High mortality among patients with positive blood cultures at a children's hospital in Tbilisi, Georgia. *J Infect Dev Ctries* **3**:267–272.

6. **Campbell J, Washington JA II.** 1980. Evaluation of the necessity for routine terminal subcultures of previously negative blood cultures. *J Clin Microbiol* **12**:576–578.

7. **Gill VJ.** 1981. Lack of clinical relevance in routine terminal subculturing of blood cultures. *J Clin Microbiol* **14**:116–118.

8. **Blazevic DJ, Stemper JE, Matsen JM.** 1974. Comparison of macroscopic examination, routine gram stains, and routine subcultures in the initial detection of positive blood cultures. *Appl Microbiol* **27**:537–539.

9. **Doern GV, Brueggemann AB, Dunne WM, Jenkins SG, Halstead DC, McLaughlin JC.** 1997. Four-day incubation period for blood culture bottles processed with the Difco ESP blood culture system. *J Clin Microbiol* **35**:1290–1292.

10. **Han XY, Truant AL.** 1999. The detection of positive blood cultures by the AccuMed ESP-384 system: the clinical significance of three-day testing. *Diagn Microbiol Infect Dis* **33**:1–6.

11. **Castaneda MR.** 1947. A practical method for routine blood cultures in brucellosis. *Proc Soc Exp Biol Med* **64**:114–115.

12. **Murray PR, Niles AC, Heeren RL, Curren MM, James LE, Hoppe-Bauer JE.** 1988. Comparative evaluation of the oxoid signal and Roche Septi-Chek blood culture systems. *J Clin Microbiol* **26**:2526–2530.

13. **Daley C, Lim I, Modra J, Wilkinson I.** 1990. Comparative evaluation of nonradiometric BACTEC and improved oxoid signal blood culture systems in a clinical laboratory. *J Clin Microbiol* **28**:1586–1590.

14. **Rohner P, Pepey B, Auckenthaler R.** 1995. Comparison of BacT/Alert with Signal blood culture system. *J Clin Microbiol* **33**:313–317.

15. **Weinstein MP, Mirrett S, Wilson ML, Harrell LJ, Stratton CW, Reller LB.** 1991. Controlled evaluation of BACTEC Plus 26 and Roche Septi-Chek aerobic blood culture bottles. *J Clin Microbiol* **29**:879–882.

16. **Welby PL, Zusag TM, Storch GA.** 1992. Comparison of the Bactec Peds Plus pediatric blood culture vial with Roche pediatric Septi-Chek for blood cultures from pediatric patients. *J Clin Microbiol* **30**:1361–1362.

17. **Culture Media Special Interest Group for the Australian Society for Microbiology.** 2012. *Guidelines for Assuring Quality of Medical Microbiological Culture Media.* The Australian Society for Microbiology, Melbourne, Victoria, Australia.

APPENDIX A   PREPARATION OF BLOOD CULTURE BOTTLES

Scope and objective

This document describes the procedure for preparation and quality control (QC) testing of blood culture bottles (adult and pediatric) for medical use.

Equipment

Equipment listed below is necessary to perform this job:

- Water still and container for distilled water
- Graduated cylinder
- Magnetic stirrer
- Magnetic hot plate
- Electronic balance
- Autoclave
- Peristaltic pump
- Blood bottle vials 50 ml (pediatric) and 100 ml (adults)
- Blood bottle cap crimper

Procedure

- Wash all the vials in clean water before using.
- Print and begin to complete "Form UHS-F03, Preparation of Blood Culture Bottles" with all available information before starting production.
- Calculate the correct amount of brain heart infusion (BHI) powder with the formula written on the powder box (X grams for 1 liter) and the SPS amount to add (0.25 g/liter of BHI media).
- Choose a bottle with a sufficient volume.
- Clean and make sure there are no small particles inside the bottle.
- Check the conductivity of the distilled water and be sure it is <1 µS/cm; otherwise adjust it with HCl 0.1N.
- Add half of the total volume of distilled water needed in the bottle with a graduated cylinder.
- Weigh the BHI powder and also the correct amount of SPS.
- Transfer the powder into the bottle and add the magnetic bar: adjust the magnetic hot plate to approximately 500 rpm and 100°C.
- Mix for 30 min.
- Add the rest of the water.
- Close the bottle and warm on the hot plate until the medium is completely dissolved.
- Set up the peristaltic pump to deliver the correct volume of the solution (25 ml or 50 ml), check the volume on the scale. Dispense 25 ml in pediatric bottles and 50 ml in adult bottles.
- Seal bottles with rubber stopper and metal cap using the crimper (Fig. 3).
- Place all the bottles in a metal basket.
- Bring the basket to the autoclave with the trolley.

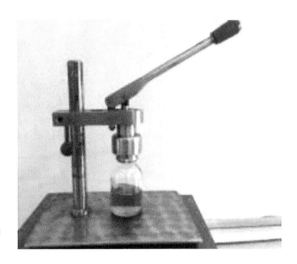

Figure 3 Blood culture bottle metal cap crimping device.

- Autoclave: fix a cycle of 20 min at 121°C and do not forget to add an autoclave control (see the SOP for autoclave use).
- When the autoclave cycle is complete, take out the bottles from the autoclave.
- Create the lot number as follows: BHI-*ddmmyy*.
    Example: Brain Heart Infusion media made on January 23, 2013, will be assigned a Lot # BHI-230113.
- Assign an expiration date of 6 months from the date of production.
- Label each batch with a lot number and expiration date.
- Store the blood bottle at room temperature 25 to 30°C.

Quality control
Internal Quality Control (IQC)
Sterility control. Depending on the batch size, follow the sampling plan as outlined in Table 1.

Growth promotion testing

Strains used as positive control

Streptococcus pneumoniae ATCC 49619	*Haemophilus influenzae* ATCC 49247

- Disinfect the bottle septum with 70% ethanol.
- Use a fresh overnight subculture of the two strains.
- Prepare a 0.5McFarland solution for each strain by using the reference tube for 0.5McFarland.

Table 1 Sampling plan for sterility control of blood culture bottles from Australian Guidelines (17)

Batch size (units made)	Sample number		First sample[a]		Second sample[b]	
	First sample	Second sample	Accept	Reject	Accept	Reject
101–150	5	5	0	2	1	2
151–280	8	8	0	2	1	2
281–500	13	13	0	2	1	2
501–1200	20	20	0	3	3	4

Interpretation: For a batch of 520 bottles, the quality control sample would be 20 bottles.

[a]First Sample: Accept the batch if none of the bottles are contaminated. If 3 bottles are contaminated, reject the batch. If 1 or 2 bottles are contaminated, collect another sample of 20 bottles as second sample. **WARNING!!** Total the number of contaminated bottles between the first and second samples!

[b]Second Sample: Accept the batch if the number of contaminated bottles (sample 1 plus sample 2) is equal to or less than 3 bottles. If the cumulative number of bottles is equal to or greater than 4, reject the batch.

- Perform a 10^{-5} dilution.
- Inoculate one bottle from each batch with:
  - 100 ml of 10^{-5} dilution of each organism
  - 5 ml of sheep blood
- Label the bottle with the date, operator name, and organism name.
- Incubate both bottles at 35°C for a maximum of 3 days.
- When bottle appears turbid, subculture:
  - *S. pneumoniae* ATCC 49619 on BAP
  - *H. influenzae* ATCC 49247 on chocolate agar
- Incubate 24 h in a candle jar.
- Check for growth.
- Record the data on QC form for: *Preparation of Blood Culture Bottles*.

Independent External Quality Control (EQC)
Performed at Sihanouk Hospital Center of Hope microbiology laboratory using SOP UHS-05, Enumeration of Microorganisms.

Safety and security

- BHI powder: use a N95 mask.
- ATCC strains: use a biosafety cabinet.

References
Brain Heart Infusion M210-5kg, HiMedia Laboratories datasheet http://www.theasm.org.au/assets/ASM-Society/Guidelines-for-the-Quality-

Assurance-of-Medical-Microbiological-culture-media-2nd-edition-July-2012.pdf

Sodium polyanethol sulfonate (S.P.S.) datasheet FD786-25G HiMedia Laboratories.

Microbiology of Food, Animal Feed and Water – Preparation, Production, Storage and Performance Testing of Culture Media. ISO 11133:2014.

Guidelines for the Quality Assurance of Medical Microbiological Culture Media, Australian Society of Microbiology (17).

Batch Life Process for Blood Culture bottles, prepared by Integrated Quality Laboratory Services.

APPENDIX B   STANDARD OPERATING PROCEDURE FOR BLOOD CULTURE

Test summary

Blood culture processing assists in the diagnosis of bacteremia and sepsis. Pathogens include *Staphylococcus aureus*, *Escherichia coli*, *Klebsiella pneumoniae*, and other *Enterobacteriaceae*, *Streptococcus pneumoniae*, and *Haemophilus influenzae*. *Salmonella enterica* subsp. *enterica* serovar Typhi, other *Salmonella*, and *Burkholderia pseudomallei* are important blood culture isolates seen in Cambodia.

Principle

Blood is a sterile fluid. Inoculation of blood in prepared media bottles and incubation may detect the presence of organisms in the blood. Growth of an organism allows us to perform identification and susceptibility testing.

Specimen Handling and Preparation

Blood samples are inoculated into blood culture media bottles.

It is encouraged to collect two separate venipuncture collections per patient.

Ten milliliters of blood for each adult collection (20 ml total in two bottles) and 2 to 5 ml in one bottle for a pediatric collection).

It is important to use aseptic technique when collecting blood for blood culture so that skin flora or environmental organisms are not introduced into the bottles.

Refer to blood culture collection procedures. DMDP document code: 084 and training material video blood culture collection procedure.

Quality Control

Appropriate QC testing should be performed for all media used, biochemical testing, Gram stain, and antimicrobial susceptibility test (AST) performed according to the laboratory QC procedures.

Reagents, materials, and equipment

- Adult and pediatric blood culture bottles
- Venting needles
- Media for subculture of blood from blood culture bottles:
  - Sheep blood agar (BAP)
  - Chocolate agar (CHOC)
  - MacConkey agar (MAC)
- Glass slides for Gram stain preparation
- Usual laboratory equipment and consumables

Procedure

1. Ensure that the information on the request form and bottle match.
2. Label each blood culture bottle from the same patient, same day and time with the same number, but differentiate each bottle with "A" or "B."
3. Record patient details on the worksheet.
4. Weigh the bottle and record weight on the bottle. Also record uninoculated weight on the worksheet.

   Note: All blood culture bottle weights are recorded on the bottle when they are received in the laboratory. Both the uninoculated weight and the inoculated weight should be recorded on the bottle and the worksheet.
5. Clean the top of the blood culture bottle with 70% alcohol.
6. Aseptically insert a venting needle.
7. Incubate bottles for 7 days at 35 to 37°C.
8. Keep the venting needle in place for the full 7 days of incubation.
9. Do not disturb the bottle, but check the bottles daily for signs of growth: turbidity, bubbles, hemolysis. If none seen, gently rotate the bottle on the bench to resuspend the blood and mix it. Reincubate until the next day.
10. Hold for 7 days before reporting final report as "negative."
11. Gram stain and subculture all bottles that show signs of growth.

12. Subculture all bottles after 1 night incubation.
13. Subculture:
        Place 1 drop of blood to CHOC and 1 drop for Gram stain.
    - If Gram-positive cocci are detected on the Gram stain, add BAP and an optochin disc to the second quadrant of the BAP plate.
    - If Gram-negative bacilli are detected on Gram stain, subculture blood to a BAP and MAC plate. Add Polymyxin B and Gentamycin, Amox/Clav to BAP plate if patient suspected of a melioidosis or thin Gram-negative rod with bipolar staining.
14. Incubate BAP and CHOC plates in a candle jar. Incubate the MAC plate and the candle jar for 3 days at 35 to 37°C.
15. Read all agar plates daily for 3 days.
16. After the visual checks of blood culture bottles, gently invert before reincubation. Examine all bottles daily for turbidity, gas, etc. If any bottles look suspicious, perform a Gram stain and CHOC agar subculture. Hold these subcultures for 3 days and examine daily.
17. At the end of the 7-day incubation period, perform Gram stain.
18. Record daily on the specimen worksheet all actions performed.

Reading Gram Stains

- Read the Gram stains the same day that they are prepared.
- A positive Gram stain result is a critical result. The result may have direct impact on the treatment of the patient. Record all Gram stain results on the specimen worksheet.
- Phone the result to the clinician or ward. Record notification on the worksheet, and document in laboratory information system as a preliminary report. Be sure to include the name of the person who took the report, have them read the report back to you, and record the time and date and your initials on both the worksheet and in the computer.

Reading Cultures

- Read all plates daily and record results on the specimen worksheet.
- If growth is detected, perform identification and susceptibility testing.
- Refer to flow charts for pathogen identification.
- Refer to the current AST Guidelines to help choose appropriate antibiotic discs for testing.
- Keep plates until a final report has been sent to the clinician.
- Inoculate a broth for storage of all blood culture isolates at −20°C.

Result Reporting

Blood culture showing "growth"

- Primary Report: Gram stain result. Example: Gram-negative bacilli
- Secondary Report: add organism identification. Example: *E. coli*
- Final Report: add Antibiotic Susceptibility Test result.
- Refer to the current AST Guidelines to help choose appropriate antibiotic discs for reporting.
- In some cases, the significance of the isolate will not be clear. In this case, add the following comment: "Significance depends on clinical assessment."

Blood culture showing "NO growth"

- Expected Values: Blood is a sterile fluid.

Note: Growth from a blood culture may indicate bacteremia or sepsis.

Notes

It is important to inoculate the correct volume of blood into a blood culture bottle. Follow the collection procedure. Insufficient blood volume decreases the sensitivity of this test. The uninoculated and inoculated weights will be used to determine the volume of blood that was collected.

Sometimes contaminants from the environment or from skin flora may be introduced to the blood culture bottles. Always report positive growth. Add the comment: "Significance depends on clinical assessment."

On visual inspection, bottles may appear turbid but show no growth on subculture.

In these circumstances, always carefully examine the Gram stain. If there is any doubt, repeat the Gram stain and subculture.

Some fastidious bacteria may not grow under the usual culture conditions. Some bacteria require a microaerophilic atmosphere (*Campylobacter* or *Helicobacter*).

In Cambodia, we do not use anaerobic blood culture bottles or culture for anaerobes.

Sometimes a bottle may not appear turbid, but the subculture will be positive.

Collection of only one blood culture bottle makes the interpretation of the significance of the isolation of skin flora difficult. Communication with clinician should be done before sending the report out.

Reference

Murray PR, Baron EJ, Jorgensen JH, Landry ML, Pfaller MA. 2007. *Manual of Clinical Microbiology*. 9th edition. ASM Press, Washington, DC.

The Dark Art of Blood Cultures
Edited by Wm. Michael Dunne, Jr. and Carey-Ann D. Burnham
© 2018 American Society for Microbiology, Washington, DC
doi:10.1128/9781555819811.ch3

Lysis-Centrifugation Methods of Blood Culture

3

Erin McElvania TeKippe[1] and Morgan A. Pence[2]

Introduction

History of Lysis-Centrifugation Blood Culture Methods

In 1917, Mildred Clough first demonstrated the usefulness of lysis-centrifugation blood culture when she used it to isolate *Mycobacterium tuberculosis* from blood (1, 2). Using this processing method, she was able to recover colonies of *M. tuberculosis* on solid agar media in just two weeks. The process was complex and time-consuming, and, despite the desirable results, lysis-centrifugation blood culture was largely abandoned until the mid-1970s.

In 1976, Gordon Dorn proposed that a lysis-centrifugation method for blood pathogen detection may have similar benefits to blood culture pathogen isolation using filtration methods, such as removal of antimicrobial compounds, ability to culture organisms on various types of media, and a reduction in the amount of time required to obtain a pure isolate. Lysis-centrifugation blood culture also improved upon the drawbacks of the filtration method, including the need to chemically solubilize microorganisms, a step that could harm many fastidious microbes and required manipulation of organisms in the open atmosphere, which was damaging to anaerobes and fastidious bacteria (3).

In brief, the process of lysis-centrifugation blood culture involved using SOLRYTH, or purified saponin, and sodium polyanethol sulfonate (SPS) to lyse red blood cells, after which a sucrose-gelatin or Ficoll-gelatin density

[1]University of Texas Southwestern and Children's Health, Dallas, TX 75390
[2]Cook Children's Medical Center, Fort Worth, TX 76104

39

gradient was used to enrich for microorganisms during centrifugation. This method increased the rate of pathogen detection in blood cultures and decreased the amount of time required to obtain colonies on solid agar. The downside of lysis-centrifugation blood culture was that the method was technically challenging, required making all reagents and consumables in house because they were not commercially available, and it involved a centrifuging processing step that required a swinging bucket rotor, not something routinely found in clinical microbiology laboratories of the day. A study of 1,000 blood specimens from 400 patients was used to compare three different blood culture methods: lysis-centrifugation, incubation in liquid broth medium with blind subculture on two and ten days postinoculation, and pour plate technique. Of the 176 specimens found to be positive by at least one method, the lysis-centrifugation technique recovered 73% of total isolates, while the comparators of broth-based culture and pour plate techniques recovered 38% and 49%, respectively (4). The lysis-centrifugation technique enhanced recovery of *Pseudomonas*, *Staphylococcus*, *Streptococcus*, and *Cryptococcus* species over the broth and pour plate techniques. The mean time to positivity for all positive cultures was shorter using the lysis-centrifugation method with an average time to positivity of 36.6 h compared with 61.3 h for blood incubated in broth medium and 47.7 h using the pour plate technique. Unfortunately, the contamination rate using the lysis-centrifugation method was markedly increased compared with the comparator methods. Shortly after the first published report describing enhanced detection of *Cryptococcus* spp. using the lysis-centrifugation method came the first report of improved recovery of the dimorphic fungi, *Coccidioides immitis* (5).

Subsequent modifications to the lysis-centrifugation method included using a fluorochemical density layer and a fixed-angle rotor for centrifugation (6). These changes retained the superior rate of organism isolation documented for the previous lysis-centrifugation method, but reduced contamination. In a clinical study of nearly 3,335 patients, 1,180 suspected of having bacteremia, the lysis-centrifugation method was able to isolate a potential pathogen in 80% of the 370 positive cultures compared with a traditional broth-based culture in which an organism was recovered from 67% of the 370 positive blood cultures (7). In agreement with previous reports, the increase in pathogen detection was notable for enhanced recovery of *Staphylococcus aureus*, *Pseudomonas aeruginosa*, and yeast. The overall time to detection of growth was shorter using the lysis-centrifugation method and the contamination rate was lower than in previous reports and comparable for both methods compared in the study. In addition, because a known blood volume was used, the lysis-centrifugation allowed quantitative measurement of the number of bacteria per ml of blood.

In clinical microbiology laboratories today, the Isolator lysis-centrifugation blood culture system (Wampole Laboratories, Cranbury, NJ) is used to enhance detection of a subset of bacterial pathogens, molds (especially dimorphic fungi), and slowly growing *Mycobacterium* spp. Historical and current uses of this blood culture methodology are described in subsequent sections.

Commercially Available Lysis-Centrifugation Testing
Isolator 10-ml Microbial Tubes

The initial work on the lysis-centrifugation method of blood culture cited above led to the first commercially available product—the Wampole Isostat Microbial System—which was manufactured by the E. I. du Pont de Nemours & Co., Inc. The system is now manufactured by Wampole (Wampole Laboratories, Cranbury, NJ) and marketed by Alere (Alere Inc., Waltham, MA) (Fig. 1). The Wampole Isostat Microbial System includes a 10-ml glass vacutainer tube, the Isolator 10, which includes the following additives: (i) saponin, a lysing agent; (ii) polypropylene glycol, an antifoaming agent; (iii) anticoagulants SPS and ethylenediaminetetraacetic acid (EDTA); and (iv) an inert fluorochemical density layer that serves as a cushion during centrifugation (8).

The laboratory workflow of the Wampole Isostat Microbial System is as follows: first, 10 ml of blood must be placed in the provided Isolator 10 vacuum tube. Volumes of <10 ml are problematic because the increased SPS concentration in a less than full tube is potentially toxic to fastidious organisms. The red blood cells are lysed by the saponin, and the Isolator tube is placed into a fixed-angle rotor and centrifuged for 30 min. After centrifugation, the tube is placed into the Isostat Rack, which can hold a maximum of 10 tubes at one time for processing. The Isostat Press is a small, hand-operated press that is used to remove the Isolator 10 septum (Fig. 2). A specialized pipette is used to remove the supernatant from the Isolator tube, after which the concentrated pellet, containing any microorganisms present, is resuspended using a vortex and aseptically removed from the tube for plating onto appropriate solid media. The initial hands-on processing steps take approximately 15 min, which does not include centrifugation. Because the system is manual and not automated, once the specimen is plated to solid media, the plates must be viewed one to two times per day for the first week and several times per week thereafter to monitor for microbial growth.

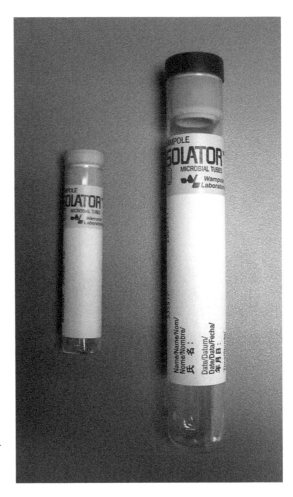

Figure 1 Wampole Isolator 1.5-ml microbial tube and Isolator 10 tube. Image courtesy of Dr. Dominick Cavuoti, used with permission from Alere.

It is recommended that Isolator tubes be processed as soon as possible following specimen collection (8). While delays in processing of 8 to 24 h showed no overall differences in microbial recovery, organisms such as *Candida* spp., *Pseudomonas* spp., and *Staphylococcus* spp. had increased numbers of organisms recovered with shorter time to detection, while fastidious organisms such as *Streptococcus pneumoniae* and *Haemophilus influenzae* had decreased numbers of organisms with increased time to detection compared with Isolator tubes that were processed immediately (9, 10). Based on these data, quantitative culture cannot be performed from Isolator tubes held for extended periods of time prior to processing, because the number of bacteria recovered is not reflective of the colony-forming units (CFU) per milliliter of blood.

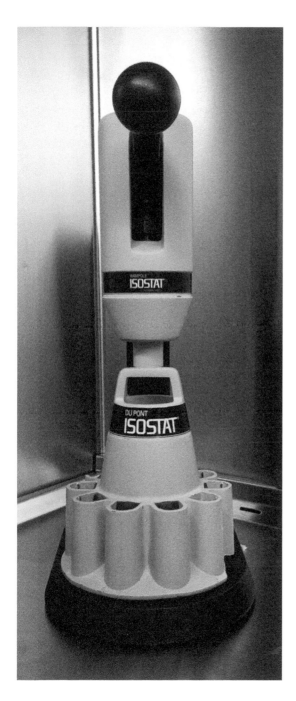

Figure 2 Isostat Press and Rack for processing of Isolator 10 tubes. Image used with permission from Alere.

Isolator 1.5-ml Microbial Tubes

Isolator 1.5 tubes are a smaller version of the Isolator 10 tubes and hold 0.5 to 1.5 ml of blood (compared with 10 ml) (Fig. 1). They contain a lower concentration of SPS compared with Isolator 10 tubes (9.6 g/liter versus 15.3 g/liter) but contain a higher concentration of saponin (40 g/liter versus 28 g/liter) (8, 11). Isolator 1.5 tubes can be held at room temperature for up to 16 h without adverse effects on organism recovery, but colony counts will not reflect the colony-forming units per milliliter of blood if held longer than 4 h (11).

In contrast to the Isolator 10 tubes, no centrifugation is required. The tube is vortexed and the stopper disinfected with 10% polyvinylpyrrolidone (PVP) iodine solution or tincture of iodine and allowed to dry. A syringe is used to withdraw blood from the tube, and the entire volume of blood is subcultured directly to solid media. Isolator 1.5 tubes are typically used in the pediatric setting where blood volume is limited. Isolator 1.5 tubes are not recommended for use in adults since organism burden is low in bacteremic patients, and the Isolator 10 tubes use a larger volume of blood (11). Additionally, the 1.5 tubes may be used for bone marrow cultures, since bone marrow aspirates are unlikely to yield the 10 ml required for Isolator 10 use.

Benefits and Drawbacks

The benefit of the Isolator system is that it requires very little equipment beyond a centrifuge. This allows testing to be performed in laboratories that do not have the resources to support an automated blood culture system. The Isolator systems also allow for recovery of organisms that are not routinely detected by routine continuously monitored blood culture systems (CMBCSs), such as filamentous fungi and mycobacteria. Unlike automated blood cultures, the amount of microorganism present can be quantified based on the 10-ml starting blood volume.

Drawbacks of the Isolator system include the manual nature of lysis-centrifugation blood culture. Processing and viewing agar plates daily is labor intensive for laboratory technicians compared with CMBCSs, in which the instrument continuously monitors the bottles for growth and only a small number of positive blood cultures require hands-on processing by laboratory personnel. Other drawbacks, discussed in detail in the sections below, include increased rates of contamination due to the hands-on processing and the physical characteristics of the Isolator tube septum, as well as the reduced viability of some microorganisms after prolonged incubation in the Isolator tube.

Uses for Isolator Microbial Tubes

Isolation of Bacteria

Prior to the development of CMBCSs, the majority of studies demonstrated greater recovery from Isolator tubes compared with routine blood cultures. Additionally, certain organisms were more frequently detected by Isolator cultures than by blood culture systems. In one study, Isolator 1.5 tubes detected 3% more positive cultures than the Bactec 6B and 7C/D bottles, and *S. pneumoniae* and *Neisseria meningitidis*, in particular, were more frequently recovered from Isolator specimens (12). Studies with the Isolator 10 tubes showed that the Isolator system allowed for greater and more rapid detection of staphylococci, *Enterobacteriaceae*, and yeasts, but recovered fewer streptococci and anaerobes (13–16).

With the evolution of CMBCSs, the use of lysis-centrifugation has fallen out of favor for the isolation of bacteria. Studies comparing the Isolator system with BacT/Alert, Bactec 9240, and ESP (predecessor to the current Thermo Fisher VersaTREK system) demonstrated equivalent or superior analytical performance of CMBCSs for recovery of Gram-positive and Gram-negative bacteria (17–22). Although there are no direct comparisons of Isolator tubes and CMBCSs for the recovery of aerobic actinomycetes, the handful of cases of *Nocardia* bacteremia reported in the literature were diagnosed using CMBCSs, and the isolates were recovered within the standard 5-day incubation period (23–26).

A recent study demonstrated that direct culturing on solid medium, using bacterial reference strains and Isolator 10 tubes, resulted in decreased time to identification and susceptibility results compared with the Bactec blood culture system (27). Seven bacterial reference strains were inoculated into human blood at concentrations of 100, 10, and 1 CFU per milliliter of blood. Plates were monitored hourly, and matrix-assisted laser desorption ionization–time of flight mass spectrometry (MALDI-TOF MS) was performed as soon as microcolonies were visible. Antimicrobial susceptibility testing (AST) from microcolonies was set up, on average, 2.5 h earlier than Bactec detected bacterial growth, and AST profiles were available 9 h after Bactec positivity. Categorical agreement was achieved for all species/concentrations tested. Although the use of Isolator tubes in this case led to decreased time to identification and susceptibility results, the workflow is not currently feasible for routine use in clinical microbiology laboratories.

Although CMBCSs are currently the preferred method for isolation of bacteria from blood, Isolator tubes are preferred for the recovery of certain bacterial species. Detection of *Bartonella* spp. is one exception where lysis-centrifugation is still recommended over CMBCSs. *Bartonella quintana* was recovered from an Isolator blood culture from a HIV-positive patient with bacillary angiomatosis, while the organism was not recovered using the corresponding biphasic Castaneda blood culture (28). Isolator blood cultures also recovered *Bartonella henselae* from three HIV patients (29, 30). On the contrary, one study using BacT/Alert bottles demonstrated growth of *B. henselae* in routine blood cultures from five patients. The bottles signaled positive over a range of 0.125 to 6.4 days, with a mean of 4 days (31). However, no organisms were detected by direct Gram stain. Gram-negative bacilli were observed on wet preparation of the positive broth, and only one of the five isolates grew from direct subculture of the bottles. Two additional isolates were recovered by transferring 7.5 ml of positive blood culture broth to Isolator tubes and subculturing to solid media, likely due to lysis and release of intracellular bacteria. Growth on subculture required up to three weeks of incubation. Because the organisms were not seen on initial Gram stain, the recovery of *Bartonella* spp. by CMBCSs may be underestimated, because many laboratories do not perform additional testing, such as wet preparations or acridine orange on cultures with negative direct Gram stains. Laboratories typically perform subcultures on such bottles, but these sub-cultures are not routinely held long enough to recover *Bartonella* spp. Although Isolator tubes have been used to recover *Bartonella* spp. from blood cultures, the preferred diagnostic methods for *Bartonella* infection are serology and/or PCR (32).

Isolator tubes also appear to provide better recovery of *Finegoldia magna* (formerly *Peptostreptococcus magnus*) and *Peptostreptococcus anaerobius* from blood. Three case reports of *F. magna* endocarditis were undetected by the Bactec 9240 and BacT/Alert FAN CMBC systems after 14 days of incubation (33, 34). All three cases were diagnosed by culturing the removed affected valve. Follow-up studies, performed with contrived specimens using the BacT/Alert system, demonstrated that five isolates of *F. magna* and three isolates of *P. anaerobius* did not grow in the BacT/Alert bottles after 14 days of incubation, while *Parvimonas micra* (formerly *Peptostreptococcus micros*) and *Peptoniphilus asaccharolyticus* (formerly *Peptostreptococcus asaccharolyticus*) grew readily in the anaerobic BacT/Alert FAN bottles (33, 34). Two isolates of *F. magna* were also inoculated into a Septi-Chek BHI-S bottle and Isolator tube and were recovered after two days of growth (33). SPS did not account for the differences in growth between media, because the isolates in the study were resistant to SPS (34). Five additional cases of *F. magna* endocarditis have been reported in the literature (35). Sterile routine blood cultures, collected before the administration of antimicrobials, were observed in three cases (35). *F. magna* was recovered in the two remaining cases. In one case, it was isolated from routine blood culture after 10 days of incubation, although the particular CMBCS was not mentioned (36). In the second case, *F. magna* was isolated after one week in three of three thioglycollate bottles and one of three bottles of Trypticase soy broth (37). Isolator cultures were not performed in last five cases.

The role of the Isolator system in cases of polymicrobial bacteremia is debated. In theory, polymicrobial bacteremia should be detected with higher sensitivity using the Isolator method, since CMBCSs provide a "survival of the fittest" environment, but studies have shown conflicting results. In one study, the Isolator system detected 21 of 25 polymicrobial infections, while 17 were detected by standard blood cultures (38). A second study showed that the Isolator system detected 21 episodes of polymicrobial bacteremia, while blood culture bottles detected 17 (39). However, a third study demonstrated no difference in detection of polymicrobial bacteremias (16). Of note, the first two studies were performed by the same authors. Differences between the first two studies and the third study, which may have contributed to opposite conclusions, include (i) 7.5 ml of blood was added to each Isolator 10 tube in the first two studies, while 10 ml was added in the third study, and (ii) comparative blood cultures consisted of a 1:10 dilution into tryptic soy broth and Columbia broth in the first two studies and a 1:6 dilution into Bactec 6B and 7C bottles in the third study.

Contamination rates are higher with the Isolator system than with CMBCSs because of the manual processing required for Isolator 10 tubes. Reported contamination rates ranged from 0.3 to 13.8% in the 1980s; however, this was before processing was consistently performed in laminar flow hoods (40). Two studies demonstrated that the use of laminar flow hoods for processing specimens decreased the contamination rates from 9.5% and 9.6% to 6.2% and 2.5%, respectively (13, 41, 42). A more recent study reported a 5.9% contamination rate for Isolator tubes (43), which is nearly twice the 3% threshold for routine blood cultures. Contaminated blood cultures lead to increased length of stay, unnecessary use of antimicrobials, and increased costs, with studies showing associated costs greater than $8,000 to $10,000 per contamination event (44, 45).

Isolation of Fungi

Although the manufacturer's instructions state that Isolator tubes can be held at room temperature for 16 h without impacting organism viability,

Stockman et al. demonstrated a significantly higher recovery of yeast and filamentous fungi in tubes processed within 9 h (46). For optimal recovery, Isolator specimens should be processed as soon as possible.

CMBCSs are the preferred method for isolation of the majority of yeasts, including *Candida* spp., *Cryptococcus* spp., and *Trichosporon* spp., but that is not the case for *Malassezia furfur* and most other *Malassezia* spp., such as *Malassezia sympodialis* (47–49). Current CBMCS blood culture bottles do not contain a high enough lipid content to support the growth of *Malassezia* spp. with the exception of *Malassezia pachydermatis*, which does not require lipid supplementation (50–53). Isolator blood cultures should be performed when *Malassezia* sp. is suspected. After processing the Isolator specimen, the plates must be overlaid with sterile olive oil to provide necessary lipid supplementation.

In addition to *Malassezia* spp., the Isolator system has demonstrated better recovery of dimorphic and filamentous fungi than CMBCSs, especially *Histoplasma capsulatum* (48, 54–56). Although the Isolator has demonstrated better recovery of these organisms, the utility and cost-effectiveness of Isolator cultures are debated because the majority of isolates recovered appear to represent clinically insignificant fungemia or pseudofungemia rather than pathogens (48, 57, 58).

Morrell and colleagues performed a 14-month study to determine the utility and cost-effectiveness of the Isolator system compared with the Bactec 460 radiometric system. Of 5,196 fungal blood cultures performed, 84 (1.6%) were positive (58). Thirty-seven were also positive by simultaneous bacterial blood culture and 15 were positive by bacterial blood culture or another bacterial culture within the previous 48 h. Of the remaining 32 cultures, five grew low quantities of *Candida albicans*, which the authors attributed to specimen sampling variance rather than to the specialized media of fungal cultures. The remaining 27 cultures were collected from 24 patients. A retrospective chart review revealed that therapy was only affected in 5 (0.1%) of the 5,196 patients. Two patients had antifungal therapy initiated based on the positive culture, although antifungal therapy was discontinued for one patient when the mold was identified as *Penicillium* sp. and deemed a contaminant. Three additional patients were already on antifungal therapy, and the positive culture resulted in a prolonged duration of antifungals.

Campigotto et al. performed a ten-year retrospective study to determine the utility of the Isolator 1.5 system compared with Bactec FX and BacT/ Alert CMBCSs for detection of fungemia in children. Over ten years, 9,442 specimens were processed with yeast or yeast-like organisms recovered in 297 (3.1%) specimens (151 clinical episodes) and dimorphic or filamentous fungi recovered in 31 (0.3%) of specimens (25 unique clinical episodes) (48). Of the 297 specimens with yeast or yeast-like organisms, only 13 (4.4%) Isolator tubes recovered a *Candida* sp. not identified by the CMBCSs, and six specimens with *M. furfur* were only detected by the Isolator culture. Of the 25 clinical episodes where dimorphic or filamentous fungi were recovered, only nine (36%) were deemed to be clinically significant. Sixteen episodes (64%) were deemed contaminants. Of the nine clinically significant fungi, only one, an isolate of *Fusarium oxysporum*, was also detected in the CMBCS. The eight other clinically significant fungi were *H. capsulatum*, *C. immitis/posadasii*, *Aspergillus* sp., *Bipolaris* sp., *Curvularia* sp., *Exserohilum* sp., *Penicillium* sp., and a nonsporulating mold. The first four were also recovered in at least one other nonblood specimen from the same patient, so detection of these fungi by the Isolator system provided supporting evidence, but not the sole diagnosis, of disseminated infection. The later four fungi were recovered solely by the Isolator system.

Isolation of Acid-Fast Bacilli

Recovery of mycobacteria from blood culture is rare, even in cases of disseminated disease; this is typically attributed to the low concentration of the organism in the bloodstream (59). Historically, poor recovery has been compounded by significant variability between clinical laboratory practices including suboptimal media and culture techniques for isolation of mycobacteria from blood specimens. The era of acquired immune deficiency syndrome (AIDS) brought increased recognition of *Mycobacterium* spp. beyond *M. tuberculosis* as being pathogens capable of causing significant disease (60, 61). Since that time, a steady increase in the number of immunosuppressed patients has amplified interest in optimal culture techniques for identifying *Mycobacterium* bacteremia (59).

Early reports found the Isolator lysis-centrifugation method of blood culture was sensitive for detection of both rapid and slowly going mycobacterial species. This method allows for concentration of 10 ml of blood onto a few agar plates, which increases the sensitivity of acid-fast bacilli (AFB) detection. Additionally, the quantitative nature of the method allows clinicians to monitor the patient's response to antimicrobial therapy throughout treatment. A case report from 1982 described lysis-centrifugation blood culture from a total of 45 blood cultures obtained from a single patient with recurrent *Mycobacterium chelonae* bacteremia (62). They found that Isolator blood culture resulted in organism detection in 60 to 65 h, while only 10 of 34 concurrently drawn conventional blood cultures were positive based on blind subculture at seven days of incubation (62). Around the same time, several case series were published describing the detection of *Mycobacterium avium-intracellulare* complex by Isolator blood culture from patients with AIDS and other immune-compromising conditions. Cellular lysis and centrifugation enhanced the CFU per ml recovered from the blood of infected patients by 2- to 5-fold. Testing revealed that 90% of bacteria were found in the pellet following centrifugation, while only 10% were in the supernatant (60, 61, 63). Another clinician used the Isolator system to identify *M. tuberculosis* from the blood of a patient with infection of the lungs, pleural cavity, and breast (64). The Isolator blood culture was able to detect growth of *M. tuberculosis* after 36 days of incubation.

Although the Isolator system increases the sensitivity of mycobacterial detection, growth of *Mycobacterium* is slower on solid agar than in broth-based media. BACTEC 13A (Becton Dickinson Diagnostic Instrument Systems, Towson, MD) broth was developed specifically for detection of mycobacteria from blood culture and contains modified Middlebrook 7H12 media, ^{14}C-labeled substrate, catalase, bovine serum albumin, SPS, and polysorbate 80 (65). In addition to being a broth-based culture system, patient blood is injected directly into the bottle, which eliminates the hazardous processing steps required by the Isolator blood culture system. In a head-to-head comparison, the BACTEC 13A medium was found to have similar sensitivity for detection of *M. avium-intracellulare* compared with the Isolator system with 58 and 61 positive cultures detected, respectively, out of a total of 70 cultures positive for *M. avium-intracellulare* (66). Three isolates of *M. tuberculosis* were detected in this study. All three were detected by the Isolator system but only one was detected by BACTEC 13A (66). On average, BACTEC 13A detected mycobacterial bacteremia two days sooner than the Isolator system. A 2002 study comparing Isolator blood culture and BACTEC 13A with CMBCSs BACTEC MYCO/F Lytic (Becton Dickinson, Sparks, MD) and BacT/ALERT MD (bioMérieux, Durham, NC) found that the CMBCSs had comparable sensitivity to the Isolator system and radiometric BACTEC 13A broth culture, but detected *M. avium-intracellulare* more quickly than either of the predicate methods (67). The difference in time to detection of *M. tuberculosis* was also reduced with CMBCSs compared with the Isolator method (68).

A limitation of the broth-based culture method is that a reduced amount of blood is cultured compared with the Isolator system, potentially resulting

in missed detection of bacteremia in patients with very low levels of mycobacteria in the blood. Therefore, the idea was born to combine lysis-
centrifugation and broth-based incubation to capitalize on the benefits of
both systems for detection of AFB from blood. Blood collected for culture
was lysed and centrifuged to concentrate any microorganisms present, and
the resulting sediment pellet was inoculated into broth media to reduce the
incubation time necessary to detect *Mycobacterium* spp. A study comparing
the Isolator system in combination with Bactec 12A broth incubation found
that the combined method was more sensitive for the detection of *M. avium-
intracellulare* bacteremia and it reduced the time to detection by nearly
two days compared with sediment obtained from the lysis-centrifugation
method being inoculated onto solid mycobacterial media (69). Another
study performed a comprehensive head-to-head comparison of five methods
of mycobacterial blood culture and found that the Isolator system with the
sediment pellet being incubated either directly to M7H11 solid media or
inoculated into Bactec 12B broth media had similar sensitivity to blood
directly incubated in specially formulated Bactec 13A mycobacterial media.
Biphasic medium had low sensitivity for detection of mycobacterial bacteremia on its own (65). In this study, the time to detection was similar
between blood incubated in Bactec 13A media and the combination of
Isolator plus Bactec 12B media at approximately 14 days. Both methods
allowed for more rapid detection of *Mycobacterium* spp. than any agar-based
culture methods, because those required a longer incubation time of
approximately three weeks (65).

For bacteria, it is recommended that Isolator tubes be processed as close
to the time of collection as possible because of the reduced viability of
fastidious bacteria (8–10). In contrast, mycobacteria can withstand prolonged periods of exposure to lysed blood and lysing agents found in the
Isolator tube without loss of viability. A study of *M. avium-intracellulare*
spiked blood incubated in Isolator tubes for 4 h to 56 days found that the
mycobacteria not only maintained viability when held at room temperature
in Isolator tubes, but the CFU per ml of blood increased during the first
four weeks of incubation, after which viability declined (70). The revelation
that mycobacteria can survive for prolonged periods of time within the
Isolator tube allowed for room temperature storage and shipment of specimens to distant laboratories for processing without concern for loss of
viability. For quantitative culture, specimens should be processed in <24 h to
more accurately measure CFU found in patients' blood specimens. Despite
the early excitement that the lysis-centrifugation method could be used to

quantify the amount of bacteria in the blood and to monitor therapy, this practice has not proven to be as useful as clinicians had initially hoped. Studies of patients with AIDS have shown that the mycobacterial burden in tissue is several logs higher than that found in the blood (61). Macrophages in the small intestinal villi often harbor a large burden of mycobacteria (71). In contrast, the quantity of mycobacteria found in the blood may not be reflective of the overall disease burden, and has not been shown to be predictive of patient outcomes. In addition, it takes two to three weeks to obtain CFU per ml data from blood culture, so clinicians are unable to obtain and use this information to alter immunosuppressive or antibiotic regimens in a timely manner (65). For these reasons, monitoring and reporting CFU per ml for Isolator cultures is not routinely performed.

An advantage of the Isolator is that it can be used in low-resource settings to culture bacteria, fungi, and AFB from blood. A study from Malawi in the year 2000 used the Isolator system in conjunction with the Septi-Chek AFB biphasic bottle (Myco-Chek; Becton Dickinson Microbiology Systems [BDMS], Cockeysville, MD). They found that injecting the Isolator pellet sediment into the bottle was a highly sensitive method for detection of slowly growing *Mycobacterium* spp. from blood specimens, and was more sensitive than plating the lysis-centrifugation pellet directly onto Middlebrook 7H11 agar (72). The Isolator system with or without the use of a second method was commonly used internationally for detection of AFB from blood around this time (73, 74). Lysis-centrifugation blood culture for AFB using the Isolator system is inexpensive compared with other methods of culture including Myco-Chek. Unfortunately, the Isolator system requires multiple processing steps that put the laboratory technician at risk for needle stick injury and exposure to *M. tuberculosis*-containing aerosols, which is a grave risk in areas where the prevalence of HIV and/or *M. tuberculosis* is high (72).

Summary

Lysis-centrifugation blood culture has played several roles in the identification of bacteremia since its conception in 1917. While this method was an improvement for blood culture pathogen detection in the 1970s and 1980s, the advent of CMBCSs has shifted the role of lysis-centrifugation to one of specialization. Currently, the Isolator system is used primarily for detection of slowly growing *Mycobacterium* spp. and fungi, especially dimorphic fungi. For bacteria, it may have utility in detection of *Bartonella, F. magna,* and *P. anaerobius.* In the future, the role of lysis-centrifugation-based pathogen detection may decrease further because of improvements in broth-based media for detection of mycobacteria and the ease of monitoring these cultures via automated incubation compared with the laborious nature of manual daily inspection of plates required for the lysis-centrifugation method. A niche where lysis-centrifugation will likely continue to play a role is the detection of blood culture pathogens in resource-limited settings because of the limited amount of equipment required. Although the role of lysis-centrifugation may be refined to focused applications, it is unlikely to completely disappear from the practice of clinical microbiology.

References

1. Clough MC. 1917. The cultivation of tubercle bacilli from the circulating blood in miliary tuberculosis. *Am Rev Tuberc* 1:598–621.
2. Dunne W, LaRocco M. 2001. Blood culture systems. *Infect Dis Ther Ser* 26:189–210.
3. Dorn GL, Haynes JR, Burson GG. 1976. Blood culture technique based on centrifugation: developmental phase. *J Clin Microbiol* 3:251–257.
4. Dorn GL, Burson GG, Haynes JR. 1976. Blood culture technique based on centrifugation: clinical evaluation. *J Clin Microbiol* 3:258–263.
5. Land G, Dorn G, Hill J. 1977. The isolation of disseminated *Coccidioides immitis* by an improved blood culture technique, p 19–30. In *Coccidioidomycosis: Current Clinical and Diagnostic Status*. Symposia Specialists Medical Books, Miami, FL.
6. Dorn GL, Smith K. 1978. New centrifugation blood culture device. *J Clin Microbiol* 7:52–54.
7. Dorn GL, Land GA, Wilson GE. 1979. Improved blood culture technique based on centrifugation: clinical evaluation. *J Clin Microbiol* 9:391–396.
8. Alere. 2000. *Wampole ISOSTAT System, Package Insert IN-050C1-03*.
9. Cashman JS, Boshard R, Matsen JM. 1983. Viability of organisms held in the isolator blood culture system for 15 h and their rapid detection by acridine orange staining. *J Clin Microbiol* 18:709–712.
10. Hamilton DJ, Amos D, Schwartz RW, Dent CM, Counts GW. 1989. Effect of delay in processing on lysis-centrifugation blood culture results from marrow transplant patients. *J Clin Microbiol* 27:1588–1593.
11. Alere. 2008. Wampole ISOLATOR 1.5 Microbial Tubes Instructions for Use and Supplementary Application Notes.
12. Carey RB. 1984. Clinical comparison of the Isolator 1.5 microbial tube and the BACTEC radiometric system for detection of bacteremia in children. *J Clin Microbiol* 19:634–638.
13. Henry NK, McLimans CA, Wright AJ, Thompson RL, Wilson WR, Washington JA II. 1983. Microbiological and clinical evaluation of the isolator lysis-centrifugation blood culture tube. *J Clin Microbiol* 17:864–869.
14. Brannon P, Kiehn TE. 1985. Large-scale clinical comparison of the lysis-centrifugation and radiometric systems for blood culture. *J Clin Microbiol* 22:951–954.
15. Washington JA. 1987. The microbiological diagnosis of infective endocarditis. *J Antimicrob Chemother* 20(Suppl A):29–39.

16. Kellogg JA, Manzella JP, McConville JH. 1984. Clinical laboratory comparison of the 10-ml isolator blood culture system with BACTEC radiometric blood culture media. *J Clin Microbiol* **20**:618–623.
17. Frank U, Malkotsis D, Mlangeni D, Daschner FD. 1999. Controlled clinical comparison of three commercial blood culture systems. *Eur J Clin Microbiol Infect Dis* **18**:248–255.
18. Hellinger WC, Cawley JJ, Alvarez S, Hogan SF, Harmsen WS, Ilstrup DM, Cockerill FR III. 1995. Clinical comparison of the isolator and BacT/Alert aerobic blood culture systems. *J Clin Microbiol* **33**:1787–1790.
19. Pickett DA, Welch DF. 1995. Evaluation of the automated Bact-Alert system for pediatric blood culturing. *Am J Clin Pathol* **103**:320–323.
20. Cockerill FR III, Reed GS, Hughes JG, Torgerson CA, Vetter EA, Harmsen WS, Dale JC, Roberts GD, Ilstrup DM, Henry NK. 1997. Clinical comparison of BACTEC 9240 plus aerobic/F resin bottles and the isolator aerobic culture system for detection of bloodstream infections. *J Clin Microbiol* **35**:1469–1472.
21. Pohlman JK, Kirkley BA, Easley KA, Washington JA. 1995. Controlled clinical comparison of Isolator and BACTEC 9240 Aerobic/F resin bottle for detection of bloodstream infections. *J Clin Microbiol* **33**:2525–2529.
22. Cockerill FR III, Torgerson CA, Reed GS, Vetter EA, Weaver AL, Dale JC, Roberts GD, Henry NK, Ilstrup DM, Rosenblatt JE. 1996. Clinical comparison of Difco ESP, Wampole isolator, and Becton Dickinson Septi-Chek aerobic blood culturing systems. *J Clin Microbiol* **34**:20–24.
23. Elsayed S, Kealey A, Coffin CS, Read R, Megran D, Zhang K. 2006. *Nocardia cyriacigeorgica* septicemia. *J Clin Microbiol* **44**:280–282.
24. Leli C, Moretti A, Guercini F, Cardaccia A, Furbetta L, Agnelli G, Bistoni F, Mencacci A. 2013. Fatal *Nocardia farcinica* bacteremia diagnosed by matrix-assisted laser desorption-ionization time of flight mass spectrometry in a patient with myelodysplastic syndrome treated with corticosteroids. *Case Rep Med* **2013**:368637.
25. Namnyak S, Uddin M, Ahmod N. 2011. *Nocardia cyriacigeorgica* bacteraemia presenting with cytomegalovirus disease and rapidly fatal pneumonia in a renal transplant patient: a case report. *J Med Case Reports* **5**:228.
26. Piau C, Kerjouan M, Le Mouel M, Patrat-Delon S, Henaux PL, Brun V, Morin MP, Gautier P, Rodriguez-Nava V, Kayal S. 2015. First case of disseminated infection with *Nocardia cerradoensis* in a human. *J Clin Microbiol* **53**:1034–1037.
27. Idelevich EA, Grünastel B, Peters G, Becker K. 2015. Direct blood culturing on solid medium outperforms an automated continuously monitored broth-based blood culture system in terms of time to identification and susceptibility testing. *New Microbes New Infect* **10**:19–24.
28. Schmidt HU, Kaliebe T, Poppinger J, Bühler C, Sander A. 1996. Isolation of *Bartonella quintana* from an HIV-positive patient with bacillary angiomatosis. *Eur J Clin Microbiol Infect Dis* **15**:736–741.
29. Regnery RL, Anderson BE, Clarridge JE III, Rodriguez-Barradas MC, Jones DC, Carr JH. 1992. Characterization of a novel *Rochalimaea* species, *R. henselae* sp. nov., isolated from blood of a febrile, human immunodeficiency virus-positive patient. *J Clin Microbiol* **30**:265–274.
30. Clarridge JE III, Raich TJ, Pirwani D, Simon B, Tsai L, Rodriguez-Barradas MC, Regnery R, Zollo A, Jones DC, Rambo C. 1995. Strategy to detect and identify

Bartonella species in routine clinical laboratory yields *Bartonella henselae* from human immunodeficiency virus-positive patient and unique *Bartonella* strain from his cat. *J Clin Microbiol* 33:2107–2113.

31. Tierno PM Jr, Inglima K, Parisi MT. 1995. Detection of *Bartonella* (*Rochalimaea*) *henselae* bacteremia using BacT/Alert blood culture system. *Am J Clin Pathol* 104:530–536.

32. Jorgensen JH. 2015. *Manual of Clinical Microbiology*, 11th ed. ASM Press, Washington, DC.

33. Bassetti S, Laifer G, Goy G, Fluckiger U, Frei R. 2003. Endocarditis caused by *Finegoldia magna* (formerly *Peptostreptococcus magnus*): diagnosis depends on the blood culture system used. *Diagn Microbiol Infect Dis* 47:359–360.

34. van der Vorm ER, Dondorp AM, van Ketel RJ, Dankert J. 2000. Apparent culture-negative prosthetic valve endocarditis caused by *Peptostreptococcus magnus*. *J Clin Microbiol* 38:4640–4642.

35. Hussein K, Savin Z, Shani L, Dickstein Y, Geffen Y, Raz-Pasteur A. 2014. Infective endocarditis caused by *Finegoldia magna* following aortic dissection repair: a case report and data evaluation. *Am J Case Rep* 15:554–558.

36. Fournier PE, La MV, Casalta JP, Richet H, Collart F, Raoult D. 2008. *Finegoldia magna*, an early post-operative cause of infectious endocarditis: report of two cases and review of the literature. *Anaerobe* 14:310–312.

37. Cofsky RD, Seligman SJ. 1985. *Peptococcus magnus* endocarditis. *South Med J* 78:361–362.

38. Kelly MT, Fojtasek MF, Abbott TM, Hale DC, Dizikes JR, Boshard R, Buck GE, Martin WJ, Matsen JM. 1983. Clinical evaluation of a lysis-centrifugation technique for the detection of septicemia. *JAMA* 250:2185–2188.

39. Kelly MT, Buck GE, Fojtasek MF. 1983. Evaluation of a lysis-centrifugation and biphasic bottle blood culture system during routine use. *J Clin Microbiol* 18:554–557.

40. Strand CL, Shulman JA. 1988. *Blood Stream Infections: Laboratory Detection and Clinical Considerations*. American Society of Clinical Pathologists, Chicago, IL.

41. Thomson RB Jr, Vanzo SJ, Henry NK, Guenther KL, Washington JA II. 1984. Contamination of cultures processed with the isolator lysis-centrifugation blood culture tube. *J Clin Microbiol* 19:97–99.

42. Washington JA II, Ilstrup DM. 1986. Blood cultures: issues and controversies. *Rev Infect Dis* 8:792–802.

43. Engler HD, Fahle GA, Gill VJ. 1996. Clinical evaluation of the BacT/Alert and isolator aerobic blood culture systems. *Am J Clin Pathol* 105:774–781.

44. Gander RM, Byrd L, DeCrescenzo M, Hirany S, Bowen M, Baughman J. 2009. Impact of blood cultures drawn by phlebotomy on contamination rates and health care costs in a hospital emergency department. *J Clin Microbiol* 47:1021–1024.

45. Surdulescu S, Utamsingh D, Shekar R. 1998. Phlebotomy teams reduce blood-culture contamination rate and save money. *Clin Perform Qual Health Care* 6:60–62.

46. Stockman L, Roberts GD, Ilstrup DM. 1984. Effect of storage of the du Pont lysis-centrifugation system on recovery of bacteria and fungi in a prospective clinical trial. *J Clin Microbiol* 19:283–285.

47. Petti CA, Zaidi AK, Mirrett S, Reller LB. 1996. Comparison of Isolator 1.5 and BACTEC NR660 aerobic 6A blood culture systems for detection of fungemia in children. *J Clin Microbiol* 34:1877–1879.

48. Campigotto A, Richardson SE, Sebert M, McElvania TeKippe E, Chakravarty A, Doern CD. 2016. Low utility of pediatric isolator blood culture system for detection of fungemia in children: a 10-year review. *J Clin Microbiol* **54**:2284–2287.

49. Patron RL. 2016. A 34-year-old man with cough, lung nodules, fever, and eosinophilia. *Clin Infect Dis* **63**:1525–1526.

50. Oliveri S, Trovato L, Betta P, Romeo MG, Nicoletti G. 2011. *Malassezia furfur* fungaemia in a neonatal patient detected by lysis-centrifugation blood culture method: first case reported in Italy. *Mycoses* **54**:e638–e640.

51. Surmont I, Gavilanes A, Vandepitte J, Devlieger H, Eggermont E. 1989. *Malassezia furfur* fungaemia in infants receiving intravenous lipid emulsions. A rarity or just underestimated? *Eur J Pediatr* **148**:435–438.

52. Al-Sweih N, Ahmad S, Joseph L, Khan S, Khan Z. 2014. *Malassezia pachydermatis* fungemia in a preterm neonate resistant to fluconazole and flucytosine. *Med Mycol Case Rep* **5**:9–11.

53. Roman J, Bagla P, Ren P, Blanton LS, Berman MA. 2016. *Malassezia pachydermatis* fungemia in an adult with multibacillary leprosy. *Med Mycol Case Rep* **12**:1–3.

54. Vetter E, Torgerson C, Feuker A, Hughes J, Harmsen S, Schleck C, Horstmeier C, Roberts G, Cockerill F III. 2001. Comparison of the BACTEC MYCO/F Lytic bottle to the isolator tube, BACTEC Plus Aerobic F/bottle, and BACTEC Anaerobic Lytic/10 bottle and comparison of the BACTEC Plus Aerobic F/bottle to the Isolator tube for recovery of bacteria, mycobacteria, and fungi from blood. *J Clin Microbiol* **39**:4380–4386.

55. Wilson ML, Davis TE, Mirrett S, Reynolds J, Fuller D, Allen SD, Flint KK, Koontz F, Reller LB. 1993. Controlled comparison of the BACTEC high-blood-volume fungal medium, BACTEC Plus 26 aerobic blood culture bottle, and 10-milliliter isolator blood culture system for detection of fungemia and bacteremia. *J Clin Microbiol* **31**:865–871.

56. Murray PR. 1991. Comparison of the lysis-centrifugation and agitated biphasic blood culture systems for detection of fungemia. *J Clin Microbiol* **29**:96–98.

57. Safdar A, Singhal S, Mehta J. 2004. Clinical significance of non-*Candida* fungal blood isolation in patients undergoing high-risk allogeneic hematopoietic stem cell transplantation (1993-2001). *Cancer* **100**:2456–2461.

58. Morrell RM Jr, Wasilauskas BL, Steffee CH. 1996. Performance of fungal blood cultures by using the Isolator collection system: is it cost-effective? *J Clin Microbiol* **34**:3040–3043.

59. Pierce PF, DeYoung DR, Roberts GD. 1983. Mycobacteremia and the new blood culture systems. *Ann Intern Med* **99**:786–789.

60. Macher AM, Kovacs JA, Gill V, Roberts GD, Ames J, Park CH, Straus S, Lane HC, Parrillo JE, Fauci AS, Masur H. 1983. Bacteremia due to *Mycobacterium avium-intracellulare* in the acquired immunodeficiency syndrome. *Ann Intern Med* **99**:782–785.

61. Wong B, Edwards FF, Kiehn TE, Whimbey E, Donnelly H, Bernard EM, Gold JW, Armstrong D. 1985. Continuous high-grade *Mycobacterium avium-intracellulare* bacteremia in patients with the acquired immune deficiency syndrome. *Am J Med* **78**:35–40.

62. Fojtasek MF, Kelly MT. 1982. Isolation of *Mycobacterium chelonei* with the lysis-centrifugation blood culture technique. *J Clin Microbiol* **16**:403–405.

63. Kiehn TE, Edwards FF, Brannon P, Tsang AY, Maio M, Gold JW, Whimbey E, Wong B, McClatchy JK, Armstrong D. 1985. Infections caused by *Mycobacterium avium* complex in immunocompromised patients: diagnosis by blood culture and fecal

examination, antimicrobial susceptibility tests, and morphological and seroagglutination characteristics. *J Clin Microbiol* **21**:168–173.

64. Kiehn TE, Gold JW, Brannon P, Timberger RJ, Armstrong D. 1985. *Mycobacterium tuberculosis* bacteremia detected by the Isolator lysis-centrifugation blood culture system. *J Clin Microbiol* **21**:647–648.

65. Agy MB, Wallis CK, Plorde JJ, Carlson LC, Coyle MB. 1989. Evaluation of four mycobacterial blood culture media: BACTEC 13A, Isolator/BACTEC 12B, Isolator/Middlebrook agar, and a biphasic medium. *Diagn Microbiol Infect Dis* **12**:303–308.

66. Kiehn TE, Cammarata R. 1988. Comparative recoveries of *Mycobacterium avium-M. intracellulare* from isolator lysis-centrifugation and BACTEC 13A blood culture systems. *J Clin Microbiol* **26**:760–761.

67. Crump JA, Tanner DC, Mirrett S, McKnight CM, Reller LB. 2003. Controlled comparison of BACTEC 13A, MYCO/F LYTIC, BacT/ALERT MB, and ISOLATOR 10 systems for detection of mycobacteremia. *J Clin Microbiol* **41**:1987–1990.

68. Crump JA, Morrissey AB, Ramadhani HO, Njau BN, Maro VP, Reller LB. 2011. Controlled comparison of BacT/Alert MB system, manual Myco/F lytic procedure, and isolator 10 system for diagnosis of *Mycobacterium tuberculosis* bacteremia. *J Clin Microbiol* **49**:3054–3057.

69. Gill VJ, Park CH, Stock F, Gosey LL, Witebsky FG, Masur H. 1985. Use of lysis-centrifugation (isolator) and radiometric (BACTEC) blood culture systems for the detection of mycobacteremia. *J Clin Microbiol* **22**:543–546.

70. von Reyn CF, Hennigan S, Niemczyk S, Jacobs NJ. 1991. Effect of delays in processing on the survival of *Mycobacterium avium-M. intracellulare* in the isolator blood culture system. *J Clin Microbiol* **29**:1211–1214.

71. Roth RI, Owen RL, Keren DF, Volberding PA. 1985. Intestinal infection with *Mycobacterium avium* in acquired immune deficiency syndrome (AIDS). Histological and clinical comparison with Whipple's disease. *Dig Dis Sci* **30**:497–504.

72. Archibald LK, McDonald LC, Addison RM, McKnight C, Byrne T, Dobbie H, Nwanyanwu O, Kazembe P, Reller LB, Jarvis WR. 2000. Comparison of BACTEC MYCO/F LYTIC and WAMPOLE ISOLATOR 10 (lysis-centrifugation) systems for detection of bacteremia, mycobacteremia, and fungemia in a developing country. *J Clin Microbiol* **38**:2994–2997.

73. Archibald LK, den Dulk MO, Pallangyo KJ, Reller LB. 1998. Fatal *Mycobacterium tuberculosis* bloodstream infections in febrile hospitalized adults in Dar es Salaam, Tanzania. *Clin Infect Dis* **26**:290–296.

74. Archibald LK, McDonald LC, Rheanpumikankit S, Tansuphaswadikul S, Chaovanich A, Eampokalap B, Banerjee SN, Reller LB, Jarvis WR. 1999. Fever and human immunodeficiency virus infection as sentinels for emerging mycobacterial and fungal bloodstream infections in hospitalized patients >/=15 years old, Bangkok. *J Infect Dis* **180**:87–92.

The Dark Art of Blood Cultures
Edited by Wm. Michael Dunne, Jr. and Carey-Ann D. Burnham
© 2018 American Society for Microbiology, Washington, DC
doi:10.1128/9781555819811.ch4

Bactec Blood Culture Systems　4

Robin R. Chamberland[1]

History

In the mid-1950s Dr. William Johnston and colleagues from Purdue University founded a company that specialized in developing instruments to detect very low levels of carbon-14, which were marketed for use in air quality testing. In the late 1950s, the company was sold to an investor who took it in the direction of seeking government contracts to study beta radiation and develop sensitive detection devices. The desire to transition the business to development of commercial products for the private sector led to a collaboration with scientists at Johns Hopkins University School of Medicine and the development of the Bactec 110 (Fig. 1A), the company's prototype bacterial detection system. The instrument accommodated 10 sample bottles on a rotary device and utilized a dual-needle adaptor to penetrate the rubber septum and sample headspace gas from bottles. The technology was based on Johnston's tritium air monitor, detecting carbon-14-labeled CO_2 produced by bacteria from radiolabeled substrates in the medium (1, 2).

　The company's first commercially available blood culture instrument, the Bactec 225 (Fig. 1B), was designed primarily for use in research settings, but was introduced to the clinical microbiology community at the American Society for Microbiology meeting in 1971. This semiautomated model incubated bottles online, and utilized sampling and detection technology similar to the 110, but accommodated 25 sample bottles in a removable tray. Bottles were moved to a platform for flushing/sampling of headspace gas and

---

[1]Saint Louis University School of Medicine, Saint Louis, MO 63104.

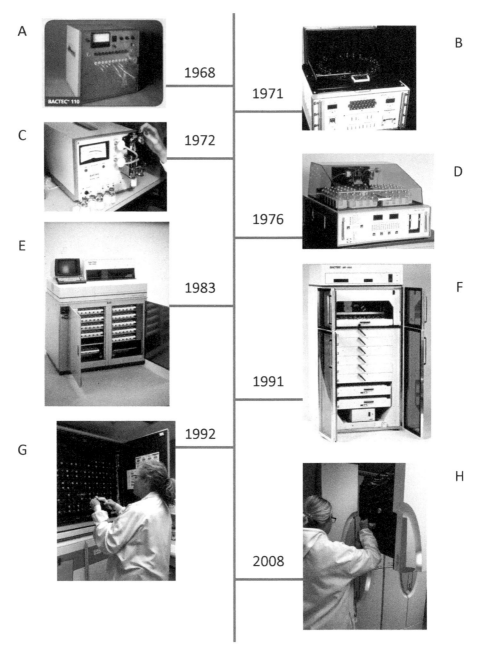

FIGURE 1 Year of introduction of Bactec blood culture instruments: 110 **(A)**, 225 **(B)**, 301 **(C)**, 460 **(D)**, NR-660 **(E)**, NR-860 **(F)**, 9240 **(G)**, and FX **(H)**.

growth detection at specified intervals. Growth was measured using an arbitrary growth index (GI) scale, with those samples registering at a pre-determined threshold progressing to Gram stain and subculture (3). Only 27 of these devices were manufactured, at a price of $35,000 each, and were followed in 1972 by the more economically appealing Bactec 301 (~$4,000) (Fig. 1C). This platform was labor intensive, in that it was capable of reading a single bottle at a time, and did not provide on-instrument incubation, but made "automated" blood culture technology accessible to smaller hospitals. The subsequent Bactec 460 (Fig. 1D), introduced in 1976, had the capacity to test 60 blood culture bottles per 1-h test cycle, with incubation performed offline. This cost-effective, semiautomated platform became the company's first widely adopted blood culture system. Three years later Becton Dickinson Diagnostic Instrument Systems (BD) purchased Johnston Laboratories and expanded production of the Bactec 460, still using radiometric detection (1, 2).

The Bactec NR-660 (Fig. 1E), introduced in 1983, was BD's first blood culture instrument to utilize nonradiometric growth detection, instead using infrared spectrometric analysis of CO_2 in headspace gases. Detection still required introduction of a probe into the headspace of the bottle for sampling purposes, although the sampling time was shortened from 60 to 35 s (1, 2).

The Bactec NR-860 (Fig. 1F), introduced in 1991, continued to utilize infrared technology for growth detection, but was the company's first fully automated platform, bringing together incubation, agitation, and micro-processor control. The 860 transported bottles between the incubator and sampling areas, allowing for continuous unattended testing (2).

Detection technology was further upgraded in 1992 with the introduction of the 9000 series instruments, which used noninvasive fluorescent technology to evaluate for CO_2 production. A fluorometric sensor incorporated into the bottom of each blood culture bottle was overlaid with a CO_2-permeable membrane, with fluorescence activated by acidification as CO_2 dissolves in the presence of water. This sensor was exposed to a light-emitting diode (LED) at 10-min intervals to detect bacterial growth. A positive result was generated by a computerized algorithm that took into account rate of change and sustained increase in CO_2 production to generate growth curves, rather than a GI threshold as in previous instruments (1, 2).

The Bactec 9240 (Fig. 1G) and 9120, named for their bottle capacity of 240 and 120, respectively, used identical technology. A smaller 50-bottle model, the 9050, differed slightly in that bottles were rotated to detectors and the computer was contained within the module (4).

The Bactec FX System (Fig. 1H) came to market in 2008, using the same detection technology as the 9000 series, but with added features meant to improve laboratory workflows, addressing areas such as ergonomics, ease of use, and instrument footprint. The addition of the EpiCenter Microbiology Data Management System expanded workflow and data management capabilities of the system (2).

Bactec Blood Culture Media

Several generations of BD media (radiometric, infrared, and fluorescence based), each with multiple iterations, have been produced for use on the Bactec platforms (Table 1). The initial aerobic and anaerobic media introduced, 6A and 7A, contained ^{14}C-labeled substrate with a total reactivity of 1.5 µCi/bottle. Using the Bactec 225 system and 6A and 7A media, Strauss et al. demonstrated that approximately 6% of positive blood cultures failed to be detected without terminal subculture, primarily enterococci and group D streptococci (5). A later evaluation demonstrated efficient detection of enterococci, but failure to detect *Streptococcus bovis* and viridans streptococci using 6A media. These organisms were recovered using 6B or 8B media, which contained 0.25% and 10% sucrose, respectively, and both of which had additional 0.5 µCi of ^{14}C-labeled substrate in comparison with their predecessor formulations for a final amount of 2.0 µCi (6). These changes in media were intended to aid in the growth and detection of streptococci, and it was subsequently reported that terminal subculture was unnecessary using these media (7).

Nonradiometric media NR6A and NR7A followed with the introduction of the NR-660 implementing infrared CO_2 detection. Aerobic (16B) and anaerobic (17D) media, introduced in the early 1980s, were the first to contain resin beads; one type that binds antimicrobial agents by creating ionic bonds with positively charged drugs and another that binds hydrophobic regions of all antimicrobial agents (2).

Standard Aerobic/F and Anaerobic/F media were introduced, containing a fluorometric sensor, and allowed fluorescent detection of CO_2 production, compatible with the technology of the Bactec 9000 series and FX instruments. Plus Aerobic and Plus Anaerobic media were introduced in the late 1980s, allowing the introduction of up to 10 ml of blood to each bottle, whereas earlier Bactec bottles were formulated to receive 3 to 5 or 5 to 7 ml of blood. BD made the Plus Aerobic/F media available in plastic bottles in 2012, and went on to offer Plus Anaerobic/F, Peds Plus/F, and Lytic/10 Anaerobic/F in plastic bottles as well.

Table 1 Comprehensive list of media types developed for BACTEC blood culture systems[a]

Medium	Blood volume, ml	Date released	Notes
Radiometric 6 Aerobic	5–7	1971	Radiometric 6 and 7 were the first pair of semi- or fully automated blood culture media.
Radiometric 7 Anaerobic	5–7	1971	Radiometric 6 and 7 media went through a number of iterations as the media manufacturing technology was developed to ensure the highest quality of product.
Radiometric 8 Hypertonic	5–7	1975	The Hypertonic medium was developed to aid in the culture of cell wall-deficient organisms.
Radiometric 16 Aerobic Resin	5–7	1980	Radiometric 16 and 17 were the first paired set of blood culture media to contain antibiotic-neutralizing resins.
Radiometric 17 Anaerobic Resin	5–7	1980	
NR 6 Aerobic	5–7	1984	The Non-Radiometric or NR technology was developed in the 1980s to eliminate the problems associated with the accumulation of radioactive waste.
NR 7 Anaerobic	5–7	1984	
NR 16 Aerobic Resin	5–7	1984	
NR 17 Anaerobic Resin	5–7	1984	
NR 26 Plus Aerobic	8–10	1985	The NR 26 and 27 blood culture pair was the first to accommodate 10 ml of blood per bottle, thus allowing the standard recommended blood culture volume (10 ml) and antibiotic removal in a single bottle.
NR27 Plus Anaerobic	8–10	1985	
Peds Plus	1–5	1989	Specifically developed for low blood volume specimens that are most commonly associated with pediatric patients.
Lytic Anaerobic	5–7	1990	Medium designed to lyse human blood, decreasing the blood background (increasing sensitivity) and releasing phagocytized organisms (increasing recovery).
Fungal	8–10	1991	Designed as a selective medium specifically for the recovery of yeast and fungi.
Standard Aerobic/F	5–7	1992	The fluorescent technology was developed to allow continuous monitoring and eliminate the need
Standard Anaerobic/F	5–7	1992	
Plus Aerobic/F	8–10	1992	

(*continued on next page*)

Table 1 (*continued*)

Medium	Blood volume, ml	Date released	Notes
Plus Anaerobic/F	8–10	1992	for extraneous culture gas. MYCO/F
Peds Plus/F	0.5–5	1994	Lytic medium was developed for the
Lytic/10 Anaerobic/F	8–10	1994	culture of primarily mycobacteria,
Standard 10 Aerobic/F	8–10	1994	yeast, and fungi
Mycosis IC/F	8–10	1997	from blood.
MYCO/F Lytic	1–5	1996	

[a]Provided courtesy of Shawn Beaty, BD Life Sciences.

Bactec 225 Studies

Thiemke and Wicher conducted one of the early studies of the semiautomated Bactec 225 system, comparing it with their conventional manual system, which consisted of 50-ml bottles of aerobic and anaerobic media plus 4 to 5 ml of blood incubated at 37°C for 14 days with daily visual examination for signs of growth (3). Gram stain and subculture to solid media occurred on day 1 if signs of growth were present and on days 2, 7, and 12 otherwise. Bactec 6A aerobic and 7A anaerobic bottles with 2 to 3 ml of blood were incubated for 7 days with sampling every 3 h for the first day, then daily through day 5, followed by subculture onto solid media on day 5. Over 3,000 blood culture samples were included, and methods were evaluated based on both detection of positive cultures and contamination rates. Conventional culture outperformed Bactec in the detection of significant Gram-negative (particularly *Escherichia coli*) and anaerobic (particularly *Bacteroides* and *Peptococcus*) organisms, while performance was similar for Gram-positive organisms, and Bactec was superior in detection of yeast. Across all organism types, time to detection was shorter with Bactec than conventional culture, and contamination rates were slightly lower.

Two additional studies reported similar findings of a greater number of positive cultures detected using conventional culture methods than with Bactec, but fewer isolates were detected during the first day of incubation using conventional methods (65% versus 4%, and 20% versus 7%) (8, 9). It should be noted that the volume of blood used in all three studies was less for the Bactec system (2 to 3 ml/bottle) than the conventional culture systems (5 to 10 ml/bottle for aerobic and 2 to 10 ml/bottle for anaerobic cultures), which likely accounted for decreased detection in comparison with conventional methods. Additional concerns included false-positive signals, frequently associated with elevated leukocyte counts, and the cost of the system given the limited degree of automation offered.

Bactec 301 Studies

The Bactec 301 instrument required offline incubation and agitation of blood culture bottles, which were then manually placed on the instrument individually for sampling of headspace gas and detection of radiolabeled CO_2. Few studies were published evaluating this labor-intensive system. A small study of 139 blood cultures comparing the Bactec 301 with 6A and 7B media bottles with conventional culture using biphasic media, 3 ml/bottle for all cultures, identified only six patients (16 cultures) with true bacteremia. The systems performed identically in detection, with each identifying 88% of positive cultures. One-third of positive cultures were detected earlier by Bactec, while one (8.3%) was earlier with conventional methods, and the remainder was detected simultaneously using twice-daily visual inspection of conventional cultures and thrice-daily Bactec detection during the initial 2 days followed by once daily thereafter. This study noted a high rate of false-positive cultures (12.2%) using a GI of 25, which added to the workload required to analyze these samples. Of concern, 75% of anaerobic bottles with growth on subculture failed to register a GI above the threshold of 25, and were therefore classified as false negatives. These subcultures of false-negative bottles grew *Propionibacterium acnes*, nutritionally variant streptococci, and *Bacillus* spp., the latter of which were detected in the concomitant aerobic bottles. Reasons for this failure were speculated to include formulation and age of the anaerobic media used and variation in metabolism under anaerobic conditions (10).

Bactec 460 Studies

The semiautomated Bactec 460 streamlined workflow in a way that made it more viable for use in higher-volume laboratories by allowing up to 60 blood culture bottles to be loaded onto the system for processing over an hour-long cycle. Bottles were moved by a conveyer system to the needle assembly for sampling, automating this previously time-consuming process, while incubation and agitation still occurred offline.

An early study conducted at Emory University compared efficiency, speed, cost, and technical time of blood culture using the Bactec 460 with conventional culture (11). Evaluated were 1,121 blood cultures from 493 patients, revealing 76 clinically significant isolates and 50 isolates classified as contaminants. Conventional culture consisted of inoculation of 5 ml of blood into 50 ml of Difco tryptic soy broth (aerobic) and Difco thiol broth (anaerobic), followed by daily visual inspection for signs of growth (turbidity, hemolysis), which led to Gram stain and subculture. Bottles were incubated for 10 days with blind subculture in the first 24 h and again at the end of incubation. Cultures evaluated by the Bactec system consisted of 10 ml of patient blood divided between three 30-ml media bottles: tryptic soy broth (6A) and hypertonic tryptic soy broth (8A) for aerobic and pre-reduced tryptic soy broth (7A) for anaerobic recovery. Aerobic Bactec bottles were tested three times in the first 24 h of incubation, then once on days 2, 3, 4, 7, and 10. Anaerobic Bactec bottles were tested on days 2, 3, 4, 7, and 10. Cultures demonstrating a GI of >30 (6A) or >20 (7A or 8A) were considered positive and followed with Gram stain and subculture.

The Bactec 460 was found to be significantly more efficient at detecting true positive cultures (92% versus 76%), demonstrating statistical significance for Gram-negative organisms, but not for Gram-positive organisms or anaerobes, both of which were present in lower numbers. The authors attribute the increased detection efficiency over conventional culture, at least in part, to the inclusion of the hypertonic medium (8A) with 10% sucrose, which detected the most isolates that were not present in other media types. Similar results were observed for time to detection, in which all organisms were detected more quickly (32 versus 46 h), but when groups were examined separately, again only Gram-negative bacilli demonstrated a significant difference.

This publication also provided the first cost analysis of the Bactec system, including an evaluation of technical time, consumables, reagent, and equipment costs, concluding that the Bactec system cost nearly twice as much per specimen as their conventional culture. The higher cost was attributed to increased technical time to perform testing, higher equipment cost, and increased reagent costs due to the use of three types of blood culture bottles.

Smith et al. compared the performance of Septi-Chek (SC) (Becton Dickinson Microbiology Systems, Sparks, MD [previously manufactured by Roche Diagnostics, Div. Hoffmann-La Roche, Inc., Montreal, Canada, at the time of publication]) with that of Bactec 460 in 903 patient blood cultures (12). The SC system combined a blood culture bottle with a paddle coated with chocolate, MacConkey, and malt agar contained in a cylinder that attached to the bottle, allowing the medium to flow over the paddle when the bottle was inverted. Cultures were conducted using 10 ml of blood per bottle with inversion of the SC system to perform subculture twice per day after inspection for turbidity in liquid medium or growth on solid medium. For Bactec 460 cultures, enriched tryptic soy broth (6B) was used for aerobic culture, and pre-reduced enriched tryptic soy broth (7C) for anaerobic culture, each with 3.5 ml of blood added. Bactec bottles were processed twice each day for the first 2 days for aerobic media, then once on days 3, 4, and 6 for both aerobic and anaerobic media, finishing with a subculture onto solid media on day 6.

The SC system detected more true positive blood cultures than the Bactec 460 in this study ($P = 0.024$), but also more contaminants ($P = 0.001$). The former was attributed to the lower blood volume used in the Bactec bottles, and the latter to the need for manual manipulation of the SC system when placing the agar paddle unit onto the bottles. Time to detection was shorter in the Bactec system, but isolated colonies were available on the agar paddle of the SC system, allowing progression to identification and susceptibility more quickly in some cases.

A third study comparing manual blood culture with the Bactec 460 reported more rapid identification of bacteremia by the latter (13). The conventional system used in this study consisted of biphasic aerobic medium and anaerobic broth. Bactec aerobic bottles (6B) were tested three times on the day of sample collection and aerobic (6B) and anaerobic (7C) bottles were tested twice on day 2 and once on days 3, 4, and 7. A GI of ≥30 in aerobic bottles, ≥15 in anaerobic bottles, or an increase in GI of ≥10 between readings in any bottle was considered positive. Manual cultures were examined visually each day. A blind early subculture was performed on the night of collection of the manual aerobic bottle by tilting to allow broth to flood over the solid media. Aerobic biphasic media were subcultured daily thereafter, and anaerobic cultures blindly subcultured onto solid media on days 1, 2, 4, and 7. A second, prospective, phase of the study added blind subculture of Bactec aerobic bottles on day 1.

The authors report no significant difference in detection of positive blood cultures within 24 h when using manual and radiometric methods across two different time periods, which they attribute to superior biphasic media and manual culture procedures. However, using early blind subculture, significantly more isolates were available for testing from solid media within 24 h ($P < 0.025$) with the manual method, leading to earlier organism identification and susceptibility testing. This study also found that 67% of Bactec bottles that were positive by blind subculture on day 1 had a negative GI at that time, but eventually went on to signal positive on day 2. This study also reports the higher cost of using the Bactec system, in addition to disadvantages of small maximum blood volume and use of radioactive materials.

A study comparing Bactec 460 with the Isolator lysis-centrifugation blood culture system examined the effect of blood volume on organism recovery by inoculating aerobic (6B) and anaerobic (7C) Bactec bottles with the minimum and maximum recommended blood volume suggested by the package inserts, 3 and 5 ml, respectively (14). Isolator tubes were filled with 10 ml of blood, and, following centrifugation and processing, the sediment was inoculated onto aerobic and anaerobic media. The Isolator system detected significantly more pathogens than either 3-ml ($P < 0.001$) or 5-ml ($P < 0.005$) Bactec bottles, primarily due to increased recovery of *Enterobacteriaceae*. The contamination rate was four times higher with the Isolator system than with Bactec, resulting in a monthly contamination rate of approximately 8%. Interestingly, there was no improvement in recovery of aerobic organisms observed in Bactec bottles inoculated with 5 ml instead of 3 ml of blood, and the authors speculated that this could be due to the less optimal blood-to-media ratio in the 5-ml cultures. There was an increased recovery of anaerobes in the 5-ml bottles, with the conclusion that a combination of 10-ml Isolator and 5-ml anaerobic Bactec bottle may provide optimal comprehensive recovery of blood-borne pathogens.

The Bactec 460 system was associated with episodes of pseudobacteremia, with one laboratory reporting 23 cases retrospectively identified over a 7-month period despite appropriate instrument maintenance including daily cleaning, sterilization, and inspection of the sampling needle (15). While this report found 22 of 23 cases to involve cultures with Gram-positive cocci, similar cross-contamination issues were reported by others involving a variety of organisms, including *Mycobacterium avium* (16, 17).

Some of the early mixed findings of efficiency of detection by conventional means versus radiometric detection could be attributed to the low volume of blood used in early Bactec culture bottles along with media formulations that were optimized over time to improve detection of a wider range of organisms.

Bactec NR-660 Studies

The introduction of the NR-660 system eliminated the need for radio-active media by using infrared spectrometry to detect CO_2 production. Other advantages included a shortened sampling test cycle from 60 to 35 s, allowing quicker completion of workload, improved sampling needle sterilization to prevent contamination, a computer database facilitating culture status inquiry, and computerized management of quality control and testing processes (18).

A multicenter trial of over 18,000 aerobic and 13,000 anaerobic paired blood cultures compared detection of bacterial growth using the 660 infrared with the 460 radiometric detection method (18). Equal volumes of blood (3.5 ml) were inoculated into aerobic 6B and NR6A bottles and anaerobic 7D and NR7A bottles, and incubated on their respective systems for 7 days. Aerobic bottles were tested twice daily for the first 2 days, then daily thereafter. Anaerobic bottles were tested once daily. There was no significant difference in ability to detect organisms overall between the systems, although there was a difference in recovery of Gram-positive cocci from aerobic media ($P = 0.04$), with better detection in the radiometric system. There was also no overall difference in time to recovery between the two systems.

A study evaluating the NR-660 for detection of bacteremia in neonates and young children utilized seeded cultures with 0.5 ml of blood to simulate common practice in this population (19). Bottles were inoculated with between 1 and 22 CFU of organism. No difference was found between Bactec radiometric and nonradiometric detection in these conditions.

Bactec NR-860 Studies

The fully automated 860 was introduced in 1991, the same year that Organon Teknika (later bioMérieux [bMx], Durham, NC) brought the BacT/Alert blood culture system, which featured "continuous" monitoring, to market. The bMx system used colorimetric CO_2 detection in 10-min cycles (20). A study comparing the NR-860 system with BacT/Alert evaluated high-volume resin-containing Bactec bottles 26A (aerobic) and 27A (anaerobic) and BacT/Alert aerobic and anaerobic nonresin bottles, each inoculated with 8 ml of blood (21). There were no significant differences in organisms recovered or time to detection. Major limitations of this study were that inoculated bottles were held outside the laboratory prior to being placed on the instruments, sometimes for extended periods; BacT/Alert bottles did not contain antimicrobial-removing resins; and the sampling interval for the Bactec instrument is not described.

Bactec 9000 Series Studies

The 860 was quickly surpassed by the launch of the 9240 in 1992, bringing Bactec into the era of continuously monitored blood cultures, as well as introducing noninvasive sampling by use of a fluorescent indicator of CO_2 detection within the bottle. A multicenter study evaluated the Bactec 9240 in comparison with the NR-660 system in a study of approximately 9,000 sets of blood cultures (22). This study used standard aerobic and anaerobic (6F,

7F, NR6A, NR7A) bottles inoculated with 2 to 5 ml of blood. Cultures incubated on the NR-660 system were tested at least twice on days 1 and 2, then daily for a total of 5 to 7 days, while bottles on the 9240 were tested automatically at 10-min intervals for 5 to 7 days, with length of incubation and performance of terminal subculture dependent on study site. The 9240 system and 6F aerobic media detected more organisms, with significant differences in overall detection ($P < 0.01$), *Staphylococcus aureus* ($P < 0.05$), and coagulase-negative staphylococci (CoNS) ($P < 0.01$), while anaerobic bottles (7F) yielded more positive cultures overall ($P < 0.001$) and for CoNS ($P < 0.001$) and *Enterobacteriaceae* ($P < 0.01$). Differences in yield were attributed to differences in media volume (30 ml for NR media versus 40 ml for 9240 media) leading to differences in blood-broth ratio, as well as media composition (sodium polyanethol sulfonate [SPS] concentration was lower in 9240 media). The average time to detection was 20.2 h for the 9240 and 27.5 h for the NR-660. In order to compensate for the delay in detection inherent in the sampling schedule with noncontinuous monitoring, cultures that became positive within 12 h of one another were considered equivalent, indicating that differences observed were due to other factors, such as the detection algorithm used by the 9240 system as opposed to the GI index.

Smith et al. evaluated the Bactec 9240 and the BacT/Alert in a direct comparison of over 6,000 blood cultures using continuously monitored blood culture systems (23). The study utilized aerobic and anaerobic bottles, with Bactec containing resin and BacT/Alert not having any antimicrobial-removing additives. All bottles were inoculated with 8 ml of blood and incubated for 6 days without terminal subculture.

The 9240 system detected more total microorganisms ($P < 0.001$), with significant differences occurring in detection of *S. aureus* ($P < 0.001$) and CoNS ($P < 0.001$). Additional analysis revealed that patients whose staphylococcal bacteremia failed to be detected by BacT/Alert were frequently receiving an antimicrobial agent at the time of culture. Among those who were known to have antibiotic present at the time of culture, there were significant differences between recovery of *S. aureus* ($P < 0.004$) and CoNS ($P < 0.0003$), but none in the absence of antimicrobials ($P = 1.0$). BacT/Alert showed a trend toward improved detection of nonenteric Gram-negative bacilli. Bactec displayed shorter time to detection for all bacterial groups, with significant differences for CoNS and nonenteric Gram-negative bacilli, while the BacT/Alert showed a trend toward more rapid detection of yeast. Costs and rates of contamination and false positives were similar between the two systems.

Shortly thereafter, a study of over 7,000 blood cultures was published comparing Bactec's aerobic resin-containing media with newly introduced aerobic FAN media for BacT/Alert containing activated carbon and Fuller's earth to absorb antimicrobials (24). Each bottle was inoculated with 10 ml of blood and incubated for 5 days with terminal subculture. Sixty-three percent of patients enrolled in the study were receiving antibiotics at the time of blood culture collection. No significant difference in recovery was observed overall or in any organism group, although there was a trend toward improved recovery of *Enterobacteriaceae* with the BacT/Alert system and CoNS with the Bactec system. BacT/Alert showed more rapid detection of *S. aureus* (mean 0.9 versus 1.1 days, $P = 0.005$), although no difference for other organisms. This publication demonstrated that the performance of these two systems was essentially equivalent when media with similar characteristics were used.

A comparison of the two systems evaluating standard aerobic media without additives for antimicrobial removal for 6,700 blood cultures reported that BacT/Alert detected more organisms overall ($P < 0.005$), as well as more clinically relevant CoNS ($P < 0.05$) and yeasts ($P < 0.001$) (25). Total organisms, and yeasts specifically, were detected more frequently by BacT/Alert in a subset of patients who were receiving antimicrobial agents at the time of culture. There were no differences detected for those patients not receiving antibiotics. The median time to detection, while similar for both systems (14 h BacT/Alert versus 13 h Bactec), was statistically significant ($P < 0.0001$), with *Enterococcus* spp., *Streptococcus* spp., *Klebsiella pneumoniae*, and nonpseudomonad, non-*Enterobacteriaceae* Gram-negative organisms detected earlier by Bactec and *Candida albicans* detected earlier by BacT/Alert. While statistically significant, difference in median time to detection for all groups was ≤3 h, while enhanced ability to detect yeast and CoNS is likely to be clinically relevant, conferring an advantage to BacT/Alert in this study. Taken together, these studies suggest that the selection of the combined system of instrument and media impacts performance.

Manometric detection of positive blood cultures has been utilized by Signal Blood Culture System (Oxoid Ltd., Basingstoke, United Kingdom) and the ESP (Difco, Detroit, MI). A report from Birmingham Children's Hospital describing the transition from the Signal system to Bactec 9240 demonstrated a significant increase in clinically relevant isolates and detection of episodes of bacteremia, particularly for CoNS and *Enterobacteriaceae*, along with shorter time to detection, after switching to Bactec (26).

A study evaluating the effect of delayed incubation compared the ESP blood culture system with the 9240 using seeded blood cultures was published in 1996 (27). Bactec aerobic and anaerobic Plus/F media and Difco ESP 80A aerobic and 80N anaerobic (high-volume, nonresin) broth were used with 8 to 10 ml of blood and approximately 45 CFU of organism. When there was no delay in time to incubation, recovery time across all organisms was similar from both platforms ($P > 0.05$), while the Bactec system detected growth more rapidly in cultures that had been held at room temperature for 24, 36, or 48 h prior to loading onto the instrument.

The system that evolved from the Difco ESP, i.e., the VersaTREK (TREK Diagnostic Systems, Cleveland, OH; currently Thermo Scientific, Waltham, MA), was compared with Bactec 9240 in a small study of 74 patients in South Africa (28). Five ml of blood was inoculated into each VersaTREK REDOX 1 (aerobic), REDOX 2 (anaerobic), and Bactec Plus Aerobic/F and Plus Anaerobic/F bottle. In this setting, VersaTREK demonstrated a false-positive rate of 7.9% compared with 0% for the Bactec. Overall, there was no difference in detection rate between the two instruments, with a positivity rate of 25% for VersaTREK and 24% for Bactec. There was a trend toward earlier time to detection with the Bactec, which detected growth 1.9 h earlier for Gram-positive organisms and 5.5 h earlier for Gram-negative organisms, but the difference was not statistically significant.

Bactec FX Studies

While the technology used in the 9000 series was carried over to the Bactec FX instrument, improvements were made in users' experience with the instrument, including better ergonomic design and features such as one-handed scanning of bottles.

The Bactec FX was compared with the BacT/Alert 3D using Bactec Plus Aerobic/F and Anaerobic/F and BacT/Alert FAN media in a study of 1,539 blood cultures from 270 intensive care unit patients, a population with especially high antimicrobial usage (87.7% in this study) (29). The recovery rate from the FX was 80.6% compared with 73.0% from the 3D system, with significant differences seen in detection of *E. coli* and *Acinetobacter baumannii*. Overall time to detection and that in aerobic bottles alone was earlier with the Bactec system ($P < 0.001$), which held true when Gram-positive cocci, Gram-negative bacilli, and CoNS were examined separately.

A similar study evaluated the performance of FA Plus (aerobic) and FN Plus (anaerobic) media for the BacT/Alert 3D, which replaced charcoal particles with adsorbent polymeric beads for antimicrobial agent removal, in comparison with Bactec Plus Aerobic/F and Anaerobic/F media (30). This study also assessed identification of organisms by matrix-assisted laser desorption ionization–time of flight mass spectrometry (MALDI-TOF MS) directly from blood culture bottles. Bactec aerobic media proved superior in detection of Gram-negative organisms ($P = 0.006$), while BacT/Alert was better able to detect *Enterococcus faecalis* ($P = 0.024$), although overall detection did not differ between the two systems. However, BacT/Alert identified more organisms overall ($P = 0.003$), and specifically *E. coli* ($P = 0.030$), *E. faecalis* ($P = 0.04$), and Gram-positive organisms as a group ($P = 0.013$) from the anaerobic media, although no difference was seen in the detection of strict anaerobes. Time to detection also did not differ overall, although BacT/Alert detected CoNS ($P = 0.003$) in aerobic media and treatment-negative organisms in anaerobic media ($P = 0.007$) more rapidly. Identification of organisms directly from broth of positive blood culture bottles was attempted using the Bruker MALDI BioTyper, with no difference between Bactec and BacT/Alert bottles, 88.1 and 88.9% of which yielded a result concordant with biochemical and/or sequence-based conventional results.

Studies comparing VersaTREK with Bactec FX largely focus on the ability to recover organisms in the presence of antimicrobial agents. An *in vitro* study using seeded bottles with antibiotics added demonstrated that VersaTREK REDOX medium, which does not contain any agents to neutralize antimicrobial agents, was inferior to Bactec media containing resins in their ability to recover a range of microorganisms in the presence of common antibiotics (31).

A small study of 20 patients with *S. aureus* bacteremia indicated that the VersaTREK system was limited in its ability to detect persistent bacteremia in patients receiving antibiotic therapy, because it recovered no organism in follow-up cultures, while Bactec FX using Plus Aerobic/F media allowed recovery of *S. aureus* from 25% of those cultures (32).

Fungal Culture Studies

Prevost and Bannister (33) reported on the superiority of the Bactec 460 system for detection of yeast from blood compared with commercially available biphasic media (BBL Microbiology Systems, Cockeysville, MD), all of which were tested with 3 to 5 ml of blood. *Candida* spp. comprised 88% of yeast recovered from 188 positive of 38,324 Bactec blood cultures, with the remainder attributed to *Cryptococcus neoformans* (10.3%) and *Rhodotorula rubra* (1.6%). The majority (84%) were detected in the aerobic bottle only, with a mean time to detection of 2.3 days. *C. albicans*, *C. tropicalis*, and *C. parapsilosis* were detected on average in <2 days, while *Candida krusei*, *Candida glabrata*, and *C. neoformans* required 5 to 7 days. Thirty positive of 668 fungal blood cultures from the biphasic media yielded 80% *Candida* spp. and 20% *C. neoformans*, with an overall mean time to detection of 7.8 days. *C. albicans*, *C. tropicalis*, and *C. parapsilosis* were detected on average in 6.5 to 9 days, while *C. krusei* required 6 days and *C. glabrata* and *C. neoformans* required an average of 10 days incubation. Only 53 cultures were performed by both methods on the same day, representing 15 separate instances, allowing a more direct comparison of methods. Yeast species were detected in the Bactec media only in 47% of these cases, and biphasic media only 20% of time, with one instance being ruled a skin contaminant, reducing this to 13% of true positives found by using biphasic media only. Mean time to detection was 2.6 days using the Bactec system and 8.5 days using the biphasic system. These findings suggested that yeast could be detected rapidly and efficiently without the added expense or workload necessary for separate blood fungal cultures, or the necessity for the physician to consider and place a second order for yeast detection.

A seeded study looked at the ability to recover *Candida* spp. from blood cultures in the presence of antifungal agents using the Bactec system with resin-containing media and the VersaTREK system with REDOX media (34). Bottles were inoculated with *C. albicans*, *C. glabrata*, *C. parapsilosis*, or *C. tropicalis*, along with peak and trough concentrations of amphotericin B, fluconazole, voriconazole, or caspofungin. Cultures without antifungal agent present showed no difference in detection between systems overall, although the detection rate for *C. glabrata* was 97.2% in VersaTREK and 86.1% in Bactec, a difference that did not reach statistical significance. Median time to detection was shorter by 2.2 h in the VersaTREK cultures ($P < 0.001$). In the presence of antifungal agents recovery from Bactec (83.1%) was superior to that from VersaTREK (50.7%), as was time to detection ($P < 0.001$) for all organisms, with the exception of *C. glabrata*.

BD's MYCO/F Lytic medium is optimized to aid in the recovery of fungi and mycobacteria from blood using Bactec 9000 or FX instruments. Fluorescence of the sensor in this medium is triggered by decreases in O_2 in the culture. BD product literature indicates that this medium supports the growth of a number of species of *Candida* as well as *C. neoformans*, *Histoplasma capsulatum*, *Aspergillus flavus* and *A. fumigatus*, *Malassezia furfur*, *Trichophyton rubrum*, as well as *Nocardia asteroides* and mycobacteria, but does not support the growth of *Blastomyces dermatitidis*. This medium does not contain any inhibitors to prevent the growth of routine bacteria.

A seeded study examining Bactec 9240 and BacT/Alert 3D's ability to detect *Candida* spp. was conducted using each company's aerobic, anaerobic, and mycology media (35). Bactec Plus Aerobic/F, Plus Anaerobic/F, and MYCO/F Lytic bottles and BacT/Alert FA (aerobic), SN (anaerobic), and MB (mycology) bottles were inoculated with blood and ~10^3 CFU of *C. albicans, C. glabrata, C. krusei, C. parapsilosis,* or *C. tropicalis* and incubated for 12 days with terminal subculture. Overall, BacT/Alert detected growth in 90% of cultures, while Bactec detected only 66%. Notably, the mycology media from both companies exhibited growth in all bottles; while bMx's other media outperformed BD's, exhibiting 100% versus 90% overall detection in aerobic bottles and 70% versus 10% overall in anaerobic bottles. Terminal subcultures of all bottles were positive, indicating growth of yeast undetected by CO_2 production in some media. Detection failures in BD aerobic media were all *C. glabrata* and *C. krusei*, while BD anaerobic media failed to detect any *Candida* species other than *C. glabrata.*

Time to detection between the two instruments for mycology media was similar, while bMx aerobic media exhibited faster detection overall ($P <$ 0.01), based on the extended period required for recovery of *C. glabrata* (mean 106.0 versus 51.8 h) in Plus Aerobic/F media. While it is not unexpected that anaerobic media from both systems performed poorly and mycology media performed well for recovery of *Candida* spp. in both systems, it is somewhat concerning that Bactec aerobic media failed to detect growth of *C. glabrata*, an important pathogen, in 40% of cases, because fungal blood cultures are not commonly ordered and physicians often rely on routine blood culture to detect candidemia.

An evaluation of MYCO/F Lytic media on the 9240 using patient samples, compared with the Isolator system, was conducted in a population of patients with AIDS and suspected fungemia or mycobacteremia (36). Seven hundred seventeen cultures were performed, consisting of 5 ml of blood in the Bactec MYCO/F Lytic bottle, and 6 to 10 ml from the Isolator tube, processed and plated per manufacturer's instructions, and incubated for 42 days. Of note, none of the patients were receiving antifungal drugs at the time of culture. Twenty-four fungal isolates were detected from patient samples. Fourteen *H. capsulatum* infections were detected, seven of which grew in both systems, and seven of which were recovered from MYCO/F Lytic media only. Ten cultures yielded *C. neoformans*, five of which were only recovered from the Isolator system. The time to detection for *H. capsulatum* did not differ between the two systems, but time to identification was shorter from the Isolator system, because colonies on solid media were available earlier. Conversely, *C. neoformans* time to detection was shorter with MYCO/F Lytic media, but there was no significant difference in time to identification, likely based on the small sample number.

Few comparative data exist regarding recovery of filamentous fungi from blood culture systems. A Mayo Clinic study comparing 8,293 patient blood cultures using MYCO/F Lytic media and the Bactec FX to Isolator system demonstrated *Candida* spp. and *H. capsulatum* as the most frequent fungal isolates recovered, and noted that 15 of 28 *H. capsulatum* isolates grew only with the Isolator system, while there were not significant differences in recovery of *Candida* spp. between the systems (37). Only seven organisms recovered in the study were filamentous fungi, representing five different genera, making any attempt to compare systems for these organisms impossible.

A 10-year pediatric hospital study also discovered very few molds in blood cultures; only 25 isolates of filamentous fungi from over 9,000 blood cultures using Isolator and either Bactec FX or BacT/Alert (depending upon laboratory site) (38). On chart review, seven of these were considered clinically relevant, with the remainder likely contaminants. Only one of the nine considered relevant, *Fusarium oxysporum*, was recovered from an automated culture system. A limitation of this study is that cultures on the automated platforms used aerobic media only and did not include specialized fungal culture media that may have aided in the recovery of additional molds.

Mycobacterial Cultures

The demand to perform blood culture for detection of mycobacteria became widespread as the need to diagnose *M. avium* complex infections in patients with AIDS increased. Lysis-centrifugation and concentration of blood, using the Isolator system or laboratory-developed methods with plating on mycobacterial solid media, was the conventional culture method. Bactec media 12B allowed concentrate to also be inoculated into broth media and analyzed by the radiometric 460 instrument. 13A media (Middlebrook 7H13) provided the advantage of direct inoculation of patient blood into the bottle without a lysis centrifugation step, and performed equally well for recovery of *M. avium* complex (MAC) from blood to the combination of 12B and solid media (39).

A later evaluation compared BD MYCO/F Lytic media for recovery of acid-fast organisms from blood using the 9240 instrument to ESP II media inoculated with concentrate from the Isolator system (36). *Mycobacterium* spp. were recovered from 64 of 717 cultures, with 18 found only using Bactec MYCO/F Lytic media, and four found only using ESP II media ($P < 0.05$). Fifty-eight of these positive cultures were MAC, of which 14 were recovered from the BD media only and three from the ESP II media only. Two cultures grew *Mycobacterium tuberculosis* complex, one in the BD media only, and four grew *Mycobacterium kansasii*, three in the BD media only, and one in the ESP II media only. Mean time to detection overall and for MAC was shorter with the Bactec system ($P < 0.05$).

A Duke University study compared BD's 13A media and 460 instrument, MYCO/F Lytic and 9240 instrument, MB media 110, and BacT/Alert, and Isolator tubes plated on Middlebrook 7H10 media for recovery of mycobacteria from blood (40). Mycobacterial species recovered in the study were: MAC (n = 85), *M. tuberculosis* complex (n = 5), *Mycobacterium chelonae* (n = 3), and *M. kansasii* (n = 1). There was no significant difference in detection of MAC between any of the media/systems tested. Time to recovery was shorter in all other methods than in Isolator ($P < 0.001$), and shorter for BacT/Alert MB (11.0 days) than for MYCO/F Lytic (12.8 days) ($P = 0.038$). Interestingly, of the five MTB isolates, no single system detected all; Isolator and 13A each recovered 80%, while MYCO/F Lytic and BacT/Alert MB yielded 60% and 40%, respectively.

An obvious limitation of these studies is the low number of isolates for any mycobacterial group other than MAC. FDA submission data for the MYCOF/Lytic medium indicate that this medium supports the growth of a wide range of species, but most of these are rarely seen clinically and thus not well represented in publications based on patient samples.

Sterile Body Fluids

Bactec aerobic and anaerobic blood culture bottles are FDA cleared for culture of blood only but are routinely validated for culture of other sterile body fluids (SBF). An evaluation of 908 SBFs, including peritoneal, synovial, pleural, amniotic, pericardial, and cerebrospinal (CSF), queried the ability of Bactec Peds Plus/F, Plus Aerobic/F, Plus Anaerobic/F, and Lytic/F media to support the recovery of organisms as compared with centrifugation and plating on solid media (41). BD media were tested with or without fastidious organism supplement (FOS) in the 9240 instrument. Cultures yielded 116 positive results, of which 72 were deemed clinically relevant. None of the positive results were detected by conventional culture alone, while 26 isolates were recovered from Bactec media only, and 22 more from Bactec with FOS added only. Mean time to detection in automated culture was 10 to 12 h, depending on media combination used, while conventional culture mean time to detection was 43 h. The Bactec system also proved superior to conventional culture when antibiotics were administered prior to fluid collection; 60% of those organisms from patients receiving therapy were recovered only from automated culture or exhibited delayed growth on conventional culture, compared with 15% of those from patients not receiving antimicrobial agents.

A similar study of SBF, including CSF, peritoneal fluid, pleural fluid, synovial fluid, bone marrow, and pericardial fluid, evaluated the Bactec 9000 series (9120) instrument using aerobic media only compared with conventional culture (42). A total of 906 specimens yielded 139 clinically relevant isolates, 80 of which were detected by the Bactec system only. This study included a large number of CSF samples (290), of which 66 were positive, and 32 of those were detected by automated culture only. Among organisms recovered in this study that failed to grow in routine cultures were five isolates of *Brucella melitensis* and one of *Neisseria meningitidis*.

Yagupsky et al. compared the Bactec 460 aerobic blood culture with conventional solid media for recovery of organisms from pediatric joint fluid (43). Similar performance was observed for the two methods for all pathogens with the exception of *Kingella kingae*, which accounted for 22.2% of positive cultures in this study. Eleven samples yielding *K. kingae* were evaluated by both methods, with 10 growing only in the Bactec system, and one by both methods, demonstrating the superiority of this automated culture system for recovery of a common cause of septic arthritis in children that may fail to grow using conventional laboratory methods.

EpiCenter
BD EpiCenter data management software was introduced in 2000, allowing interfacing with Bactec blood culture instruments as well as BD's other testing platforms and a variety of laboratory information systems (LIS). Patient demographic information and orders can be downloaded from the LIS into EpiCenter, and results uploaded from EpiCenter to the LIS. Depending on what instruments are interfaced through EpiCenter, and what data are being collected, it can be used in a number of ways. One of the blood culture-specific tools available is monitoring of bottle fill volumes, along with the ability to generate reports for quality assurance purposes broken down by unit, phlebotomist, etc. (Fig. 2). This is a valuable resource

A.

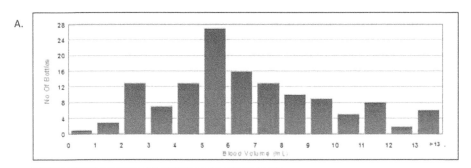

B.

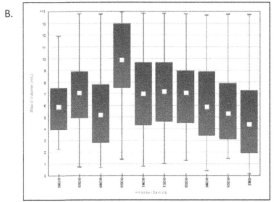

C..

	Mean (mL)	Conf - 95% (mL)	Conf + 95% (mL)	Std Dev (mL)	n
PHLEBOTOMIST1	9.7	8.5	10.9	4.0	40
PHLEBOTOMIST2	10.7	9.4	12.0	4.7	49
PHLEBOTOMIST3	4.4	3.9	5.0	1.5	33
PHLEBOTOMIST4	6.5	5.4	7.5	3.1	32
PHLEBOTOMIST5	7.4	6.2	8.6	4.2	44
PHLEBOTOMIST6	5.5	5.0	5.9	2.2	101
PHLEBOTOMIST7	3.9	3.5	4.4	2.1	84
All Groups:	6.9	6.0	7.8	3.1	383

'-' = Not enough Data to display (n<25)

FIGURE 2 Examples of reports available using EpiCenter. Blood Volume Distribution Histogram **(A)** returns number of bottles (*y* axis) for each blood volume estimate (*x* axis), shown for two hospital services. Blood Volume Box Plot **(B)** displays median (square), minimum, maximum, 25th, and 75th percentile blood collection volume (*y* axis) by hospital service (*x* axis). Volume Summary **(C)** contains mean volume by group or individual, along with standard deviation, confidence interval, and number of events during the chosen timeframe.

for targeting coaching opportunities to improve pathogen detection through collection of adequate blood volume and optimal blood-to-broth ratios. Fill volumes are based on red blood cell metabolism, so cultures from patients with low hemoglobin would appear to be underfilled. The system does not report data for individual cultures, but rather requires a minimum of 25 cultures per entity (ward, phlebotomist, etc.) being analyzed, then reports means and medians. While this should prevent the occasional anemic patient from skewing results, it should be noted that if patients in a particular unit, hematology/oncology wards, for example, are frequently anemic, data from that area can falsely indicate bottle underfilling.

Conclusion

BACTEC blood culture systems have demonstrated innovation in product design for nearly 50 years, ranging from radiometric technology to infrared and fluorescent detection with continuous improvements in media formulation over time. These systems have proven their value in timely and accurate infection diagnosis, and helped to secure BD's place as one of the leaders in the production of blood culture technology.

References

1. **Dunne W, LaRocco M.** 2001. Blood culture systems, p 189–209. *In Laboratory Diagnosis of Bacterial Infections.* CRC Press, Boca Raton, FL.
2. **BD Diagnostics.** 2008. TechniTopics BD BACTEC Blood Culture Systems celebrating 40 years of leadership in blood culturing. *BD LabO* **19:**2. https://www.bd.com/ds/learningCenter/labo/nl_labo_222788.pdf
3. **Thiemke WA, Wicher K.** 1975. Laboratory experience with a radiometric method for detecting bacteremia. *J Clin Microbiol* **1:**302–308.
4. **Murray PR, Hollick GE, Jerris RC, Wilson ML.** 1998. Multicenter comparison of BACTEC 9050 and BACTEC 9240 blood culture systems. *J Clin Microbiol* **36:**1601–1603.
5. **Strauss RR, Throm R, Friedman H.** 1977. Radiometric detection of bacteremia: requirement for terminal subcultures. *J Clin Microbiol* **5:**145–148.
6. **Beckwith DG.** 1979. Detection of group D and viridans streptococci in blood by radiometric methods. *J Clin Microbiol* **9:**20–22.
7. **McLaughlin JC, Evers JL, Officer JL.** 1981. Lack of requirement for blind subcultures of BACTEC blood culture media. *J Clin Microbiol* **14:**567–570.
8. **DeBlanc HJ Jr, DeLand F, Wagner HN Jr.** 1971. Automated radiometric detection of bacteria in 2,967 blood cultures. *Appl Microbiol* **22:**846–849.
9. **Renner ED, Gatheridge LA, Washington JA II.** 1973. Evaluation of radiometric system for detecting bacteremia. *Appl Microbiol* **26:**368–372.
10. **Wood NG.** 1976. Comparative study of two systems for detecting becteraemia and septicaemia. *J Clin Pathol* **29:**530–533.

11. Strand CL, Jones MC, Daniel WD. 1980. Comparison of a radiometric and a conventional blood culture system: efficiency of recovery, speed of recovery, cost and technical time. *Lab Med* **11**:41–46.

12. Smith JA, Roberts FJ, Ngui-Yen J. 1983. Comparison of a radiometric and a broth-slide system for aerobic blood culture. *J Clin Microbiol* **18**:217–218.

13. Ganguli LA, Keaney MG, Hyde WA, Fraser SB. 1985. More rapid identification of bacteraemia by manual rather than radiometric method. *J Clin Pathol* **38**:1146–1149.

14. Kellogg JA, Manzella JP, McConville JH. 1984. Clinical laboratory comparison of the 10-ml isolator blood culture system with BACTEC radiometric blood culture media. *J Clin Microbiol* **20**:618–623.

15. Craven DE, Lichtenberg DA, Browne KF, Coffey DM, Treadwell TL, McCabe WR. 1984. Pseudobacteremia traced to cross-contamination by an automated blood culture analyzer. *Infect Control* **5**:75–78.

16. Griffin MR, Miller AD, Davis AC. 1982. Blood culture cross contamination associated with a radiometric analyzer. *J Clin Microbiol* **15**:567–570.

17. Vannier AM, Tarrand JJ, Murray PR. 1988. Mycobacterial cross contamination during radiometric culturing. *J Clin Microbiol* **26**:1867–1868.

18. Jungkind D, Millan J, Allen S, Dyke J, Hill E. 1986. Clinical comparison of a new automated infrared blood culture system with the BACTEC 460 system. *J Clin Microbiol* **23**:262–266.

19. Anderson JD, Trombley C, Cimolai N. 1989. Assessment of the BACTEC NR660 blood culture system for the detection of bacteremia in young children. *J Clin Microbiol* **27**:721–723.

20. Thorpe TC, Wilson ML, Turner JE, DiGuiseppi JL, Willert M, Mirrett S, Reller LB. 1990. BacT/Alert: an automated colorimetric microbial detection system. *J Clin Microbiol* **28**:1608–1612.

21. Riest G, Linde HJ, Shah PM. 1997. Comparison of BacT/Alert and BACTEC NR 860 blood culture systems in a laboratory not continuously staffed. *Clin Microbiol Infect* **3**:345–351.

22. Nolte FS, Williams JM, Jerris RC, Morello JA, Leitch CD, Matushek S, Schwabe LD, Dorigan F, Kocka FE. 1993. Multicenter clinical evaluation of a continuous monitoring blood culture system using fluorescent-sensor technology (BACTEC 9240). *J Clin Microbiol* **31**:552–557.

23. Smith JA, Bryce EA, Ngui-Yen JH, Roberts FJ. 1995. Comparison of BACTEC 9240 and BacT/Alert blood culture systems in an adult hospital. *J Clin Microbiol* **33**:1905–1908.

24. Pohlman JK, Kirkley BA, Easley KA, Basille BA, Washington JA. 1995. Controlled clinical evaluation of BACTEC Plus Aerobic/F and BacT/Alert Aerobic FAN bottles for detection of bloodstream infections. *J Clin Microbiol* **33**:2856–2858.

25. Mirrett S, Reller LB, Petti CA, Woods CW, Vazirani B, Sivadas R, Weinstein MP. 2003. Controlled clinical comparison of BacT/ALERT standard aerobic medium with BACTEC standard aerobic medium for culturing blood. *J Clin Microbiol* **41**:2391–2394.

26. Gray J, Brockwell M, Das I. 1998. Experience of changing between signal and Bactec 9240 blood culture systems in a children's hospital. *J Clin Pathol* **51**:302–305.

27. Chapin K, Lauderdale TL. 1996. Comparison of Bactec 9240 and Difco ESP blood culture systems for detection of organisms from vials whose entry was delayed. *J Clin Microbiol* **34**:543–549.

28. Dreyer AW, Ismail NA, Nkosi D, Lindeque K, Matthews M, van Zyl DG, Hoosen AA. 2011. Comparison of the VersaTREK blood culture system against the Bactec9240 system in patients with suspected bloodstream infections. *Ann Clin Microbiol Antimicrob* **10**:4. doi:10.1186/1476-0711-10-4.

29. Roh KH, Kim JY, Kim HN, Lee HJ, Sohn JW, Kim MJ, Cho Y, Kim YK, Lee CK. 2012. Evaluation of BACTEC Plus aerobic and anaerobic blood culture bottles and BacT/Alert FAN aerobic and anaerobic blood culture bottles for the detection of bacteremia in ICU patients. *Diagn Microbiol Infect Dis* **73**:239–242.

30. Fiori B, D'Inzeo T, Di Florio V, De Maio F, De Angelis G, Giaquinto A, Campana L, Tanzarella E, Tumbarello M, Antonelli M, Sanguinetti M, Spanu T. 2014. Performance of two resin-containing blood culture media in detection of bloodstream infections and in direct matrix-assisted laser desorption ionization-time of flight mass spectrometry (MALDI-TOF MS) broth assays for isolate identification: clinical comparison of the BacT/Alert Plus and Bactec Plus systems. *J Clin Microbiol* **52**:3558–3567.

31. Miller NS, Rogan D, Orr BL, Whitney D. 2011. Comparison of BD Bactec Plus blood culture media to VersaTREK Redox blood culture media for detection of bacterial pathogens in simulated adult blood cultures containing therapeutic concentrations of antibiotics. *J Clin Microbiol* **49**:1624–1627.

32. Bonilla H, Zervos M, Saravolatz LD. 2011. Comparison of BACTEC™ plus Aerobic/F and VersaTREK REDOX(®) blood culture media for the recovery of *Staphylococcus aureus* from patients with suspected persistent bacteremia. *J Infect* **63**:89–90.

33. Prevost E, Bannister E. 1981. Detection of yeast septicemia by biphasic and radiometric methods. *J Clin Microbiol* **13**:655–660.

34. Riedel S, Eisinger SW, Dam L, Stamper PD, Carroll KC. 2011. Comparison of BD Bactec Plus Aerobic/F medium to VersaTREK Redox 1 blood culture medium for detection of *Candida* spp. in seeded blood culture specimens containing therapeutic levels of antifungal agents. *J Clin Microbiol* **49**:1524–1529.

35. Horvath LL, George BJ, Murray CK, Harrison LS, Hospenthal DR. 2004. Direct comparison of the BACTEC 9240 and BacT/ALERT 3D automated blood culture systems for *Candida* growth detection. *J Clin Microbiol* **42**:115–118.

36. Waite RT, Woods GL. 1998. Evaluation of BACTEC MYCO/F lytic medium for recovery of mycobacteria and fungi from blood. *J Clin Microbiol* **36**:1176–1179.

37. Ramanan P, Vetter EA, Milone AA, Patel R, Wengenack NL. 2016. Comparison of BACTEC MYCO/F Lytic bottle to the Wampole Isolator for recovery of fungal and mycobacterial organisms. *Open Forum Infect Dis* **3**:1557. doi:10.1093/ofid/ofw172.1258

38. Campigotto A, Richardson SE, Sebert M, McElvania TeKippe E, Chakravarty A, Doern CD. 2016. Low utility of pediatric isolator blood culture system for detection of fungemia in children: a 10-year review. *J Clin Microbiol* **54**:2284–2287.

39. Strand CL, Epstein C, Verzosa S, Effatt E, Hormozi P, Siddiqi SH. 1989. Evaluation of a new blood culture medium for mycobacteria. *Am J Clin Pathol* **91**:316–318.

40. Crump JA, Tanner DC, Mirrett S, McKnight CM, Reller LB. 2003. Controlled comparison of BACTEC 13A, MYCO/F LYTIC, BacT/ALERT MB, and ISOLA-TOR 10 systems for detection of mycobacteremia. *J Clin Microbiol* **41**:1987–1990.

41. Fuller DD, Davis TE. 1997. Comparison of BACTEC plus Aerobic/F, Anaerobic/F, Peds Plus/F, and Lytic/F media with and without fastidious organism supplement to conventional methods for culture of sterile body fluids. *Diagn Microbiol Infect Dis* **29**: 219–225.

42. Akcam FZ, Yayli G, Uskun E, Kaya O, Demir C. 2006. Evaluation of the Bactec microbial detection system for culturing miscellaneous sterile body fluids. *Res Microbiol* 157:433–436.

43. Yagupsky P, Dagan R, Howard CW, Einhorn M, Kassis I, Simu A. 1992. High prevalence of *Kingella kingae* in joint fluid from children with septic arthritis revealed by the BACTEC blood culture system. *J Clin Microbiol* 30:1278–1281.

The Dark Art of Blood Cultures
Edited by Wm. Michael Dunne, Jr. and Carey-Ann D. Burnham
© 2018 American Society for Microbiology, Washington, DC
doi:10.1128/9781555819811.ch5

The bioMérieux BacT/Alert: Automation at Last in the Black Box

5

Bradley Ford[1] and George Kallstrom[2,3]

Introduction and Historical Context

This chapter introduces the BacT/Alert, the first automated blood culture system, and its descendants. The first part of the chapter covers the historical context in which the system was developed and some of the key design considerations that were intended to close gaps in blood culture practice in the early 1990s. The second part of the chapter outlines the evolution of the BacT/Alert culture media, their performance, and design changes to subsequent instruments in the BacT/Alert family tree.

The beginning of this chapter is primarily an oral history supplied by Thurman Thorpe, a microbiologist for General Diagnostics (later Organon Teknika and bioMérieux), and James DiGuiseppi, who started his involvement at Organon Teknika and ended his career at bioMérieux. Between the two of them, and with the help of a relatively small development team, much of the research and development for what became the BacT/Alert blood culture system was performed in the late 1980s. This system's core principles remained relatively static through the BacT/Alert 3D system and the BacT/Alert VIRTUO system.

General Diagnostics was a company owned by Warner Lambert in Morris Plains, NJ. The idea to create an improved externally monitored blood culture system originated in the marketing department of General Diagnostics, a company otherwise focused on biochemical identification

[1]Department of Pathology, University of Iowa Carver College of Medicine, Iowa City, IA 52242
[2]Department of Pathology and Laboratory Medicine, Summa Health System, Akron, OH 44304
[3]Department of Pathology, Northeast Ohio Medical University (NEOMED), Rootstown, OH 44272

tests. As a pure marketing exercise, General Diagnostics went into the field to ask customers about their unmet needs. A common response was a request for an alternative to the Bactec 460 (Becton Dickinson, Sparks, MD, see chapter 4), which, while not ubiquitous, was essentially the only option for a semiautomated blood culture system (distinguished from manual monitoring and paddle systems) commercially available at the time. The Bactec 460 had several notable disadvantages, many of which are seen in the schematic diagram in Fig. 1 (1):

1. Carrying racks of bottles and manually loading them onto the machine several times a day was labor intensive. The rubber septa sealing the bottles had to be cleaned with 70% ethanol, and the lack of scrupulous attention to technique could introduce contamination. Each bottle took 30 to 60 s to read. In a large laboratory, this could be extremely time-consuming and cumbersome.
2. To obtain a measurement, the Bactec 460 system required the rubber septa at the tops of the bottles to be pierced with two needles to draw headspace gas for analysis, routinely exposing the user to sharp objects.

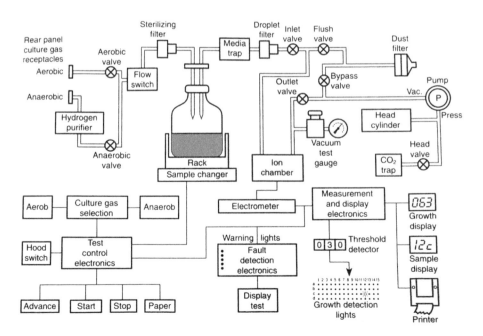

Figure 1 Bactec 460 schematic illustrating the complex gas flow, bottle piercing, and analysis of positivity versus the BacT/Alert. Reproduced from (1), with permission.

The needles frequently required replacement by hand, further in-creasing the risk of injury.

3. The electrical sterilizer element heating the needles did not work especially well and cross-contamination occasionally occurred between bottles.

4. Each bottle contained 2 μCi of carbon-14, a weakly radioactive beta-emitter. Carbon-14 disposal required capture of the waste stream in barrels and disposal as radioactive waste, adding to the cost and labor intensity of the system.

5. Gas canisters had to be stocked to flush headspace gas through the system.

6. The instruments were not fully computerized or automated; paper reports were generated, and positive bottles had to be manually sorted.

Later, the Bactec 660 (Becton Dickinson) resolved some of these issues by using an infrared spectrophotometer to detect carbon dioxide production. The 660 was touted to include a more efficient sterilization heater, coupled with ultraviolet sterilization of the loading area. It was claimed that the 660 had the ability to puncture the rubber septa at different points with each sample, although in practice this ability was questionable. However, the overall workflow and lack of continuous monitoring were still points of dissatisfaction for clinical laboratories. In 1985, a group at General Diagnostics consisting of one microbiologist (Thorpe), one engineer, and an organic chemist was formed. This group was funded for 1 year and focused on fluorescent methods to detect microbial growth but did not pursue a complete continuously monitored blood culture system at the time.

In the 1980s, Organon Teknika was the human diagnostics arm of a large Dutch conglomerate, Akzo Nobel. Akzo's U.S. headquarters was in Winston-Salem, NC. In 1986, Organon Teknika relocated several U.S. companies it had purchased, including General Diagnostics, to Durham, NC. Organon Teknika specialized in enzyme immunoassay technology (EIA) and was marketing EIA technology as their primary product (reviewed in reference 2, with examples of early kits). The company had minimal interest in microbiology *per se*. It was not until the partially developed idea of a continuous-monitoring blood culture system emerged from research and marketing that efforts expanded to build such a system at its Durham campus.

In November 1986, a group formed at the Durham site that included Thurman Thorpe and James DiGuiseppi under the direction of the head of research, Richard Driscoll, who had come from Dade. At the time, Organon Teknika was exiting the clinical microbiology space and had only one primary product, the Autobac MTS, which was a system inherited from General Diagnostics used for screening urine for clinically significant bacteriuria. This system was generally unpopular and was being discontinued after a long period of dwindling support. Driscoll insisted on autonomy and adequate funding to pursue new projects as a condition of his employment. The group was therefore largely left alone to rapidly develop a prototype of an entirely new system. This inventive spirit was facilitated by the Dutch culture at Organon Teknika, which accepted individual independence in incubating ideas without micromanaging through top-down control of development.

Technical Challenges and Construction of the BacT/Alert

Starting to address the issues of needle-based bottle sampling inherent to the Bactec 460 system, the team first tackled the problem of fluorescent detection of bacteria using techniques originated at General Diagnostics. In the original formulation, the team attempted to place fluorescent molecules in the broth with the ability to respond to changes in the liquid environment. This was a challenging approach because of the many factors that can quench fluorescence in solution, and because microorganisms require a stable environment for growth (especially with respect to pH). Fluorophores were nevertheless chosen based on a robust response to changing pH, setting the stage for failure of the fluid-phase approach and development of an improved solid-phase system.

Thorpe realized by analogy to a CO_2 pH electrode that a pH indicator could be placed behind a silicone wall permeable to CO_2, essentially making the indicator independent of the solution. At the time, Thorpe had also been working on an instrument to diagnose urinary tract infections by filtering urine and dyeing bacteria and white blood cells on a filter material able to change color if certain analytes were present. He was, therefore, familiar with a large array of pH-responsive dyes able to bind to filters. The group settled on xylenol blue, which bound to filter material and worked in the pH range of 9 to 10 (where CO_2 could effectively produce a change of pH). Dye filter plugs were manufactured (with difficulty, because of the need for humidity control and uniform charge to ensure uniform xylenol blue binding) (Fig. 2). This chemistry was changed to an emulsion of the same dye with silicon about 10 years later to alleviate some of the problems in getting dye to bind

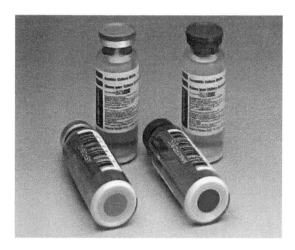

Figure 2 Original BacT/Alert media (aerobic at left and anaerobic at right) containing a disk of membrane with bound dye at their bases. Compare with the positive and negative modern emulsion bottles in Figure 3B. The bottle on the right is negative but is gassed with 2.5% CO_2, which, combined with a difference in equilibrium from being bound to a membrane, results in a greenish color relative to the bottle at left in Figure 3B. The bottle at left is positive; the increase in reflected red light from the instrument's LEDs would be interpreted as growth. Image courtesy of bioMérieux, used with permission.

to filter surfaces (Fig. 3B). DiGuiseppi then focused on light-emitting diodes (LEDs) to detect color changes on a solid-phase surface, greatly reducing the technical difficulties of detecting changes in a fluid phase while maintaining a high dynamic range because of the white filter background.

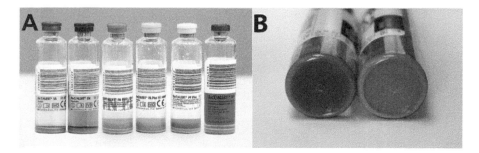

Figure 3 (A) An array of modern BacT/Alert bottles (left to right: SA, SN, FN Plus, FA Plus, PF Plus, and MP). **(B)** A negative (left) and positive (right) bottle, demonstrating the dye emulsion medium and the color change detected by the BacT/Alert system. Image courtesy of bioMérieux, used with permission.

Because the filter and dye were separated from the fluid within the bottles by a membrane impervious to most ions but freely permeable to CO_2, bottles with different formulations could be created without concern of liquid components interfering with the signal being detected by the instrument. As microorganisms grew, they produced CO_2, which diffused across the membrane and interacted with water impregnated in the membrane to produce hydrogen ions ($CO_2 + H_2O \leftrightarrow H_2CO_3 \leftrightarrow H^+ + HCO_3^-$), thereby decreasing the pH of the indicator and changing its color from blue/green to yellow. An increase in reflected red light from positive bottles was therefore easily observed through the membrane at the bottom of the bottles (Fig. 2, 3B, and 4).

LEDs were a relatively recent invention at the end of the 1980s. In the Bactec 460 model, bottles were individually transported to a reader which did not lend the machine to continuous monitoring. To circumvent the transport of bottles to a detector, the new Organon Teknika instrument required a large array of relatively inexpensive individual sensors and detectors to monitor bottles individually, and all of them needed to be individually calibrated for equivalence. At the time, only red and green LEDs were readily available. Red wavelengths were not optimal for detection of color changes associated with the dye, but the very high output of red LEDs versus alternative colors was adequate, so they were chosen for the detectors.

Another limitation of the Bactec 460 was the intermittent draining of the headspace gas, which was not sensitive for detection of some slower

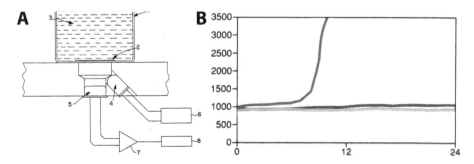

Figure 4 (**A**) Mechanism of detection of growth detection in the BacT/Alert from the original patent (47). 1, vessel; 2, sensor; 3, culture medium; 4, light source; 5, photodetector; and associated electronics including 6, current source; 7, current to voltage converter; and 8, low-pass filter. (**B**) BacT/Alert reflectance curves for blood with *E. coli* (red), blood without organisms (blue, demonstrating baseline drift), and an uninoculated bottle (yellow).

growth kinetics and limited the analytical sensitivity of the instrument. Continuous monitoring of a closed system by this new instrument generated large quantities of data. To analyze this large data set, innovative calculus-based algorithms were designed by DiGuiseppi. These algorithms needed to be insensitive to noise but sensitive to the growth of organisms generating a small amount of CO_2. They, therefore, examined first and second derivatives of data monitored every 10 min, accounting for the gradual background drift in pH from the human cells inoculated into the bottle (blue line in Fig. 4B). Of note, bottles with high absolute levels of signal suggested that growth may have occurred before kinetics began to be measured. The initial software and interfaces were written by a single Organon Teknika software engineer, and the algorithms encoded in this software remained essentially unchanged through the introduction of the BacT/Alert 3D. An initial prototype of the BacT/Alert is shown in Fig. 5: the hardware and software

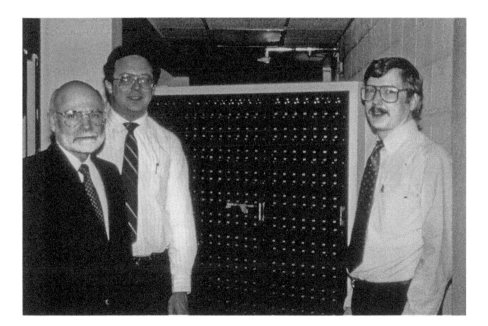

Figure 5 The first prototype BacT/Alert, one of two built at Durham, NC, during placement in the laboratory of Barth Reller at Duke. Left to right are James Turner (director of the Durham group), James DiGuiseppi, and Thurman Thorpe. Note the differences in the instrument compared with the production instrument in Fig. 6. Doors evolved from clear plastic prone to light leakage and interference to clear/dark (but infrared transparent) in initial production, then opaque doors.

remain largely recognizable through subsequent iterations of the instrument (Fig. 6 to 8).

Continuous monitoring presented one additional challenge. Classically, bacterial cultures were vigorously shaken to support growth of aerobic

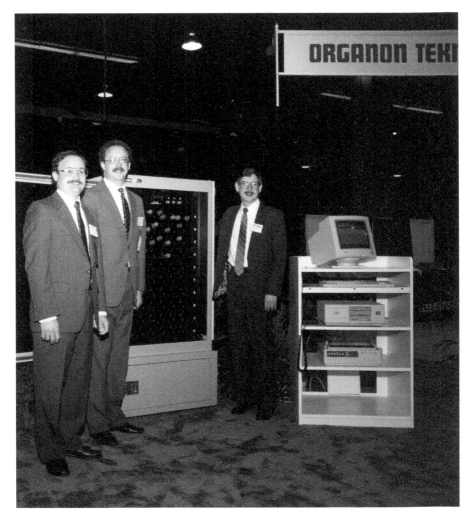

Figure 6 Larry Pope (manager of the instrument development group at Organon Teknika, where the production instrument was designed and manufactured), Thurman Thorpe, and James DiGuiseppi at the American Society for Microbiology general meeting, New Orleans, 1989, with a production model of the BacT/Alert. This instrument was produced for more than 10 years before it was succeeded by the BacT/Alert 3D system.

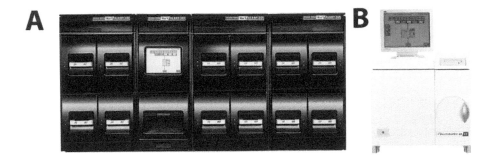

Figure 7 BacT/Alert 3D system in modular form with touchscreen and integrated bar coder **(A)** and the standalone BacT/Alert/3D 60 system **(B)**. Image used with permission from bioMérieux.

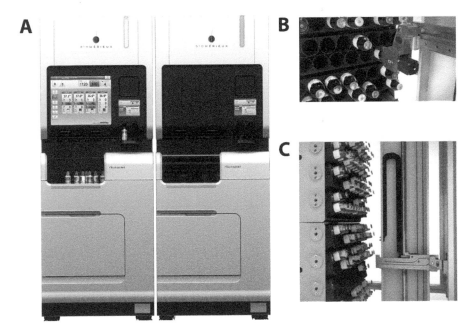

Figure 8 (A) The BacT/Alert VIRTUO system in dual-unit format. The touchscreen at upper left can be used to automatically unload positive bottles (yellow "button" at upper right of screen), which are automatically deposited in the two slots at middle right. Bottles are robotically accessioned in groups of up to 40 at a time (center), and placed in internal racks by a robotic arm **(B)**, allowing the bottles to be rocked **(C)**. Negative bottles are automatically removed and placed in a waste receptacle at the bottom of each unit. Image used with permission from bioMérieux.

organisms. The design team realized that shaking of large numbers of bottles was physically impractical and would shorten the life of an instrument in continuous use for long periods of time. To overcome this problem they developed a gentle rocking motion able to provide complete mixing and adequate aeration. This was a new way of thinking within the microbiological community, and through careful experiments documenting mixing with glycerol and other tracers, the team proved complete mixing occurred in rocked bottles. Time to detection and recovery studies demonstrated the rocking motion was very effective, especially for anaerobes, making blind subculture at the end of incubation unnecessary (3).

Business Environment and Initial Commercial Success

The first BacT/Alert system was in clinical trials for about 2 years and FDA approval was obtained within 2 years after their completion. The BacT/Alert was the product of a small group of experts combining different complementary skill sets, and accelerated by a relatively permissive regulatory environment at the time.

The synergy between regulatory environment, new technology, and a company new to the blood culture arena was evident in internal marketing surveys at the time. Per James DiGuiseppi, a series of blinded laboratory manager focus panels was held well before the launch of the BacT/Alert. These potential customers were presented with the instrument concept, which generated expected enthusiasm. When asked "Who is bringing this to market?" Organon Teknika ranked last, behind even fictitious companies inserted as internal controls for the survey.

The release of the instrument, now named the BacT/Alert, at the American Society for Microbiology general meeting in New Orleans (1989) (Fig. 6) was met with surprise by the public and rival companies. Becton Dickinson sent a contingent from New Jersey to inspect the Organon Teknika floor display. Between customers and rivals, the Organon Teknika booth was one of the most well-attended points of interest on the meeting floor that year.

Much of the enthusiasm had been anticipated when the business case was originally made for a continuously monitored blood culture system. Organon Teknika was unsurprisingly not the only company working on such a system. MicroScan (then a division of Baxter Diagnostics) had been developing a rival instrument, subsequently demonstrated the year after the New Orleans meeting, which worked by a very similar mechanism and fell under the same patents. It is unknown how long the larger, more well-established microbiology company had been working on this technology only to be scooped by an upstart. The MicroScan instrument was subsequently lost to history and little more public information is known about it. Another rival, Becton Dickinson (BD), had developed the Bactec 9000 and its associated blood culture bottles during a slightly later time period, and this system closely resembled the BacT/Alert and its bottles (chapter 4). BD's failure to recognize Organon Teknika's intellectual property resulted in a lawsuit in late 1992 over patent and trade secret infringement that resulted in an undisclosed settlement plus a royalty-bearing nonexclusive license to the Organon patents that allowed the market survival of the Bactec system (4).

A major contributor to the speed of the clinical trials was the involvement of Barth Reller. Dr. Reller dedicated a long career to clinical microbiology after coming to Duke University with the goal of improving the art and science of blood culture. Reller organized the "Consortium," a group of clinical microbiology laboratories around the country, to pool efforts and data. Dr. Reller and Organon Teknika found themselves with common goals and fortuitous timing. The initial clinical trials included a wide variety of patients, clinical isolates, and geographic variability, yet were completed in relatively short order (5). The compliance, record keeping, and organization between sites were a model for many future blood culture studies as well as countless other similar clinical trials.

Manufacturing and design of the BacT/Alert were done in Oklahoma City. Before manufacturing the BacT/Alert, the technical group in Oklahoma City focused on repair and redesign of dialysis machines. Much of the culture at the Oklahoma City site derived from the engineers' experience in the oil industry, where "When you design an instrument to drop a couple of miles down a hole, reliability is at the top of your mind" (per J. DiGuiseppi). Given the opportunity to design something new, they threw themselves at the task with great enthusiasm, and because the development group at the site was relatively powerless, design focused on the things important to a conservative group focused on redesign, manufacturing, and repair for a living: reliability, durability, ease of repair, cost, and availability of materials. While rapidly prototyped, the BacT/Alert proved to be very durable, cementing its position as a market leader in the 1990s as clinical microbiology groups slowly adopted this new technology. The Bactec 460 and 660 persisted long after the introduction of continuously monitored blood culture systems, and any lack of reliability in the BacT/Alert would almost certainly have set the adoption of new systems back for many years because this was a prominent concern at the time (6).

Evolution of BacT/Alert and VIRTUO Blood Culture Systems

The original BacT/Alert system had a modular design with room for 240 bottles per incubator. It had tape backup for data storage and 2 h of battery backup for power outages. Specimens were bar-coded into the system at a freestanding computer next to the instrument (seen at the right in Fig. 6).

The second generation of the BacT/Alert, the BacT/Alert 3D, was introduced in the early 2000s. The Bact/Alert 3D upgrades included an integral graphical computer interface and a modular design. There are three versions of the BacT/Alert 3D, the 240, the 120, and the 60, named for the bottle capacity of individual modules (Fig. 7). Incubation modules can be added to a single central core module in the 240/120 systems to increase capacity (Fig. 7A). The BacT/Alert 240 can run five additional 240 incubation modules from a single central processor for a maximum of 1,440 bottles. The 120 system is more compact than the 240 system. The 120 system can add up to three 240 incubator modules for a maximum capacity of 840 bottles. The 60 is a smaller version of the 120 without expansion capability and is designed for smaller laboratories with volumes no greater than 3,600 cultures per year (Fig. 7B). Detection algorithms and indicator chemistry remained unchanged apart from conversion to silicon emulsion of the dye at the bottoms of the bottles.

The latest generation of blood culture instrument developed by bioMérieux is called the VIRTUO. The VIRTUO automates more of the blood culture processing steps and limits the temperature changes associated with opening the drawers to provide consistent temperature incubation. This constant temperature, along with improved detection algorithms, reduces time to detection by up to 20% (7). In addition to the reduction of time to detection, the VIRTUO automates bottle loading and unloading. Each VIRTUO system is scalable to handle between 216 and 432 cultures. The VIRTUO system's robotics include bottle-scanning functions that allow (i) hands-free accessioning and troubleshooting of bottle loading and unloading, (ii) bar code scanning, with distinction between the patient accessioning sticker and the bottle sticker, and (iii) the ability to detect the fill level of bottles for quality control purposes. A dual-unit VIRTUO system and its operation are shown in Fig. 8.

The BacT/Alert 3D and VIRTUO can connect via middleware software (Myla) to provide statistical analysis and remote viewing of blood cultures. Myla can track contaminants, bottle fill, the presence of positive and negative bottles, and other metrics. Myla middleware is also able to connect to other bioMérieux instruments for integrated microbiology management of blood cultures and the isolates generated from blood culture instruments. In contrast to legacy systems, Myla is a server-based system allowing for remote access without the need for a physical presence for all operations.

The BacT/Alert is the only automated instrument cleared by the FDA for platelet sterility testing, and even early data regarding its use in platelet sterility testing were favorable (8). Because platelets are stored at room temperature, bacterial contamination and subsequent overgrowth is a particular problem. Furthermore, because platelet units must be used within a week, there is an inherent tension between the ability to detect low-level contamination and the need to use platelet units before they expire. This results in transfusion of some platelet units to patients before subsequently flagging positive on the BacT/Alert despite its relatively short time to positivity for most common contaminating organisms (9). Because of this, pathogen inactivation rather than culture is becoming a more general approach to the contamination problem. Inactivation can destroy a variety of known (and unknown) viral and bacterial pathogens (reviewed in reference 10).

Still, the application of blood culture techniques to other sterile fluids has many promising applications. Because of the inactivation of antibiotics by charcoal or resin, blood culture bottles may recover organisms not otherwise able to survive routine incubation on plates (11). Blood culture bottles are capable of culturing very large amounts of fluid relative to routine methods, vastly increasing the yield of pathogens from fluid clinical samples other than blood (12, 13), including fastidious and difficult-to-culture organisms such as *Kingella kingae* from pediatric joint infections (14).

In addition to clinical product sterility testing, the BacT/Alert has commercial applications in culture of a variety of other matrices of liquid products such as vaccines, foodstuffs, and other commercial products (15, 16). The solid-phase detection system renders many fluids amenable to culture in the various formulations of BacT/Alert media. Some examples include culture of total parenteral nutrition (TPN) fluid, which detected TPN contamination by *Candida parapsilosis* using unspecified aerobic BacT/Alert bottles (17). Parveen and colleagues (16) explored the BacT/Alert 3D as an alternative to sterility testing using tryptic soy broth and thioglycollate media incubated at 20 to 25°C and 30 to 35°C for 2 weeks to recover aerobes, anaerobes, and yeast. Influenza vaccine matrix spiked with 1 or 10 CFU/ml standard organisms exhibited greatly reduced time to detection over plate-based culture. These authors also evaluated growth in the presence of the preservative thimerosal and found that membrane filtration was superior to the BacT/Alert for recovering a variety of organisms as membrane filtration removes toxic compounds, and the bottles used presumably did not, although the bottle types used were unfortunately not specified. Bugno and colleagues (15) used the BacT/Alert 3D with SA and SN media to culture a metronidazole solution, dialysate solution, and normal saline and compared the results with the standard Brazilian pharmacopoeia method. These authors observed equivalent recovery of a variety of organisms with significantly decreased time to recovery with the BacT/Alert 3D. One unusual aspect of this study was the inclusion of a filamentous fungus, *Aspergillus brasiliensis*, making it one of only a few studies to show efficient recovery of any filamentous fungus in routine blood culture media.

Direct Detection Using Molecular Technologies and Future Applications

Several studies have shown that one can perform matrix-assisted laser desorption ionization–time of flight (MALDI-TOF) mass spectrometry from positive bioMérieux blood bottles after manual processing (multiple centrifugation, washing) of the positive blood culture broth. Integrating rapid pathogen identification and antimicrobial stewardship significantly decreases hospital costs (18).

These methods reduce the time to detection to a couple of hours. In addition to MALDI-TOF, several molecular assays have been developed to identify microorganisms directly from BacT/Alert bottles, including the Biofire Film Array (19), Nanosphere (20), peptide nucleic acid fluorescent *in situ* hybridization (PNA FISH) (21), and Cepheid (22). Molecular techniques for detection of pathogens from positive blood cultures or blood samples are addressed in chapter 7.

Although the BacT/Alert was the first automated self-contained blood culture system, complete automation, processing, and identification were demonstrated in a recent article (23). This automated system used a VIRTUO blood culture system connected to a spectrofluorometer with a robotic system to process blood cultures. This prototype could identify bacteria without human intervention in less than 15 min by using intrinsic fluorescence spectroscopy.

Media Formulations

Appendix 1 contains media formulations of blood culture bottles.

Original Aerobic/Anaerobic Media (SA/SN/Pedi-BacT)

Paralleling the evolution of Organon Teknika/bioMérieux blood culture instruments, several media were developed over the years by these companies. Adult aerobic media included "Standard" tryptic soy broth "SA" (aerobic, blue cap) and "SN" (anaerobic, purple top); "FAN" (Fastidious Antimicrobial Neutralization) bottles with adsorbent charcoal and enriched with peptone and brain heart infusion solids, including "FA" aerobic and "FN" anaerobic; and "FAN plus" aerobic and anaerobic versions (pale green top, with polymeric beads substituted for charcoal). Pediatric media formulations were called Pedi-BacT, PF, and PF Plus. Mycobacterial "MP" media contained supplemented Middlebrook 7H9 broth. These various media compositions in addition to new media and instrumentation from competitors led to many comparison studies of BacT/Alert media versus previous versions of the BacT/Alert media. Over the past two and a half decades, multitudes of publications have described comparison studies between the BacT/Alert and various versions of media and instruments of the two major blood culture competitors, the BD Bactec and Difco/TREK ESP/VersaTREK. Many of the larger comparison studies regarding BacT/Alert were performed through the aforementioned collaboration between microbiology laboratories at Duke University Medical Center, Robert Wood Johnson University Hospital, University of Utah School of Medicine, and the Denver General Hospital (under the leadership of Barth Reller).

The initial media pairing (SA/SN) contained 40 ml of supplemented (amino acids, carbohydrates, and other proprietary compounds) tryptic soy broth with 0.035% sodium polyanethol sulfonate (SPS) as an anticoagulant. The atmosphere in BacT/Alert aerobic bottles contained CO_2 and ambient air. Anaerobic bottles were similar in composition to the aerobic composition, with the addition of reducing agents and an atmosphere of CO_2 and nitrogen. Vacuum pressure was sufficient in both aerobic and anaerobic bottles to draw up to 10 ml of blood. The original description of the system used a combination of spiked and clinical samples comparing detection with a manual sampling radiometric Bactec 460 instrument. The results demonstrated that the BacT/Alert was comparable to the radiometric instrument in detecting bacterial growth in both spiked and clinical specimens (5).

Pediatric Media

Pediatric media were developed for use with the BacT/Alert system. The original pediatric (Pedi-BacT/PF) blood culture bottles (aerobic only) contained 20 ml of brain heart infusion broth with 0.020% SPS and other proprietary compounds with an atmosphere of CO_2 in nitrogen under vacuum.

The first publication describing pediatric medium was in 1993 (24). Six thousand six hundred twenty-eight comparisons were conducted by using a manual BD vacutainer/peptone broth tube system. Data from this study demonstrated the BacT/Alert Pedi-BacT bottles recovered more pathogens than the manual BD system. The Pedi-BacT system significantly increased recovery of *Enterobacteriaceae*, nonfermenting Gram-negative rods, and *Candida* spp. Time to detection was superior for all organism types, with the exception of enterococci and fastidious Gram-negative rods, which were equivalent. Labor was dramatically reduced. There were fewer false positives (0.2% versus 0.5%) and false negatives (0.02% versus 0.3%) with BacT/Alert incubation than with the manual BD system.

FAN (FA-FAN, FN-FAN, PF): Charcoal Media

A new media offering was developed and released in 1995 named FAN. FAN media used brain heart infusion instead of tryptic soy broth and initially included a proprietary mixture named Escorb. Escorb contains charcoal and clay compounds (Fuller's earth) to sequester inhibitory compounds and antibiotics and enhanced the recovery of fastidious organisms. Several large studies evaluated FAN media showing favorable recovery rates. One negative aspect of FAN media was the inclusion of charcoal, which made reading Gram stains from positive bottles more difficult.

A comparison study in 1995 using FAN versus standard aerobic media showed FAN media to be superior to traditional media (25). Increased recovery of all microorganisms was noted with significant increases in *Staphylococcus aureus*, coagulase-negative *Staphylococcus* spp., and yeast. Time to detection did not change between FAN and standard BacT/Alert media, although patients receiving antibiotics were more likely to generate a positive culture. There were fewer false positives with FAN than with standard aerobic BacT/Alert media (0.6% versus 1.8%).

Glass to Plastic

A plastic version of the BacT/Alert blood bottles was introduced in 2003 to minimize breakage and sharps waste in the interest of reducing staff exposure to blood-borne pathogens and overall safety. Several studies demonstrated equivalent performance to glass bottles for multiple plastic bottle types (26–28).

No Venting

Although the original FAN medium demonstrated improved recovery of microorganisms, one drawback was that the original aerobic FAN bottles required transient venting prior to incubation. To address the venting issue, bioMérieux developed a FAN medium containing extra oxygen that allowed for bottles to be incubated without venting. A large study with 5,256 comparisons was published in 2001 from the Reller group at Duke University Medical Center (29) demonstrating that the nonvented aerobic bottles were in large part comparable to the vented bottles, with increased recovery of some yeasts and *Burkholderia cepacia*.

Between the development of FAN and FA Plus media, some quality control issues raised by complaints to the FDA plagued bioMérieux. The FDA cited bioMérieux in 2009, and again in August 2012, for failing to comply with good manufacturing practice rules (30). bioMérieux had several production shortages during this period while the company revamped its quality control and manufacturing process, which included implementation of additional production at the Durham site where all BacT/Alert bottles are manufactured. These issues have since been fully resolved.

FA Plus (FA Plus, FN Plus, PF Plus): Polymeric Resin

As technology advanced between 1995 and 2015, newer technologies were released, resulting in reduced time to positivity, the addition of polymeric resin to absorb inhibitors and antibiotics, and also products to achieve direct detection of pathogens from positive blood culture bottles (BD resin, MALDI-TOF, PNA FISH, Cepheid, BioFire, Nanosphere). One issue with the initial charcoal formulations was the interference with Gram stain interpretation. In addition to Gram stain problems, the charcoal in the FAN-containing bottles also inhibited some molecular amplification assays and MALDI-TOF mass spectrometry applications, in part, because of its tendency to absorb small molecules required for chemical reactions and/or mechanical clogging. In response to these difficulties and several studies demonstrating Bactec resin bottle superiority (31–33), bioMérieux modified its FAN and Pediatric FAN media formulations to include polymeric resin beads to neutralize antibiotics, adsorb inhibitory compounds, and provide a cleaner background for Gram staining purposes (11). In addition to polymeric resin, the formulation of the media was optimized. The new FA Plus medium composition contains peptones, yeast extracts, supplements, and 1.6 g adsorbent resins in a 30-ml volume. BacT/Alert FA Plus (aerobic) and FN Plus (anaerobic) media differ in their compositions as well as their relative contents of two different polymeric resins designed for neutralization of antibiotics and additional inhibitory substances. The anaerobic formulation includes a complex amino acid component not contained in the aerobic formulation.

In premarket trials for the FDA, antibiotic neutralization was demonstrated for several antibiotics, including clarithromycin, clindamycin, gentamicin, linezolid, tigecycline, vancomycin, and fluconazole. Ciprofloxacin and piperacillin-tazobactam were incompletely neutralized, while ceftriaxone and cefotaxime were not neutralized (34, 35). Several studies have demonstrated detection and shorter time to detection in patients on and off antibiotics (36–40). Lovern and colleagues (11) published a thorough assessment of the growth kinetics of common organisms in BacT/Alert FA Plus resin bottles spiked with commonly used antibiotics. This revealed similar performance to the FDA studies cited above, performance superior to Aerobic/F Plus bottles for every drug but linezolid, and failure of both the FA Plus and Aerobic/F Plus bottles to neutralize ceftriaxone and cefepime.

System Comparisons
BacT/Alert versus Bactec
The first large clinical trial comparing the BacT/Alert with the Bactec 660/730 nonradiometric system was published in 1992 and compared approximately 6,000 paired blood cultures (41). Three large academic institutions used paired sets of two bottles from each blood culture system (four bottles total), each filled with 5 ml of blood from the same blood draw. Recovery and time to detection were evaluated. Time to detection was faster for several common organisms recovered using the standard BacT/Alert (not called SA until FAN came along) aerobic bottle. The number of isolates detected earlier with the BacT/Alert versus Bactec were as follows: *S. aureus* (61 versus 10, $P \leq 0.001$), coagulase-negative *Staphylococcus* spp. (24 versus 9, $P \leq 0.01$), *Streptococcus* spp. (14 versus 1, $P \leq 0.001$), *Pseudomonas aeruginosa* (6 versus 0, $P \leq 0.05$), *Escherichia coli* (16 versus 3, $P \leq 0.01$), and other *Enterobacteriaceae* (17 versus 5, $P \leq 0.02$) were detected earlier in the aerobic BacT/Alert SA bottles versus the Bactec. Total organism detection was faster in BacT/Alert versus Bactec (173 versus 46, $P \leq 0.001$). For the standard anaerobic medium (not called SN until after FAN media were introduced), *S. aureus* (62 versus 7, $P \leq 0.001$), coagulase-negative *Staphylococcus* spp. (16 versus 6, $P \leq 0.05$), enterococci (10 versus 0, $P = 0.01$), *Streptococcus pneumoniae* (8 versus 0, $P \leq 0.02$), viridans group streptococci (6 versus 0, $P \leq 0.05$), *Klebsiella pneumoniae* (9 versus 0, $P \leq 0.01$), and other

Enterobacteriaceae (19 versus 1, $P \leq 0.001$) were detected sooner in BacT/Alert versus Bactec. Overall, BacT/Alert recovered organisms faster than Bactec (176 versus 25, $P \leq 0.001$). Additionally, significantly fewer false-positive results were seen in the BacT/Alert system than in the Bactec (40 versus 1,183). The Bactec 660 detected more Gram-positive cocci than the BacT/Alert.

Another study used 7,190 culture sets to compare FAN with BACTEC Plus Aerobic/F (42). This study showed increased recovery of *Enterobacteriaceae* and *P. aeruginosa* with the FAN media. *S. aureus* was recovered more quickly with FAN media. There was no difference in the overall number of positive cultures or recovery of organisms from patients on antibiotics.

DifcoTREK ESP/VersaTREK versus BacT/Alert

A 1994 multicenter comparison study was completed from a Veterans Affairs Medical Center, Durham, NC; Duke University, Durham NC; and the University of Michigan, Ann Arbor, MI. In this comparison, the Difco ESP versus the BacT/Alert (43) made approximately 5,000 comparisons. This study used the first generation of medium (BacT/Alert SA-SN, ESP 80A-80N). Statistically, more organisms were recovered with the ESP versus BacT/Alert overall (of 405 clinically relevant isolates, 272 recovered in both, 86 in ESP only versus 47 BacT/Alert, $P \leq 0.005$). When clinically significant isolates were evaluated individually, there was no statistical difference in overall recovery with the exception of increased *S. aureus* detection by the ESP (18 versus 6, $P \leq 0.025$). For the aerobic bottles, ESP had a more rapid time to detection for all organisms (18.3 h versus 22.0 h, $P \leq 0.001$), with *S. aureus* (17.5 h versus 24.2 h, $P \leq 0.02$) and yeast (32.8 h versus 46.2 h, $P \leq 0.05$) reaching statistical significance. ESP detected more anaerobic infections than the BacT/Alert in a side-by-side panel of seeded anaerobes (17/20 versus 10/20, $P \leq 0.025$). The BacT/Alert recovered streptococci more rapidly than the ESP (12.0 h versus 13.5 h, $P \leq 0.05$).

An approximately 5,000 set comparison in 2007 by Reller and colleagues (44) evaluated a new formulation of the VersaTREK system (REDOX 1 aerobic and REDOX 2 anaerobic) with standard aerobic (SA) and anaerobic (SN) BacT/Alert media on the BacT/Alert 3D system. The VersaTREK recovered more isolates of streptococci/enterococci (16 versus 6, $P \leq 0.05$) as well as more isolates from patients on antimicrobial therapy (25 versus 10, $P \leq 0.025$). Charcoal or resin media were not compared, but the authors hypothesized those media would perform better than standard media as supported by numerous other publications, such as a study from 1998 comparing

FAN media with VersaTREK ESP 80 medium (45). In this study, Doern et al. compared approximately 5,000 blood culture sets and demonstrated significant enhanced recovery of *S. aureus, Enterobacteriaceae*, and other Gram-negative rods with FAN media, while the ESP 80A media showed increased recovery of streptococci. Time to detection was equivalent in the two systems. Patients receiving antibiotics had enhanced detection in the BacT/Alert cohort presumably because of the Escorb in the FAN medium.

In 2015, a trial of approximately 1,000 paired sets was published comparing resin media from the BacT/Alert Plus with Bactec Plus media. There were 128 unique bloodstream infections identified. FA Plus aerobic medium was superior in recovering Gram-positive cocci ($P = 0.024$). Bactec Plus aerobic medium was superior in recovering more Gram-negative bacilli ($P = 0.006$). For anaerobic media, the recovery rates were higher for FN Plus media for recovery of total organisms ($P = 0.003$), Gram-positive cocci ($P = 0.013$), and *E. coli* ($P = 0.03$). Both Bactec and BacT/Alert Plus media were comparable when evaluating detection of bloodstream infections overall (46).

Conclusion

In conclusion, the evolution of the BacT/Alert represented major advancements in the field of blood culture technology. The BacT/Alert eliminated the need for invasive sampling of the bottle by using cost-effective integrated sensors. The elimination of radioactive isotopes, development of novel CO_2 semipermeable membranes for colorimetric detection, and continuous monitoring all contributed to the success of the first automated system for blood culturing.

Acknowledgments

The authors thank James DiGuiseppi, Ph.D., and Thurman Thorpe, Ph.D., for their assistance in the preparation of this chapter.

References

1. Ward KM, Lehmann CA, Leiken AM. 1993. *Clinical Laboratory Instrumentation and Automation: Principles, Applications, and Selection.* Saunders, Philadelphia, PA.
2. Lequin RM. 2005. Enzyme immunoassay (EIA)/enzyme-linked immunosorbent assay (ELISA). *Clin Chem* 51:2415–2418.
3. Hardy DJ, Hulbert BB, Migneault PC. 1992. Time to detection of positive BacT/Alert blood cultures and lack of need for routine subculture of 5- to 7-day negative cultures. *J Clin Microbiol* 30:2743–2745.
4. Organon Teknika v Becton Dickinson. United States Courts Archive. https://www .unitedstatescourts.org/federal/ncmd/15175/. Accessed 22 December 2016.

5. Thorpe TC, Wilson ML, Turner JE, DiGuiseppi JL, Willert M, Mirrett S, Reller LB. 1990. BacT/Alert: an automated colorimetric microbial detection system. *J Clin Microbiol* **28**:1608–1612.

6. Wilson ML, Weinstein MP, Reller LB. 1994. Automated blood culture systems. *Clin Lab Med* **14**:149–169.

7. Altun O, Almuhayawi M, Lüthje P, Taha R, Ullberg M, Özenci V. 2016. Controlled evaluation of the new BacT/Alert Virtuo blood culture system for detection and time to detection of bacteria and yeasts. *J Clin Microbiol* **54**:1148–1151.

8. Brecher ME, Means N, Jere CS, Heath D, Rothenberg S, Stutzman LC. 2001. Evaluation of an automated culture system for detecting bacterial contamination of platelets: an analysis with 15 contaminating organisms. *Transfusion* **41**:477–482.

9. Munksgaard L, Albjerg L, Lillevang ST, Gahrn-Hansen B, Georgsen J. 2004. Detection of bacterial contamination of platelet components: six years' experience with the BacT/ALERT system. *Transfusion* **44**:1166–1173.

10. Schlenke P. 2014. Pathogen inactivation technologies for cellular blood components: an update. *Transfus Med Hemother* **41**:309–325.

11. Lovern D, Katzin B, Johnson K, Broadwell D, Miller E, Gates A, Deol P, Doing K, van Belkum A, Marshall C, Mathias E, Dunne WM Jr. 2016. Antimicrobial binding and growth kinetics in BacT/ALERT® FA Plus and BACTEC® Aerobic/F Plus blood culture media. *Eur J Clin Microbiol Infect Dis* **35**:2033–2036.

12. Bourbeau P, Riley J, Heiter BJ, Master R, Young C, Pierson C. 1998. Use of the BacT/Alert blood culture system for culture of sterile body fluids other than blood. *J Clin Microbiol* **36**:3273–3277.

13. Simor AE, Scythes K, Meaney H, Louie M. 2000. Evaluation of the BacT/Alert microbial detection system with FAN aerobic and FAN anaerobic bottles for culturing normally sterile body fluids other than blood. *Diagn Microbiol Infect Dis* **37**:5–9.

14. Høst B, Schumacher H, Prag J, Arpi M. 2000. Isolation of *Kingella kingae* from synovial fluids using four commercial blood culture bottles. *Eur J Clin Microbiol Infect Dis* **19**:608–611.

15. Bugno A, Lira RS, Oliveira WA, Almodovar AAB, Saes DPS, Pinto TJ, Bugno A, Lira RS, Oliveira WA, Almodovar AAB, Saes DPS, de Jesus Andreoli Pinto T. 2015. Application of the BacT/ALERT^R 3D system for sterility testing of injectable products. *Braz J Microbiol* **46**:743–747.

16. Parveen S, Kaur S, David SAW, Kenney JL, McCormick WM, Gupta RK. 2011. Evaluation of growth based rapid microbiological methods for sterility testing of vaccines and other biological products. *Vaccine* **29**:8012–8023.

17. Marais E, Stewart R, Dusé AG, Rosekilly IC, de Jong G, Aithma N. 2004. *Candida parapsilosis* detected in TPN using the BacT/Alert system and characterized by randomly amplified polymorphic DNA. *J Hosp Infect* **56**:291–296.

18. Perez KK, Olsen RJ, Musick WL, Cernoch PL, Davis JR, Land GA, Peterson LE, Musser JM. 6 December 2012. Integrating rapid pathogen identification and anti-microbial stewardship significantly decreases hospital costs. *Arch Pathol Lab Med* **137**:ek1247–1254. doi:10.5858/arpa.2012-0651-OA.

19. Salimnia H, Fairfax MR, Lephart PR, Schreckenberger P, DesJarlais SM, Johnson JK, Robinson G, Carroll KC, Greer A, Morgan M, Chan R, Loeffelholz M, Valencia-Shelton F, Jenkins S, Schuetz AN, Daly JA, Barney T, Hemmert A, Kanack KJ. 2016.

Evaluation of the FilmArray Blood culture identification panel: results of a multicenter controlled trial. *J Clin Microbiol* **54**:687–698.

20. **Wojewoda CM, Sercia L, Navas M, Tuohy M, Wilson D, Hall GS, Procop GW, Richter SS.** 2013. Evaluation of the Verigene Gram-positive blood culture nucleic acid test for rapid detection of bacteria and resistance determinants. *J Clin Microbiol* **51**:2072–2076.

21. **Oliveira K, Procop GW, Wilson D, Coull J, Stender H.** 2002. Rapid identification of *Staphylococcus aureus* directly from blood cultures by fluorescence in situ hybridization with peptide nucleic acid probes. *J Clin Microbiol* **40**:247–251.

22. **Wolk DM, Struelens MJ, Pancholi P, Davis T, Della-Latta P, Fuller D, Picton E, Dickenson R, Denis O, Johnson D, Chapin K.** 2009. Rapid detection of *Staphylococcus aureus* and methicillin-resistant *S. aureus* (MRSA) in wound specimens and blood cultures: multicenter preclinical evaluation of the Cepheid Xpert MRSA/SA skin and soft tissue and blood culture assays. *J Clin Microbiol* **47**:823–826.

23. **Hyman JM, Walsh JD, Ronsick C, Wilson M, Hazen KC, Borzhemskaya L, Link J, Clay B, Ullery M, Sanchez-Illan M, Rothenberg S, Robinson R, van Belkum A, Dunne WM Jr.** 2016. Evaluation of a fully automated research prototype for the immediate identification of microorganisms from positive blood cultures under clinical conditions. *MBio* **7**:e00491-16. doi:10.1128/mBio.00491-16.

24. **Krisher KK, Whyburn DR, Koepnick FE.** 1993. Comparison of the BacT/Alert pediatric blood culture system, Pedi-BacT, with conventional culture using the 20-milliliter Becton-Dickinson supplemented peptone broth tube. *J Clin Microbiol* **31**:793–797.

25. **Weinstein MP, Mirrett S, Reimer LG, Wilson ML, Smith-Elekes S, Chuard CR, Joho KL, Reller LB.** 1995. Controlled evaluation of BacT/Alert standard aerobic and FAN aerobic blood culture bottles for detection of bacteremia and fungemia. *J Clin Microbiol* **33**:978–981.

26. **Mirrett S, Joyce MJ, Reller LB.** 2005. Validation of performance of plastic versus glass bottles for culturing anaerobes from blood in BacT/ALERT SN medium. *J Clin Microbiol* **43**:6150–6151.

27. **Petti CA, Mirrett S, Woods CW, Reller LB.** 2005. Controlled clinical comparison of plastic and glass bottles of BacT/ALERT FA medium for culturing organisms from blood of adult patients. *J Clin Microbiol* **43**:1960–1962.

28. **Petti CA, Mirrett S, Woods CW, Reller LB.** 2005. Controlled clinical comparison of plastic versus glass bottles of BacT/ALERT PF medium for culturing blood from children. *J Clin Microbiol* **43**:445–447.

29. **Mirrett S, Everts RJ, Reller LB.** 2001. Controlled comparison of original vented aerobic fan medium with new nonvented BacT/ALERT FA medium for culturing blood. *J Clin Microbiol* **39**:2098–2101.

30. **Food and Drug Administration Inspections.** 23 August 2012. bioMérieux, Inc. Compliance, Enforcement, and Criminal Investigations Warning Letter. http://www.fda.gov/ICECI/EnforcementActions/WarningLetters/2012/ucm318709.htm.

31. **Flayhart D, Borek AP, Wakefield T, Dick J, Carroll KC.** 2007. Comparison of BACTEC PLUS blood culture media to BacT/Alert FA blood culture media for detection of bacterial pathogens in samples containing therapeutic levels of antibiotics. *J Clin Microbiol* **45**:816–821.

32. Smith JA, Bryce EA, Ngui-Yen JH, Roberts FJ. 1995. Comparison of BACTEC 9240 and BacT/Alert blood culture systems in an adult hospital. *J Clin Microbiol* **33**:1905–1908.

33. Zadroga R, Williams DN, Gottschall R, Hanson K, Nordberg V, Deike M, Kuskowski M, Carlson L, Nicolau DP, Sutherland C, Hansen GT. 2013. Comparison of 2 blood culture media shows significant differences in bacterial recovery for patients on antimicrobial therapy. *Clin Infect Dis* **56**:790–797.

34. US Food and Drug Administration. 2013. 510(k) Premarket Notification: BACT/ALERT FA Plus Culture Bottle. https://www.accessdata.fda.gov/scripts/cdrh/cfdocs/cfpmn/pmn.cfm?ID=K121461

35. bioMérieux, Inc. 2013. BacT/ALERT FA Plus package insert (English), revision 9305048 C, 2013-04. bioMérieux, Inc., Marcy-l'Étoile, France.

36. Mitteregger D, Barousch W, Nehr M, Kundi M, Zeitlinger M, Makristathis A, Hirschl AM. 2013. Neutralization of antimicrobial substances in new BacT/Alert FA and FN Plus blood culture bottles. *J Clin Microbiol* **51**:1534–1540.

37. Lee D-H, Kim SC, Bae I-G, Koh E-H, Kim S. 2013. Clinical evaluation of BacT/Alert FA plus and FN plus bottles compared with standard bottles. *J Clin Microbiol* **51**:4150–4155.

38. Sullivan KV, Turner NN, Lancaster DP, Shah AR, Chandler LJ, Friedman DF, Blecker-Shelly DL. 2013. Superior sensitivity and decreased time to detection with the Bactec Peds Plus/F system compared to the BacT/Alert Pediatric FAN blood culture system. *J Clin Microbiol* **51**:4083–4086.

39. Nutman A, Fisher Even-Tsur S, Shapiro G, Braun T, Schwartz D, Carmeli Y. 2016. Time to detection with BacT/Alert FA Plus compared to BacT/Alert FA blood culture media. *Eur J Clin Microbiol Infect Dis* **35**:1469–1473.

40. Kirn TJ, Mirrett S, Reller LB, Weinstein MP. 2014. Controlled clinical comparison of BacT/alert FA plus and FN plus blood culture media with BacT/alert FA and FN blood culture media. *J Clin Microbiol* **52**:839–843.

41. Wilson ML, Weinstein MP, Reimer LG, Mirrett S, Reller LB. 1992. Controlled comparison of the BacT/Alert and BACTEC 660/730 nonradiometric blood culture systems. *J Clin Microbiol* **30**:323–329.

42. Pohlman JK, Kirkley BA, Easley KA, Basille BA, Washington JA. 1995. Controlled clinical evaluation of BACTEC Plus Aerobic/F and BacT/Alert Aerobic FAN bottles for detection of bloodstream infections. *J Clin Microbiol* **33**:2856–2858.

43. Zwadyk P Jr, Pierson CL, Young C. 1994. Comparison of Difco ESP and Organon Teknika BacT/Alert continuous-monitoring blood culture systems. *J Clin Microbiol* **32**:1273–1279.

44. Mirrett S, Hanson KE, Reller LB. 2007. Controlled clinical comparison of VersaTREK and BacT/ALERT blood culture systems. *J Clin Microbiol* **45**:299–302.

45. Doern GV, Barton A, Rao S. 1998. Controlled comparative evaluation of BacT/Alert FAN and ESP 80A aerobic media as means for detecting bacteremia and fungemia. *J Clin Microbiol* **36**:2686–2689.

46. Fiori B, D'Inzeo T, Di Florio V, De Maio F, De Angelis G, Giaquinto A, Campana L, Tanzarella E, Tumbarello M, Antonelli M, Sanguinetti M, Spanu T. 2014. Performance of two resin-containing blood culture media in detection of bloodstream infections and in direct matrix-assisted laser desorption ionization-time of flight mass

spectrometry (MALDI-TOF MS) broth assays for isolate identification: clinical comparison of the BacT/Alert Plus and Bactec Plus systems. *J Clin Microbiol* **52**:3558–3567.
47. Turner JE, Thorpe TC, Di Guiseppi JL, Driscoll RC. 1990. *Device for detecting microorganisms.* US4945060 A. https://www.google.com/patents/US4945060

APPENDIX 1 MEDIA FORMULATIONS
SA 40 ml
Pancreatic digest of casein (1.7% w/v)

Papaic digest of soybean meal (0.3% w/v)

Sodium polyanethol sulfonate (0.035% w/v)

Pyridoxine hydrochloride (0.001% w/v)

Other complex amino acid and carbohydrate substrates in purified water

Atmosphere is carbon dioxide and oxygen under vacuum.

SN 40 ml
Pancreatic digest of casein (1.36% w/v)

Papaic digest of soybean meal (0.24% w/v)

Sodium polyanethol sulfonate (0.035% w/v)

Menadione (0.00005% w/v)

Hemin (0.0005% w/v)

Yeast extract (0.376% w/v)

Pyridoxine hydrochloride (0.0008%)

Pyruvic acid (0.08% w/v)

Reducing agents

Other complex amino acid and carbohydrates in purified water

Atmosphere is carbon dioxide and nitrogen under vacuum.

FA-FAN BacT/Alert FA (color-coded pale green)
8 ml of a charcoal suspension with an average density of 1.0155 g/ml

22 ml of complex media

Soybean-casein digest (2.0% w/v)

Brain heart infusion solids (0.1% w/v)

Sodium polyanethol sulfonate (0.05% w/v)

Pyridoxine hydrochloride (0.001% w/v)

Menadione (0.0000725% w/v)

Hemin (0.000725% w/v)
L-Cysteine (0.03% w/v)
Other complex amino acid and carbohydrate substrates in purified water
The atmosphere is carbon dioxide and oxygen under vacuum.

FN-FAN BacT/Alert FN (color-coded orange) BacT/Alert
8 ml of a charcoal suspension with an average density of 1.0215 g/ml
32 ml of complex media
Soybean-casein digest (2.0% w/v)
Brain heart infusion solids (0.1% w/v)
Sodium polyanethol sulfonate (0.044% w/v)
Pyridoxine hydrochloride (0.001% w/v)
Menadione (0.0000625% w/v)
Hemin (0.000625% w/v)
L-Cysteine (0.025% w/v)
Other complex amino acid and carbohydrate substrates in purified water
Atmosphere is nitrogen under vacuum.

PF BacT/Alert PF Pedi-BacT (color-coded yellow) BacT/Alert
4 ml of a charcoal suspension with an average density of 1.0215 g/ml.
16 ml of complex media
Soybean-casein digest (2.0% w/v)
Brain heart infusion solids (0.1% w/v)
Sodium polyanethol sulfonate (0.025% w/v)
Pyridoxine hydrochloride (0.001% w/v)
Menadione (0.0000625% w/v)
Hemin (0.000625% w/v)
L-Cysteine (0.025% w/v)
Other complex amino acid and carbohydrate substrates in purified water.
Atmosphere is carbon dioxide, oxygen, and nitrogen under vacuum.

PF-Plus
BacT/Alert PF Plus (color-coded yellow) BacT/Alert
1.6 g adsorbent polymeric beads
30 ml of complex media

Casein peptone (1.0% w/v)

Yeast extract (0.45% w/v)

Soybean peptone (0.3% w/v)

Meat peptone (0.1% w/v)

Sodium polyanethol sulfonate (0.083% w/v)

Menadione (0.00005% w/v)

Hemin (0.0005% w/v)

L-Cysteine (0.03% w/v)

Pyruvic acid (0.1% w/v)

Pyridoxine hydrochloride (0.001% w/v)

Nicotinic acid (0.0002% w/v)

Pantothenic acid (0.002% w/v)

Thiamine hydrochloride (0.00001% w/v)

Other complex amino acid and carbohydrate substrates in purified water

Atmosphere is nitrogen, oxygen, and carbon dioxide under vacuum.

FN-Plus BacT/Alert FN Plus (color-coded orange)
1.6 g adsorbent polymeric beads

40 ml medium

Peptones (1.48% w/v)

Yeast extract (0.5% w/v)

Sodium polyanethol sulfonate (0.083% w/v)

Menadione (0.00005% w/v)

Hemin (0.001% w/v)

Pyridoxine hydrochloride (0.0008% w/v)

Pyruvic acid (0.1% w/v)

Reducing agents (0.38% w/v)

Other complex amino acid and carbohydrate substrates in purified water

Atmosphere is nitrogen and carbon dioxide under vacuum.

FA Plus 30 ml
1.6 g polymeric beads

30 ml complex medium

Casein peptone (1.0% w/v)

Yeast extract (0.45% w/v)

Soybean peptone (0.3% w/v)
Meat peptone (0.1% w/v)
Sodium polyanethol sulfonate (0.083% w/v)
Menadione (0.00005% w/v)
Hemin (0.0005% w/v)
L-Cysteine (0.03% w/v)
Pyruvic acid (0.1% w/v)
Pyridoxine hydrochloride (0.001% w/v)
Nicotinic acid (0.0002% w/v)
Pantothenic acid (0.00002% w/v)
Thiamine hydrochloride (0.0001% w/v)
Other complex amino acid and carbohydrates in purified water
Atmosphere is nitrogen, oxygen, and carbon dioxide under vacuum.

The Dark Art of Blood Cultures
Edited by Wm. Michael Dunne, Jr. and Carey-Ann D. Burnham
© 2018 American Society for Microbiology, Washington, DC
doi:10.1128/9781555819811.ch6

TREK Blood Culture Systems   6

Neil W. Anderson[1] and Melanie L. Yarbrough[1]

Introduction and Historical Perspective

Over the past three-plus decades, Difco Laboratories (Detroit, MI) and then TREK Diagnostic Systems (Thermo Scientific Microbiology, Waltham, MA) have developed several iterations of continuous-monitoring blood culture systems (CMBCSs). Similar to other CMBCSs, these systems allow for incubation of inoculated blood culture bottles with simultaneous monitoring of positivity by indirect measurement of bacterial growth. However, the unique approach toward monitoring growth distinguishes the TREK systems from other CMBCSs.

A common theme with most commercially available CMBCSs is the utilization of biochemical carbon dioxide detection as an indirect measurement of bacterial growth. The Difco/TREK systems differ in that growth is indirectly monitored through manometry. This approach had previously been utilized in research settings to indirectly monitor the respiration of bacteria by measuring changes in gaseous pressure within a closed system over time. The Difco ESP system was among the first CMBCSs to widely apply the diagnostic utility of this approach, which is advantageous for its ability to detect gas consumption (i.e., O_2) as well as gas production (i.e., CO_2, H_2, and N_2).

While the first and only FDA-approved manometric blood culture systems for clinical use were produced by Difco starting in 1992, prior manometric CMBCSs had been described. In 1987, the Signal Blood Culture

[1]Washington University School of Medicine, Saint Louis, MO 63110

System (Oxoid Ltd., Basingstoke, United Kingdom) was described by Trombley et al (1). This system utilized a reservoir attached to the head of the blood culture bottle, which was permeable to atmospheric air. Pressure within the bottle would cause medium to flow into the reservoir following atmospheric equilibration, allowing for the optical identification of positive bottles. This process was manual, and the overall sensitivity compared with other methods available at the time was low (2–4). A second manometric system, the Oxoid Automated Septicaemia Investigation System (OASIS), was described by Stevens et al. (5). This system detected changes in bottle pressure by measuring movements of a flexible septum. While initial studies of this system were promising, subsequent data and follow-up studies are lacking. In 1992, the Difco ESP Blood Culture System (Difco, Detroit, MI) became the first manometric CMBCS available for clinical use. This system and its successor, the VersaTREK, are the only FDA-approved manometric CMBCSs and are among the most widely used blood culture systems in the world. A summary of the developmental history of manometric CBCMSs is given in Fig. 1.

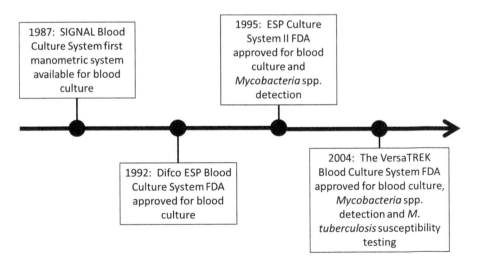

Figure 1 Developmental history of manometric continuous-monitoring blood culture systems. This timeline highlights the major historical developments leading to the widespread utilization of manometric continuous-monitoring systems for blood culture monitoring, *Mycobacterium* spp. detection and *Mycobacterium* spp. resistance testing.

DIFCO ESP

The Difco ESP blood culture system was originally developed by Difco Laboratories (Detroit, MI) in 1992 (Fig. 2). This system utilized the same manometry-based detection technology as its successor. Patient blood was inoculated into an airtight glass blood culture bottle, and, prior to incubation, a specialized disposable connector was attached to the top of the bottle. This connector had a needle that pierced the septum of the bottle, eliminating residual pressure or vacuum. Upon loading the blood culture bottle and attaching the connector into the instrument, the top of the connector was placed in contact with an electronic sensor capable of measuring pressure. Pressure was indirectly measured as millivolts at defined time points throughout the length of incubation. Measurements were taken from aerobic bottles every 12 min and from anaerobic bottles every 24 min. Measurements were stored throughout the lifetime of a culture and could be graphically viewed by

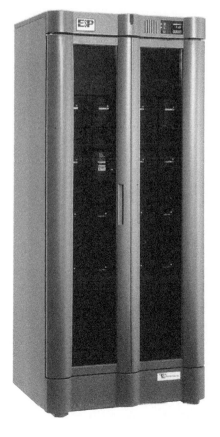

Figure 2 ESP continuous-monitoring blood culture system. This figure depicts the Difco ESP continuous-monitoring blood culture system. Incubator sizes ranged from 128 to 384 bottle capacities and were arranged as drawers that could be pulled open from the front to reveal bottle stations. Lower drawers would continuously agitate the bottles and were reserved for aerobic bottles. Upper drawers did not agitate the bottles and were used for anaerobic bottles.

the user. Bottles with pressure changes suggestive of bacterial growth were flagged as positive, which was indicated by red lights on the front of the instrument and at the bottle location within the instrument.

The Difco ESP blood culture bottles utilized two basic media types, the ESP 80A (aerobic media) and the ESP80N (anaerobic media). These bottles contained 80 ml of medium, with room for an optimum volume of 10 ml of blood. The same aerobic and anaerobic media were also available in smaller bottles containing 40 ml of medium, allowing for lower-volume pediatric blood draws. The aerobic media present in both bottle sizes contained 0.006% sodium polyanethol sulfonate (SPS) to prevent coagulation as well as the following supplements to support growth: soy-casein peptone A, yeast extract, sodium chloride, glucose, divalent salts, and supplemental oxygen (6). In contrast to the aerobic media, the anaerobic media lacked SPS anti-coagulant (which can be inhibitory to the growth of some bacteria) and was more nutritionally fortified, containing proteose peptone N, polysorbate 80, glucose, yeast extract, sodium chloride, supplemental AN, trisodium citrate, hemin, cysteine, and vitamin K. The lack of SPS and the additional nutritional fortification made these media ideal for isolation of both anaerobic bacteria as well as more fastidious facultative aerobic bacteria (6). The lack of oxygen in this medium formulation allowed for an oxygen gradient to form from the broth surface to the bottom of the bottle. Resazurin was also added to the medium formulation to indicate the presence of oxygen within the bottle. Notably, resins for the deactivation of antibiotics were not present in either medium type.

Similar to the workflow for other CMBCSs, ESP80A and ESP80N blood culture bottles were typically inoculated at the patient's bedside by staff trained in phlebotomy. Given the amount of medium present in the bottle, the optimal volume of inoculation per bottle was 10 ml. While pediatric protocols have been described using inoculations of approximately 1 ml, lower inoculation volumes were best avoided in patients with adequate blood volume to maintain sensitivity. Connectors were typically applied by laboratory staff prior to loading the bottles into the ESP incubator. This added step was unique to the ESP when compared with the other commercially available CMBCSs, and is still a feature of its successor. Although the actual process of connector placement was relatively rapid (<10 s), this additional step created an opportunity for specimen contamination if performed inappropriately (i.e., without prior sterilization of bottle septum). Furthermore, since the connector accessed the bottle by using a needle, it was a potential sharps hazard that required proper disposal. While the actual process of piercing the bottle septum with the connector created the possibility of blood exposure (particularly if any gas pressure had built up during transit), a filter was built into each connector to prevent this. Once the connector was applied, the bottle was placed on the instrument and continuously monitored as described above. Incubator sizes ranged from 128 to 384 bottle capacities and were arranged as drawers that could be pulled open to reveal bottle stations (7). The lower drawers would continuously agitate the bottles at 160 rpm and were reserved for aerobic bottles. The upper drawers did not agitate the bottles and were used for anaerobic bottles. For quality control purposes, an acceptable pressure increase was required once the bottle warmed up in the incubator. The instrument stored all pressure readings and, on a positive signal based on internal algorithms, a graphical readout of the information was available to the user.

An initial multicenter study regarding the performance of the ESP system was published by Morello et al. in 1994 (6). This group prospectively compared the recovery of organisms from aerobic (n = 7,532) and anaerobic (n = 6,007) blood cultures using the ESP and the Bactec NR-6600 systems. False-positive results were seen more frequently using the ESP system than the Bactec system (46 [0.3%] versus 12 [0.1%], respectively). Contamination rates were also higher for the ESP system than for the Bactec (2.0% versus 1.5%), although a possible explanation for this may be the higher sensitivity of the ESP system. While the Bactec NR-6600 outperformed the ESP in these regards, the overall false positivity and contamination rates were low for both systems. Furthermore, the overall sensitivity of the ESP system appeared to be greater. Although the total number of organisms recovered by each system did not differ significantly, there was a statistically significant difference between the number of clinically significant organisms detected by ESP alone compared with Bactec (63 [21% of total isolates] versus 32 [11% of total isolates]). The ESP system detected significantly more *Streptococcus pneumoniae* and clinically significant episodes of anaerobic and *Staphylococcus epidermidis* bacteremia. The ESP system also exhibited an overall quicker time to detection, likely secondary to the higher frequency of monitoring of the ESP (every 12 to 24 min) compared with the Bactec NR-6600 (every 12 to 24 h).

A second large-scale study was published in 1994 by Zwadyk et al. to examine how the ESP system compared with a CMBCS with a more comparable monitoring frequency—the BacT/Alert system (Durham, NC), which monitors for growth by CO_2 detection every 10 min (8). The study was performed using 5,421 aerobic and 5,035 anaerobic blood cultures obtained from adults at two major hospitals. Results demonstrated a statistically significant difference between the time to detection for both aerobic (18.3 h ESP versus 22.0 h BacT/Alert) and anaerobic bottles (21.6 h ESP versus 50.8 h BacT/Alert), supporting earlier detection of the ESP system. Similar to findings in the Morello study, the ESP system detected more clinically significant organisms than the BacT/Alert system (86 versus 47).

Several publications compared the ESP with the Isolator (Alere, Waltham, MA), a lysis-centrifugation system designed for the processing and direct plating of blood specimens. Kirkley et al. compared these two methodologies in a large-scale prospective study (10,535 blood cultures with 1,150 positives) (9). The Isolator recovered significantly more *Staphylococcus aureus*, *Enterococcus* spp., *Escherichia coli*, *Alcaligenes* (*Achromobacter*) *xylosoxidans*, *Xanthomonas* (*Stenotrophomonas*) *maltophilia*, *Candida albicans*, and *Candida glabrata*. While some of the extra organisms identified by the Isolator system could be explained by contamination, there were several instances of true bacteremia (as evaluated by chart review) that were detected exclusively by the Isolator. However, during the study period, seven instances of anaerobic bacteremia were detected by the ESP alone secondary to the fact that Isolator specimens were not cultured anaerobically. Thus, although the ESP might not have been as sensitive as the Isolator, the added ability to detect anaerobes remained an important benefit. In an effort to obtain a more even-handed comparison, Kellogg et al. compared organism recovery by the ESP with a combination of Isolator and Thiol broth to facilitate recovery of anaerobes and aerobes (10). From 7,070 culture sets, 149 (24.5%) organisms were detected only by the Isolator/Thiol combination, whereas 65 (10.7%) were detected only by the ESP system. However, the Isolator/Thiol combination resulted in a contamination rate greater than six times that of the ESP system. A third study performed by Cockerill et al. compared the ESP, Isolator, and Becton Dickinson Septi-Chek blood culture systems for the recovery of aerobic organisms (11). Similar to previous studies, the Isolator had better recovery of key aerobic organisms. There was no significant difference in time to detection between the Isolator and the ESP, although both had significantly shorter time to detection than the Septi-Chek. The authors of the study also specifically noted the ESP system required far less processing and manipulation than the other two systems.

To summarize early comparison studies, the Difco ESP system generally performed as good as or better than most blood culture systems available at the time. The exception appeared to be with the Isolator system, which appeared to have better overall organism recovery, although this system was more technically demanding, limited to aerobic organisms, and prone to contamination. Although these comparison studies found that the ESP performed similarly to other available blood culture systems, a noncomparison study by Tinghitella et al. sought to further explore limitations of the instrument (12). This group used blind subculture of negative bottles (n = 1,162) following a full 5 days of incubation to identify organisms that went undetected by the system. They found that 16 (1.4%) of the negative bottles exhibited growth on subculture. These consisted of *Cryptococcus neoformans* (n = 8, 50% of total positives), *C. albicans* (n = 1, 6% of total positives), *S. aureus* (n = 2, 13% of total positives), coagulase-negative *Staphylococcus* (n = 3, 19% of total positives), *Bacillus* spp. (n = 1, 6% of total positives), and *Corynebacterium* spp. (n = 1, 6% of total positives). While many of these proved to be clinically insignificant, the overrepresentation of *C. neoformans* is an important observation, calling into question the ability of the system to detect this organism.

Other groups sought to further test the limitations of the ESP system by examining how it performed in less than ideal situations. Although the manufacturer recommended a blood volume per bottle of 10 ml, Welby et al. examined the performance of the ESP system with suboptimal volumes of blood from pediatric specimens (13). Using inoculations ranging from 0.2 to 1.0 ml from 10,726 individual blood draws, the ESP system was found to perform similarly to the Septi-Chek system, having recovered 237 and 221 probable pathogens, respectively. The time to detection and time to final identification were both decreased for the ESP system. The same group published another comparison study between the BacT/Alert FAN media and the ESP system using low-volume blood cultures (14). While the BacT/Alert detected more isolates of *S. aureus*, the ESP system detected more isolates of *Streptococcus* spp. and *Enterococcus* spp. Similar to the group's previous study, the ESP system had a more rapid time to detection (13.6 h versus 15.7 h).

Chapin et al. conducted a study in 1995 that challenged the ESP system in a different way (15). Ideally, inoculated bottles should be placed on the instrument as soon as possible. In their study, they examined the ability of the ESP to detect a variety of organisms from vials with delayed entry. It was determined that delays up to 8 h did not affect organism recovery, although delays of 24 h or greater had a negative impact on organism recovery (regardless of whether delayed bottles were held at room temperature or 35°C). *Streptococcus* spp. were most affected by this delay. Another study examined the effect of reducing the bottle incubation recommendation of the manufacturer from 5 days to 4 days (16). This involved a retrospective review of 7,362 blood cultures positive for bacteria or yeast. The authors found that only 2.2% of isolates were recovered on day 5. The vast majority of these isolates were classified as probable contaminants (156/164), which led to the conclusion that only 0.1% of likely significant isolates would be missed with 4-day incubation. An added benefit of this practice would be a decrease in the amount of potential contaminants.

A second iteration of the ESP system, the ESP Culture System II, expanded the capabilities of its predecessor by providing the ability to culture mycobacteria. The recovery of mycobacteria utilized the same manometric technology. Specimens for culture were inoculated to an ESP II vial containing 12.5 ml of broth media. Additionally, a 1.0-ml growth supplementation solution was added (Middlebrook oleic acid, albumin, and dextrose) as well as a 0.5-ml solution of antibiotics (polymyxin B, vancomycin, nalidixic acid, and amphotericin B). Tholcken et al. evaluated this system for the recovery of mycobacteria from blood (17). Rather than using direct blood inoculation, the group used sediments from blood specimens collected in Isolator tubes. Compared with culture on Middlebrook 7H11 agar, the ESP II system recovered more mycobacteria than the agar-based method (66 versus 60 of 1,704 cultures). The mean time to detection was also lower for the ESP II system (15.6 versus 19.0 days). A second study by Woods et al. compared the ESP II system with the Bactec TB 460 and Middlebrook 7H11 methodologies for the culture of mycobacteria from respiratory specimens (18). In this study, 149 of 2,283 specimens were positive for mycobacteria by at least one method. The ESP II system had the highest recovery rate, at 87%. However, the authors pointed out that better recovery rates were obtained when a combination of ESP II and solid media was used.

VersaTREK

In 2004, TREK Diagnostics (Cleveland, OH) released an updated CMBCS, the VersaTREK system (Fig. 3). This system utilized the same manometric detection as the ESP and ESP II systems without any major changes in detection technology. However, a significant improvement in the VersaTREK system compared with its predecessors was added overall versatility. No longer separated into top and bottom drawers, aerobic and anaerobic bottles could be placed in the instrument in any available location. Furthermore, *Mycobacterium* spp. detection and *Mycobacterium tuberculosis* resistance testing could also be performed by placing specialized bottles into any available location on the same instrument. Another added feature of

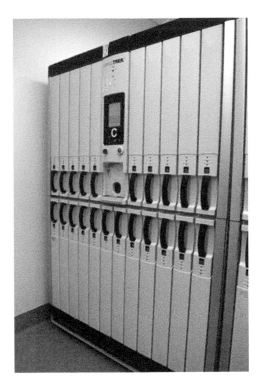

Figure 3 VersaTREK continuous-monitoring blood culture system. This figure depicts the VersaTREK continuous-monitoring blood culture system. Individual drawers are opened by pulling forward on the handles present on the front of the instrument, revealing a series of bottle-loading stations. Each bottle-loading station is capable of accommodating aerobic, anaerobic, *Mycobacterium* spp. isolation, and *Mycobacterium tuberculosis* susceptibility testing media. Thermo Scientific VersaTREK Automated Microbial Detection System is owned by Thermo Fisher Scientific. Copying is prohibited.

the VersaTREK system was the availability of aerobic blood culture bottles with incorporated stir bars, allowing for better agitation and oxygenation of aerobic cultures. The VersaTREK system quickly became one of the three most commonly used CBCMSs, and remains so at the time of this writing. An analysis of market share data based on participation in blood culture surveys from the College of American Pathologists (CAP) indicates that the Thermo Fisher TREK system is used by about 6% of laboratories, while the BD Bactec and bioMérieux BacT/Alert systems possess about 50% and 44% of the market share, respectively (19).

Instrument Specifications of the VersaTREK System
The VersaTREK instrument is a modular system made up of units containing drawers with a capacity of 24 bottles each. The system is scalable, and, currently, the system is available in units with a capacity of 96 bottles (1 to 4 drawers), 240 bottles (4 to 10 drawers), or 528 bottles (14 to 22 drawers). The drawers can be added to the different systems two at a time to meet the testing needs of the laboratory. As an example, a laboratory using

a unit with a bottle capacity of 240 bottles that holds blood cultures for 5 days has the ability to test 17,520 bottles a year.

REDOX Media for VersaTREK System

Culture bottles for the VersaTREK system are made up of paired aerobic and anaerobic bottles that are available in two different media volumes (Fig. 4). The REDOX 1 (aerobic) and REDOX 2 (anaerobic) bottles contain 80 ml of medium and can accommodate 0.1 to 10 ml of blood or sterile body fluids. The REDOX 1 EZ Draw and REDOX 2 EZ Draw bottles contain 40 ml of medium and can accommodate 0.1 to 5 ml of blood or sterile body fluids (20). Because the bottles can accommodate as little as 0.1 ml of blood volume, there are no separate bottles available for pediatric specimens, although this suboptimal volume of blood is not likely to reliably detect a culprit organism in the significant proportion of pediatric patients with low-level bacteremia (21). All bottles are compatible for use with

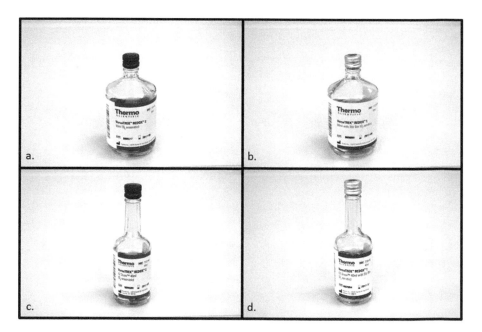

Figure 4 VersaTREK blood culture media. This figure depicts uninoculated blood culture media available for use on the VersaTREK instrument: **(a)** Aerobic REDOX 1 bottle, **(b)** Anaerobic REDOX 2 bottle, **(c)** Aerobic REDOX 1 EZ Draw bottle, and **(d)** Anaerobic REDOX 2 bottle. Thermo Scientific VersaTREK REDOX Media is owned by Thermo Fisher Scientific. Copying is prohibited.

commonly used blood collection techniques. In addition, the EZ Draw (EZD) bottles are FDA cleared for direct draw, which uses vacuum flow for controlled measure of 5 ml of blood into the bottle without the need for a separate collection device.

The performance of the EZDraw and REDOX blood culture bottles was evaluated using simulated blood cultures to compare time to positivity (TTP) for 15 different clinically significant pathogens (22). Bacterial suspensions were added to each bottle type so that organism concentration and the blood-to-broth ratio remained the same. The study found that the EZD bottles had decreased TTP for 13 of 15 microorganisms tested. The difference in TTP was significant for only four of the isolates tested and was less than 1 h for three of these four. Overall, the average TTP was lower for the EZD bottles for both the aerobic (14.4 versus 15.1 h) and anaerobic (17.8 versus 18.2 h) media. The authors speculated that the smaller headspace of the EZD bottles may permit earlier detection of changes in pressure by the instrument. However, the difference in TTP may not be clinically significant and the additional sets of blood cultures necessary for the EZD bottles to meet the CLSI standard of at least 20 ml per set (23) must be a consideration before use of the EZD media.

When the maximum amount of blood is added to either bottle type, a blood-to-broth ratio of 1:9 is maintained. This is the highest specimen dilution of the available CMBCSs and allows for dilution of host-specific inhibitors, antimicrobial compounds, and other deleterious agents that may interfere with organism growth (24). The higher dilution necessitates a larger volume of blood per bottle, which increases the sensitivity of blood culture for detection of clinically significant organisms (25–27).

The formulation of the media is different between the aerobic REDOX 1 and anaerobic REDOX 2 bottles (Table 1). The REDOX 1 media consist of a soy-casein peptone broth that is formulated to support growth of aerobic and facultative anaerobic organisms, while the REDOX 2 bottles contain proteose-peptone broth to support growth of obligate and facultative anaerobes. In addition, the REDOX 1 bottles contain a stir bar that is driven by a motor housed within the base of each slot of the instrument to provide aeration for aerobic growth. This is in contrast to the older ESP system, which continuously agitated all aerobic bottles in a dedicated drawer.

A major difference in the VersaTREK media bottles in comparison with other CMBCSs is the composition of the bottles. The VersaTREK bottles are made of molded glass, and no alternative material such as plastic is available, as in other systems. Thus, bottle breakage is a concern because of

Table 1 VersaTREK media components (20)

Contents of VersaTREK REDOX 1 and REDOX 2 media	
REDOX 1	
Processed water	40/80 ml
Soy-casein peptone A	2.1% w/v
Sodium chloride	0.5% w/v
Yeast extract	0.1% w/v
Dextrose	0.25% w/v
Divalent salts A	0.009% w/v
Supplement O	0.33% w/v
Sodium polyanethol sulfonate	0.0125% w/v
REDOX 2	
Processed water	40/80 ml
Proteose-peptone N	1.5% w/v
Yeast extract	0.5% w/v
Sodium chloride	0.23% w/v
Dextrose	0.5% w/v
Polysorbate 80 10%	0.075% w/v
Supplement AN	0.8% w/v
Trisodium citrate	0.07% w/v
Saponin	0.045% w/v
Hemin	0.0005% w/v
Cysteine	0.05% w/v
Vitamin K	0.0001% w/v
Resazurin	0.0001% w/v

the potential for injuries sustained to laboratory workers when a bottle breaks or during cleanup of a broken bottle and for exposures to blood-borne pathogens. Of note, the clinical microbiology laboratory at our institution handles over 45,000 sets of VersaTREK blood cultures per year but has had no adverse event reports filed that were attributed to the use of glass media bottles. A survey by the International Sharps Injury Prevention Society found that almost 30% of hospitals surveyed that used glass blood culture bottles from any manufacturer experienced greater than six bottle breakages per year (28). However, a subsequent survey conducted by the manufacturer of the VersaTREK instrument found that only 0.13% of sites surveyed experienced more than six breakages per year. In addition, none of these breakages resulted in injuries to laboratory workers (29). A special carrier is used to prevent bottle breakage within pneumatic tube systems. This survey attributed most of these breaks to noncompliance with the use of this carrier and highlights the importance of proper education of personnel involved with blood culture process. The glass composition of the VersaTREK bottles also adds to the weight of the bottle, which subsequently adds to the cost for waste disposal. While this should be a consideration, the decreased cost of

VersaTREK consumables in comparison with other CMBCSs typically offsets the increased costs of disposal.

Blood Culture Workflow on the VersaTREK Blood Culture System

While similarities exist between the ESP and VersaTREK workflows, several enhancements have been made to the VersaTREK workflow. Similar to the ESP, prior to loading the bottle to the VersaTREK instrument, the septum of the bottle is disinfected and a connector is added to the top of the bottle. The connector contains a needle that will pierce the septum to vent the bottle and link it to a sensor in the instrument. Unique to the VersaTREK is an electronic one-touch ordering system. Prepared bottles are scanned or manually entered into the system and loaded onto the instrument. If the system detects the addition of a REDOX 1 bottle with a stir bar, a motor activates to provide rotary aeration of the bottle. See Fig. 5 for a summary of the workflow.

When the system detects a change in pressure that indicates logarithmic growth of bacteria in the REDOX bottle, the system alerts the user with a light on the appropriate drawer and above the bottle, in addition to an optional audible alarm. Positive bottles are removed from the instrument, but the spot will remain reserved for the bottle if nothing is seen on examination. Reserved spots and negative bottles are cleared from the system when finalized using the instrument software.

Data collection and management of the instrument are handled by a computer that can connect with up to six VersaTREK instruments. The computer runs VersaTREK software that monitors the system for errors and positive signals. The touch-screen system also allows the user to view system status and bottle information, such as number of available bottle locations and pressure graphs of positive bottles (Fig. 6). The system is capable of unidirectional or bidirectional flow of data to many laboratory information systems (LIS). Importantly, connection to the LIS is not a requirement for usability, and data are still accessible when the LIS is nonfunctional.

Performance of the VersaTREK Blood Culture System

The first study to evaluate the performance of the VersaTREK blood culture system compared standard VersaTREK medium with aerobic and anaerobic 3D media incubated on the BacT/Alert 3D blood culture system (bioMérieux) (30). The BacT/Alert system detects the presence of microorganisms using a colorimetric indicator that detects CO_2 production during microbial growth. Overall, there was no difference in the time to positivity

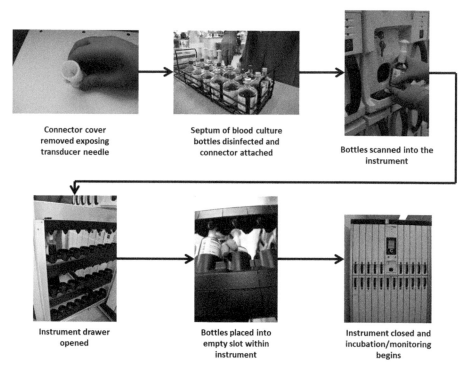

Connector cover
removed exposing
transducer needle

Septum of blood culture
bottles disinfected and
connector attached

Bottles scanned into the
instrument

Instrument drawer
opened

Bottles placed into
empty slot within
instrument

Instrument closed and
incubation/monitoring
begins

Figure 5 Summary of VersaTREK workflow. This figure illustrates the typical workflow for the preparation and loading of inoculated blood cultures onto the VersaTREK instrument. The described steps are the same for all available blood culture media, regardless of formulation. All bottle-loading stations are capable of incubating both aerobic and anaerobic media.

between the two instruments, but the VersaTREK system did have a higher rate of false-positive signals (1.6% versus 0.7% for aerobic media and 0.9% versus 0.8% for anaerobic media). The study found no significant difference in yields of many clinically significant pathogens from either blood culture system. However, the recovery of *Streptococcus* spp. and *Enterococcus* spp. was significantly improved by using the VersaTREK instrument and media. The increased blood-broth dilution in the VersaTREK bottles may explain this, because inhibitory factors such as antimicrobials are further diluted with these media. This is supported by the significantly increased recovery rates of isolates from patients on antimicrobial therapy with the VersaTREK media (30).

Several studies have compared the performance of the VersaTREK blood culture system with the Bactec 9240 and the newer Bactec FX blood culture systems (BD Diagnostics, Sparks, MD) for the recovery of clinically

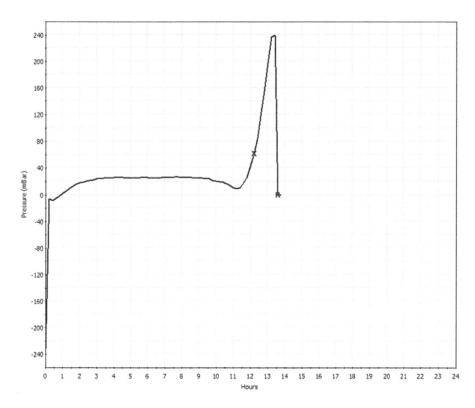

Figure 6 Example of pressure readings obtained over time for a positive blood culture by the VersaTREK system. Growth of microorganisms results in changes in headspace pressure that is detected by the instrument. The user can graphically view changes in pressure using the VersaTREK software (solid line on graph). Bottle events, such as a positive signal, are indicated in red.

significant bacteria and yeast (31–34). The Bactec blood culture systems monitor CO_2 production from growing microorganisms via an internal fluorimetric sensor. One study of clinical specimens from patients with suspected bloodstream infections found that the recovery rate of organisms was comparable for the VersaTREK and Bactec 9240 instruments (32). However, the VersaTREK instrument had a false-positive signal rate of 7.9%, which is higher than a previous study that reported a false-positive rate of 1.6% for REDOX 1 and 0.9% for REDOX 2 bottles (30). The authors speculated that this may be due to a delay in postincubation processing that was prohibitive to growth of fastidious organisms or failure to use culture media that supported growth of fastidious organisms. False positives were also attributed to prior antibiotic use and possible pressure changes due to vortexing of the aerobic bottles by the instrument, although no evidence was given to support these claims.

A very small prospective study of 20 patients with *S. aureus* bacteremia found that the VersaTREK system failed to detect five cases of persistent infection from repeat blood cultures that were detected by the Bactec FX system in patients treated with appropriate antibiotic therapy for greater than 4 days (31). Decreased recovery rates for specimens containing antimicrobials by the VersaTREK system compared with the Bactec FX system were also noted in a study of seeded blood cultures in which antimicrobials were added at trough, midlevel, and peak concentrations (33). In this study, the VersaTREK system recovered only 18.6% of aerobic isolates in the presence of antibiotics compared with a recovery rate of 58.7% for the Bactec FX system, suggesting that the inclusion of antibiotic resin in the Bactec media allowed greater analytical sensitivity. However, the same inoculum of bacteria and volume of blood were added to the VersaTREK REDOX bottles containing 80 ml of media and the Bactec Plus bottles containing 30 ml of media. This may have resulted in differences in bacterial growth kinetics that negatively affected the growth rate of organisms in the REDOX bottles.

Fastidious organisms such as *Haemophilus* and *Kingella* species are causes of infrequent yet serious bacteremia. However, recovery of these organisms by CMBCS is complicated by the fact that many fastidious bacteria produce CO_2 at a volume that is inadequate for detection by the CMBCSs. One advantage of the VersaTREK system is the ability to detect production or consumption of any gas, which makes the system more useful for recovery of fastidious bacteria. Using blood culture bottles seeded with 10 different fastidious organisms, one study showed that the overall recovery from aerobic and anaerobic bottles on the VersaTREK system was 100% compared with 97% of isolates recovered from the BacT/Alert system (35). The REDOX 1 bottle recovered 35 of 37 organisms compared with 26 of 37 isolates from the aerobic bottle of the BacT/Alert system, with decreased time to positivity with the VersaTREK instrument for all the organisms tested. Thus, it is likely that the enriched media formulation of the VersaTREK REDOX blood culture bottles and the ability to detect production or consumption of gas permit enhanced recovery of fastidious organisms from blood specimens. This is supported by a small study of five *Helicobacter cinaedi* isolates that were all detected by the VersaTREK system within 3 days, while other automated systems needed increased incubation time or failed to detect this fastidious organism (36, 37).

Many anaerobic organisms, such as *Bacteroides* and *Clostridium* species, are important causes of bloodstream infections. There is a paucity of data on the comparison of recovery of anaerobes from VersaTREK and other blood culture systems. One study, which included only one isolate of *Bacteroides fragilis*, found that the REDOX 2 bottle on the VersaTREK was able to recover this organism in a shorter period of time than the BacT/Alert system (28.0 h versus 55.2 h) (35). Another study found no significant difference in the recovery of anaerobes from either of these systems, although there was a trend toward increased episodes of recovery of anaerobes by the VersaTREK system (30).

Bloodstream infections with *Candida* species are common in hospitalized patients. Thus, detection of *Candida* in blood specimens is a high priority in many clinical microbiology laboratories. One study evaluated recovery rates and TTP of several clinically significant *Candida* spp. using simulated blood cultures with and without antifungal agents (34). Overall, there was no significant difference in the recovery rate for *Candida* species in the absence of antifungals between the VersaTREK and Bactec FX systems. However, when bottles were spiked with commonly used antifungals, the recovery rate of *Candida* organisms was significantly higher for the Bactec FX system (83.1%) than for the VersaTREK (50.7%). In the absence of antifungal agents, the overall average TTP was significantly decreased for *Candida* species in blood cultures incubated on the VersaTREK instrument. The opposite was seen in the presence of antifungals, when average TTP was significantly shorter with the Bactec FX system, which uses media containing resins for antimicrobial inactivation. The poor performance of the VersaTREK media in the presence of antifungals in this study may indicate that dilution is inadequate to permit growth of *Candida* species in the presence of even trough concentrations of antifungal agent. Clinical microbiology laboratories should be aware of the use of empiric therapy for candidemia in the patient population served by the laboratory.

Potential Causes of False-Positive Signals

False-positive signals on the VersaTREK instrument may result from preanalytical variables such as bacterial contamination and nonmicrobial causes of pressure changes within the media. The introduction of contaminants into blood culture media is a potential confounder in the diagnosis of bloodstream infections. The CAP recommends that the laboratory track contamination rates and establish an acceptable threshold, which is generally accepted to be approximately 2 to 3% (38). Excluding specimens collected from catheters, the overall contamination rate of blood cultures collected annually from inpatient locations at our institution and incubated on the VersaTREK instrument was 1.8% from inpatient locations and 4.1% from the emergency department in one recent year. A retrospective study that analyzed more than 100,000 blood culture sets from three clinical microbiology laboratories found that the contamination rate of the VersaTREK REDOX media was comparable to the frequency of contamination for the standard, resin, and lytic media available on the Bactec 9240 system. The contamination rates cited in the study range from 1.70 to 2.93% (39).

One cause of nonmicrobial pressure changes that may result in a false-positive signal is a high white blood cell (WBC) count in a blood specimen, likely as a result of carbon dioxide generation by the WBCs (40). Although theoretically possible, there is a lack of published data supporting or refuting this mechanism in the VersaTREK system. In our experience, rare false-positive signals have been noted in blood culture specimens collected from patients with leukemia and in cultures of stem cell products.

Because the VersaTREK system monitors the atmospheric pressure in the headspace of the bottles, inconsistencies in barometric pressure readings may cause a false-positive signal on the instrument. A recent Class 2 Device Recall by the FDA acknowledged the rare occurrence of this event after improper conduction of pressure readings from the bottle to the sensor due to improperly placed labels (41). Additionally, overfilling bottles may result in a false-positive signal due to increased pressure in the resultant reduced headspace of the bottle. Regardless of the cause of a false-positive signal, if growth is not confirmed upon Gram stain of a potentially positive bottle, the technical insert for the REDOX media recommends equilibration of the previously incubated bottle to ambient temperature before reincubation on the VersaTREK instrument.

Potential Causes of False-Negative Signals

A false negative on a CMBCS is arguably worse than a false positive because of the repercussions of a missed bloodstream infection. It is generally recommended that a blood-to-broth ratio between 1:5 and 1:10 is maintained in blood culture media to promote microbial recovery through dilution of inhibitory factors (42). Further dilution of specimen, for instance, because of underfilling of a bottle, may lead to reduced organism recovery and thus a false-negative result. Overfilling the bottle can also lead to false negatives because of the less than ideal dilution of specimen in the media. While no study has specifically addressed false negatives due to blood volume on the VersaTREK system, one study noted that blood culture bottles associated with the BacT/Alert system were underfilled more often than REDOX media for the VersaTREK, while the incidence of overfilled bottles was similar between the two systems (30).

The REDOX media for VersaTREK do not contain additives such as resins or charcoal for antibiotic inactivation. Instead, the system relies on proper filling of bottles to maintain an optimal blood-to-broth ratio and dilution of antimicrobials. Even with adequate specimen volume, prior treatment with antimicrobials is a potential cause for false-negative blood cultures. Using simulated cultures, one study found decreased recovery of organisms from the VersaTREK system in comparison with the Bactec system, even at trough levels of many common antimicrobials (33).

Another potential cause of falsely negative blood cultures is a prolonged delay between the addition of specimen to the REDOX media and incubation on the VersaTREK instrument. An extended period of time outside the instrument may permit enough growth of microorganisms to alter the gas pressure inside the bottle prior to entry into the instrument. Thus, when the bottle is finally added to the instrument, the subsequent change in gas pressure will not be enough that it is detectable by the system.

VersaTREK Applications Other Than Blood Culture

When compared with other commercially available CBCMSs, a potential limitation of the VersaTREK is the lack of a dedicated fungal blood culture bottle. Clinical microbiology laboratories in need of fungal blood culture must therefore adopt alternative means. While this may be a significant deficit for some laboratories, there are other applications of the VersaTREK system that some laboratories may find particularly beneficial. In addition to standard blood culture, the VersaTREK system is also FDA approved for bacterial detection in sterile body fluids other than blood (i.e., pleural, peritoneal, and pericardial fluids). These can be inoculated into the standard VersaTREK REDOX bottles and incubated in the same wells as aerobic and anaerobic blood cultures. In addition to sterile body fluids, investigators have further explored the utility of the instrument beyond the testing of clinical specimens. Dunne et al. described the use of the VersaTREK for sterility testing of platelet units. This group used dilutions of common bacterial platelet contaminants to assess the analytical sensitivity of the system. They demonstrated that the system had an analytical sensitivity of <10 CFU/ml for most bacterial contaminants, similar to other bacterial detection systems

FDA cleared for platelet monitoring (43). Although the VersaTREK is not FDA cleared for this purpose, the data from this study suggest it can be used successfully. In a similar study, Burnham et al. described the use of the VersaTREK for sterility testing of apheresis hematopoietic progenitor cell (HPC) products (44). This group spiked apheresis HPC products with different concentrations of four aerobic bacteria, five anaerobic bacteria, and one yeast. They were able to demonstrate that, at concentrations as low as 10 CFU/ml, the VersaTREK was capable of detecting all aerobic bacteria within 24 h, all anaerobic bacteria within 5 days, and *C. albicans* within 30 h. The group compared this approach with 16S rRNA gene amplification, which failed to detect any bacterial or yeast targets at the highest spiked concentrations used (10,000 CFU/ml).

Yet another unique quality of the VersaTREK compared with other CMBCSs is the ability to perform mycobacterial detection and susceptibility testing. Mycobacteria media formulations similar to those available on the ESP II are available for use with the VersaTREK. These include media with added mycobacteria growth supplement and media with added inhibitory antibiotics designed for culturing contaminated specimens. When compared with other broth-based mycobacteria detection systems, the VersaTREK is unique because of the addition of a cellulose sponge into the media bottle. This porous sponge simulates the parenchyma of lung tissue, helping promote the growth of mycobacterial respiratory pathogens. Similar to blood cultures performed on the VersaTREK, growth is detected through manometry with pressure readings occurring every 24 min.

A 2008 study by Falconi et al. compared the recovery rate and time to detection of *Mycobacterium* spp. using the VersaTREK versus traditional Lowenstein-Jensen solid media (45). While recovery rates of mycobacteria were not statistically different between the two (84.8% for VersaTREK versus 89.4% for solid media), contamination rates were significantly higher from solid media (7.4% versus 4.2%). However, the VersaTREK allowed for detection of *Mycobacterium* spp. 7.1 days faster on average and allowed for the detection of *M. tuberculosis* 9.7 days faster on average. A 2011 study demonstrated similar decreases in the amount of time to detection (46).

The diagnosis and care of patients with mycobacteria infections are further facilitated by the ability to perform *M. tuberculosis* susceptibility testing on the VersaTREK. Media bottles are available for the testing of resistance to rifampin, isoniazid, ethambutol, pyrazinamide, and strepto-mycin. A 2012 comparison of the VersaTREK system with another broth-based *M. tuberculosis* susceptibility testing system, the Bactec MGIT 960, showed great agreement of results among 67 tested strains for resistance to all five drugs (47). The only discrepancies were strains susceptible to streptomycin by VersaTREK although resistant by Bactec MGIT (n = 3) and strains susceptible to pyrazinamide by VersaTREK but resistant by Bactec MGIT (n = 2).

Conclusion

Over the past 20 years, the TREK blood culture systems have been commonly used in many microbiology laboratories. The use of manometry for organism detection, the media formulation, and the blood-to-broth ratio likely contribute to the high analytical sensitivity of these systems, particularly for fastidious organisms. The ability to perform sterile body fluid testing, mycobacterial isolation, and *M. tuberculosis* susceptibility testing may also be highly beneficial features for certain laboratories, depending on their needs. However, the lack of plastic bottles and media with antibiotic resins may cause other laboratories to consider alternative CMBCSs. Nonetheless, an abundance of data supports the robust performance of both the Difco ESP and the VersaTREK, making it little surprise that both systems have been among the most widely used CBCMSs worldwide.

References

1. Trombley C, Anderson JD. 1987. SIGNAL blood culture system for detection of bacteremia in neonates. *J Clin Microbiol* **25**:2098–2101.
2. Roberts G, Kaczmarski E. 1987. Comments on Oxoid Signal blood culture system. *J Clin Pathol* **40**:813. doi:10.1136/jcp.40.7.813-a
3. Rohner P, Pepey B, Auckenthaler R. 1995. Comparison of BacT/Alert with Signal blood culture system. *J Clin Microbiol* **33**:313–317.
4. Rimmer K, Cabot M. 1988. Comparison of Bactec NR-660 and Signal systems. *J Clin Pathol* **41**:676–678.
5. Stevens CM, Swaine D, Butler C, Carr AH, Weightman A, Catchpole CR, Healing DE, Elliott TS. 1994. Development of o.a.s.i.s., a new automated blood culture system in which detection is based on measurement of bottle headspace pressure changes. *J Clin Microbiol* **32**:1750–1756.
6. Morello JA, Leitch C, Nitz S, Dyke JW, Andruszewski M, Maier G, Landau W, Beard MA. 1994. Detection of bacteremia by Difco ESP blood culture system. *J Clin Microbiol* **32**:811–818.
7. Dunne WM Jr, LaRocco M. 2001. Blood culture systems, p 189–209. *In* Cimolai N (ed), *Laboratory Diagnosis of Bacterial Infections*. CRC Press, Boca Raton, FL.
8. Zwadyk P Jr, Pierson CL, Young C. 1994. Comparison of Difco ESP and Organon Teknika BacT/Alert continuous-monitoring blood culture systems. *J Clin Microbiol* **32**:1273–1279.

9. Kirkley BA, Easley KA, Washington JA. 1994. Controlled clinical evaluation of Isolator and ESP aerobic blood culture systems for detection of bloodstream infections. *J Clin Microbiol* **32**:1547–1549.

10. Kellogg JA, Bankert DA, Manzella JP, Parsey KS, Scott SL, Cavanaugh SH. 1994. Clinical comparison of isolator and thiol broth with ESP aerobic and anaerobic bottles for recovery of pathogens from blood. *J Clin Microbiol* **32**:2050–2055.

11. Cockerill FR III, Torgerson CA, Reed GS, Vetter EA, Weaver AL, Dale JC, Roberts GD, Henry NK, Ilstrup DM, Rosenblatt JE. 1996. Clinical comparison of difco ESP, Wampole isolator, and Becton Dickinson Septi-Chek aerobic blood culturing systems. *J Clin Microbiol* **34**:20–24.

12. Tinghitella TJ, Lamagdeleine MD. 1995. Assessment of Difco ESP 384 blood culture system by terminal subcultures: failure to detect *Cryptococcus neoformans* in clinical specimens. *J Clin Microbiol* **33**:3031–3033.

13. Welby PL, Keller DS, Storch GA. 1995. Comparison of automated Difco ESP blood culture system with biphasic BBL Septi-Chek system for detection of bloodstream infections in pediatric patients. *J Clin Microbiol* **33**:1084–1088.

14. Welby-Sellenriek PL, Keller DS, Ferrett RJ, Storch GA. 1997. Comparison of the BacT/Alert FAN aerobic and the Difco ESP 80A aerobic bottles for pediatric blood cultures. *J Clin Microbiol* **35**:1166–1171.

15. Chapin K, Lauderdale TL. 1996. Comparison of Bactec 9240 and Difco ESP blood culture systems for detection of organisms from vials whose entry was delayed. *J Clin Microbiol* **34**:543–549.

16. Doern GV, Brueggemann AB, Dunne WM, Jenkins SG, Halstead DC, McLaughlin JC. 1997. Four-day incubation period for blood culture bottles processed with the Difco ESP blood culture system. *J Clin Microbiol* **35**:1290–1292.

17. Tholcken CA, Huang S, Woods GL. 1997. Evaluation of the ESP Culture System II for recovery of mycobacteria from blood specimens collected in isolator tubes. *J Clin Microbiol* **35**:2681–2682.

18. Woods GL, Fish G, Plaunt M, Murphy T. 1997. Clinical evaluation of difco ESP culture system II for growth and detection of mycobacteria. *J Clin Microbiol* **35**:121–124.

19. Anonymous. 2016. *IVD Insights: Market Tracking Reports from MDxI, Microbiology 2015 Cycle 2.* Market Diagnostics International, Dallas, TX.

20. Thermo Scientific. 2014. *VersaTREK™ REDOX™ 1 and VersaTREK REDOX 2 media. Package Insert.*

21. Kellogg JA, Manzella JP, Bankert DA. 2000. Frequency of low-level bacteremia in children from birth to fifteen years of age. *J Clin Microbiol* **38**:2181–2185.

22. Samuel LP, Pimentel JD, Tibbetts RJ, Martin R, Hensley R, Meier FA. 2011. Comparison of time to positivity of the VersaTREK® REDOX 80-mL and the REDOX EZ draw 40-mL blood culture bottles for common bacterial bloodstream pathogens. *Diagn Microbiol Infect Dis* **71**:101–105.

23. CLSI. 2007. *Principles and Procedures for Blood Cultures; Approved Guideline*, vol M47-A. CLSI, Wayne, PA.

24. Bryan CS. 1989. Clinical implications of positive blood cultures. *Clin Microbiol Rev* **2**:329–353.

25. Gonsalves WI, Cornish N, Moore M, Chen A, Varman M. 2009. Effects of volume and site of blood draw on blood culture results. *J Clin Microbiol* **47**:3482–3485.

26. Hall MM, Ilstrup DM, Washington JA II. 1976. Effect of volume of blood cultured on detection of bacteremia. *J Clin Microbiol* **3**:643–645.

27. Mermel LA, Maki DG. 1993. Detection of bacteremia in adults: consequences of culturing an inadequate volume of blood. *Ann Intern Med* **119**:270–272.

28. Stoker R. 2010. *Microbiology Laboratory Risk Assessment of Blood Culture Bottle Breakage*. International Sharps Injury Prevention Society. http://www.biomerieuxconnection.com/12-10-10-blood-culture-bottle.html. Accessed August 1, 2016.

29. Anonymous. 2011. *VersaTREK® REDOX® Glass Bottle Survey*. https://www.thermofisher.com/content/dam/tfs/SDG/MBD/MBD%20Marketing%20Material/Clinical/Blood%20Culture/Documents/VersaTREK-REDOX-Glass-Bottle-Survey-EN.pdf. Accessed August 1, 2016.

30. Mirrett S, Hanson KE, Reller LB. 2007. Controlled clinical comparison of VersaTREK and BacT/ALERT blood culture systems. *J Clin Microbiol* **45**:299–302.

31. Bonilla H, Zervos M, Saravolatz LD. 2011. Comparison of BACTEC™ plus Aerobic/F and VersaTREK REDOX(®) blood culture media for the recovery of *Staphylococcus aureus* from patients with suspected persistent bacteremia. *J Infect* **63**:89–90.

32. Dreyer AW, Ismail NA, Nkosi D, Lindeque K, Matthews M, van Zyl DG, Hoosen AA. 2011. Comparison of the VersaTREK blood culture system against the Bactec9240 system in patients with suspected bloodstream infections. *Ann Clin Microbiol Antimicrob* **10**:4. doi:10.1186/1476-0711-10-4.

33. Miller NS, Rogan D, Orr BL, Whitney D. 2011. Comparison of BD Bactec Plus blood culture media to VersaTREK Redox blood culture media for detection of bacterial pathogens in simulated adult blood cultures containing therapeutic concentrations of antibiotics. *J Clin Microbiol* **49**:1624–1627.

34. Riedel S, Eisinger SW, Dam L, Stamper PD, Carroll KC. 2011. Comparison of BD Bactec Plus Aerobic/F medium to VersaTREK Redox 1 blood culture medium for detection of *Candida* spp. in seeded blood culture specimens containing therapeutic levels of antifungal agents. *J Clin Microbiol* **49**:1524–1529.

35. Mirrett S, Reller LB. 2005. *Comparison of the VersaTREK® and the BacT/ALERT® Blood Culture Systems for the Growth of Fastidious Microorganisms*. American Society for Microbiology meeting, 2005, poster C-214.

36. Tomida J, Tsurunaga M, Hosoda T, Hayakawa S, Suematsu H, Sawamura H. 2012. Evaluation of automated blood culture systems about the detection capability for *Helicobacter cinaedi*. *J Jpn Soc Clin Microbiol* **22**:233. [in Japanese.]

37. Kawamura Y, Tomida J, Morita Y, Fujii S, Okamoto T, Akaike T. 2014. Clinical and bacteriological characteristics of *Helicobacter cinaedi* infection. *J Infect Chemother* **20**:517–526.

38. Baron E, Weinstein M, Dunne W, Yagupsky P, Welch D, Wilson D. 2005. *Cumitech 1C, Blood Cultures IV*. Baron EJ, co-ordinating ed. ASM Press, Washington, DC.

39. Chapin KC, Napert DA, Miller JM, Whitehead V. 2008. Conversion to the VersaTREK® automated microbial detection system from the BACTEC™ 9240 system: retrospective analysis of data from three hospitals. American Society for Microbiology meeting, 2008, abstr C-177.

40. Martinez RM, Martinez R, Partal Y, Casas J, Llosa J, Almagro M. 1993. An infrequent cause of false-positive blood cultures. *Clin Microbiol Newsl* **15**:7–8.

41. **Anonymous.** 2015. *Class 2 Device Recall VersaTREK Automated Microbial Detection System, Recall number Z-1841-2015.* http://www.accessdata.fda.gov/scripts/cdrh/cfdocs/cfRes/res.cfm?ID=137244. Accessed August 8, 2016.

42. **Reimer LG, Wilson ML, Weinstein MP.** 1997. Update on detection of bacteremia and fungemia. *Clin Microbiol Rev* **10:**444–465.

43. **Nanua S, Weber C, Isgriggs L, Dunne WM Jr.** 2009. Performance evaluation of the VersaTREK blood culture system for quality control testing of platelet units. *J Clin Microbiol* **47:**817–818.

44. **Liu C, Weber C, Sempek DS, Grossman BJ, Burnham CA.** 2013. Sterility testing of apheresis hematopoietic progenitor cell products using an automated blood culture system. *Transfusion* **53:**2659–2666.

45. **Falconi FQ, Suárez LI, López MJ, Sancho CG.** 2008. Comparison of the VersaTREK system and Löwenstein-Jensen medium for the recovery of mycobacteria from clinical specimens. *Scand J Infect Dis* **40:**49–53.

46. **Gravet A, Souillard N, Habermacher J, Moser A, Lohmann C, Schmitt F, Delarbre JM.** 2011. [Culture and susceptibility testing of mycobacteria with VersaTREK]. *Pathol Biol (Paris)* **59:**32–38.

47. **Espasa M, Salvadó M, Vicente E, Tudó G, Alcaide F, Coll P, Martin-Casabona N, Torra M, Fontanals D, González-Martín J.** 2012. Evaluation of the VersaTREK system compared to the Bactec MGIT 960 system for first-line drug susceptibility testing of *Mycobacterium tuberculosis*. *J Clin Microbiol* **50:**488–491.

The Dark Art of Blood Cultures
Edited by Wm. Michael Dunne, Jr. and Carey-Ann D. Burnham
© 2018 American Society for Microbiology, Washington, DC
doi:10.1128/9781555819811.ch7

Molecular Methods for Detection of Pathogens Directly from Blood Specimens

7

Mark D. Gonzalez[1] and Robert C. Jerris[1]

Sepsis is a global problem and laboratory methods must be optimized to effect rapid, positive patient outcomes. The proverbial reference standard method for diagnosis, the actual culture of blood, suffers from a variety of preanalytical issues such as sufficient blood volume, prior antimicrobial treatment, time from sampling to incubation, and analytical issues of prolonged turnaround time until final identification and availability of antimicrobial susceptibility testing results. Advancements have occurred in molecular methods to provide rapid microorganism identification and resistance gene detection (e.g., *mecA* in *Staphylococcus* spp.) from positive blood culture broths. In a meta-analysis of these new methods, a significant reduction in time to targeted treatment was observed (1). However, these methods are dependent on having a positive blood culture, which is subject to the preanalytical issues described above. The ability to directly identify pathogens from blood specimens would greatly reduce the time to identification and time to optimization of therapy, as well as potentially contributing to avoiding unnecessary antimicrobials and/or discontinuation of treatment in patients with negative testing results. Direct detection methods for viruses from patient specimens have benefited from advances in molecular methods, which is largely because of the high viral loads present in those specimens. In contrast, the majority of septic patients have a paucity of bacteria or fungi per milliliter of blood, necessitating the need for larger blood volumes to increase blood culture sensitivity (2–4).

[1]Department of Pathology and Laboratory Medicine, Children's Healthcare of Atlanta, Atlanta, GA 30322

Nonetheless, recent advances in molecular methods have resulted in commercially available methods for the direct detection of bacterial and/or fungal pathogens from blood specimens. In this chapter, we highlight the currently available commercial tests (i.e., CE-marked *in vitro* device [CE-IVD] and FDA-cleared) for direct detection, which are listed in Table 1. As of the writing of this chapter, only one assay, the T2Candida Assay, was FDA cleared for use with whole-blood specimens.

LightCycler SeptiFast

The LightCycler SeptiFast (SF) assay from Roche Diagnostics (Mannheim, Germany) is a commercially available (CE-IVD, non-FDA cleared) multiplex real-time PCR assay able to detect and differentiate various Gram-negative and Gram-positive bacteria, and some fungi, commonly involved in systemic infections. The 25 targets on the SF panel are listed in Table 2. The targets for amplification are the internal transcribed sequences between the bacterial 16S and 23S rRNA genes, and the fungal 18S and 5.6S rRNA genes. Pathogen DNA is extracted from a 1.5-ml whole-blood specimen and amplified by the LightCycler instrument, where a positive detection occurs if the fluorescent signal of the internal hybridization probes reaches the threshold. An internal control can be included with specimens to detect PCR inhibition events. Subsequently, species identification occurs after a melting curve analysis. The manufacturer states that the analytical sensitivity is 100 colony forming units (CFU)/ml for *Candida glabrata*, *Streptococcus* spp., and coagulase-negative *Staphylococcus* spp. group (CoNS), and 30 CFU/ml for the other targets (5).

As to performance of the assay, Chang et al. (5) reported the diagnostic accuracy of SF compared with blood culture in a systematic review of published literature from 2006 to 2012. Studies were assessed using the Quality Assessment of Diagnostic Accuracy Studies tool (QUADAS) (6) with a focus on appropriate study design, data preparation and collection, and analysis. Of key note in the analysis was the fact that, while SF was used as the index test, there were multiple reference standards that were used to determine the composite accuracy. A total of 34 primary studies were assessed, which included 8,438 comparator episodes with a confirmed fungal or bacterial infection in 22.8% (n = 1,920) of all episodes. For detection of bacteremia and fungemia, the overall sensitivity and specificity of SF was 75% (95% confidence interval [CI], 65 to 83%) and 92% (95% CI, 90 to 95%), respectively. Further analysis for bacteremia alone demonstrated a sensitivity of 80% (95% CI, 70 to 88%) and specificity of 95% (95% CI, 93 to

TABLE 1 Comparison of preanalytic and analytic factors for commercially available direct-from-blood multiplex assay

Test parameter	SF[a]	ST[b]	VYOO[c]	IRIDICA[d]	T2C[e]
			System		
Regulatory clearance	CE-IVD	CE-IVD	CE-IVD	CE-IVD	CE-IVD, FDA
Volume of blood, ml	1.5	1 or 10	1–5	5	~3
Method of detection	PCR, LightCycler/melt curve analysis	PCR, gel electrophoresis, DNA sequencing	PCR, microarray analysis	PCR, ESI-MS[f]	PCR amplification, T2MR detection
Turnaround time	6 h	4 h, initial result + ~3 h, sequencing ID	7 h	6 h	3–5 h
References	5, 7–9	10, 11	12, 13	14, 15	16–19

[a]SF, LightCycler SeptiFast, Roche Diagnostics (Mannheim, Germany).
[b]ST, SepsiTest, Molzym (Bremen, Germany).
[c]VYOO, Analytikjena (Jena, Germany).
[d]IRIDICA, Inc., (Marlborough MA).
[e]T2C, T2Candida, (Lexington, MA).
[f]ESI-MS, electrospray ionization–time of flight mass spectrometry

Table 2 Comparison of targets on commercially available multiplex assays

| | System | | |
Organisms	SF[a]	VYOO[b]	T2C[c]
Gram-negative			
Acinetobacter baumannii	√	√	
Bacteroides fragilis		√	
Burkholderia cepacia		√	
Enterobacter aerogenes		√	
Enterobacter cloacae		√	
Enterobacter cloacae/Enterobacter aerogenes group	√		
Escherichia coli	√	√	
Haemophilus influenzae		√	
Klebsiella oxytoca		√	
Klebsiella pneumoniae		√	
Klebsiella pneumoniae/Klebsiella oxytoca group	√		
Morganella morganii		√	
Neisseria meningitidis		√	
Prevotella buccae		√	
Prevotella intermedia		√	
Prevotella melaninogenica		√	
Proteus mirabilis	√	√	
Pseudomonas aeruginosa	√	√	
Serratia marcescens	√	√	
Stenotrophomonas maltophilia	√	√	
Gram-positive			
Clostridium perfringens		√	
CoNS group[d]	√		
Enterococcus faecalis	√	√	
Enterococcus faecium	√		
Staphylococcus aureus	√	√	
Staphylococcus epidermidis		√	
Staphylococcus haemolyticus		√	
Staphylococcus hominis		√	
Staphylococcus saprophyticus		√	
Streptococcus agalactiae		√	
Streptococcus bovis		√	
Streptococcus dysgalactiae		√	
Streptococcus mutans		√	
Streptococcus pneumoniae	√	√	
Streptococcus pyogenes		√	
Streptococcus sanguinis		√	
Streptococcus spp. group[e]	√		
Fungi			
Aspergillus fumigatus	√	√	
Candida albicans	√	√	√
Candida dubliniensis		√	
Candida glabrata	√	√	√

(continued on next page)

Table 2 (*continued*)

Organisms	System		
	SF[a]	VYOO[b]	T2C[c]
Candida krusei	√	√	√
Candida parapsilosis	√	√	√
Candida tropicalis	√	√	√
Resistance markers			
bla$_{CTX-M}$ (several variants)		√	
bla$_{SHV}$ (several variants)		√	
mecA		√	
vanA		√	
vanB		√	

[a]SF, LightCycler SeptiFast, Roche Diagnostics (Mannheim, Germany).

[b]VYOO, Analytikjena (Jena, Germany).

[c]T2C, T2Candida, T2BioSystems (Lexington, MA).

[d]CoNS group includes *Staphylococcus epidermidis, Staphylococcus haemolyticus, Staphylococcus hominis, Staphylococcus pasteuri, Staphylococcus warneri, Staphylococcus cohnii, Staphylococcus lugdunensis, Staphylococcus capitis, Staphylococcus caprae, Staphylococcus saprophyticus,* and *Staphylococcus xylosus.*

[e]*Streptococcus* spp. group includes *Streptococcus agalactiae, Streptococcus pyogenes, Streptococcus anginosus, Streptococcus bovis, Streptococcus constellatus, Streptococcus cristatus, Streptococcus gordonii, Streptococcus intermedius, Streptococcus milleri* group, *Streptococcus mitis, Streptococcus mutans, Streptococcus oralis, Streptococcus parasanguinis, Streptococcus salivarius, Streptococcus sanguinis, Streptococcus thermophilus, Streptococcus vestibularis,* and viridans group streptococci.

97%), and for fungemia alone a sensitivity of 61% (95% CI, 48 to 72%) and specificity of 99% (95% CI, 99 to 99%). The authors concluded that SF is of high rule-in value for early detection of sepsis, and in populations with low pretest probability could be valuable for ruling out bacteremia and fungemia. They further noted, however, that there is no evidence that SF improved patient clinical outcomes and emphasized the suboptimal sensitivity of the SF assay. The authors reinforced the need to combine the SF results with patient biomarkers and clinical history to enhance diagnostic accuracy.

In one of the first phase III studies, Warhurst et al. (7) conducted a prospective multicenter study designed to detail the accuracy of SF versus blood cultures that focused on health care-associated bloodstream infections (BSIs). There were 1,006 episodes of BSI in 853 patients, of which 795 met criteria of a new episode of suspected BSI. The mean hospital length of stay (LOS) was 8 days (range 4 to 16) and the blood culture positivity rate was 9.2%. The sensitivity of SF was 50% (95% CI, 39 to 61%) and the specificity was 86% (95%, CI 83 to 86%). The posttest probability for a positive and negative result was 26.3% and 5.6%, respectively, and the authors concluded that the SF was of limited utility in this patient population, despite the more rapid turnaround time relative to blood culture.

In contrast, Markota et al. (8) found value in the test in a single-site study comparing SF with blood culture. Of 63 sample sets (57 patients), they detected 51 (89%) concordant negatives and 7 (11.1%) concordant positive results. Discrepancies included one blood culture positive with negative SF results, and three SF positives with negative blood cultures. The overall sensitivity in their study was 87.5% with a specificity of 92.6%. The time to final identification was 32 ± 23 h for SF compared with 97 ± 28 h for blood culture. Antimicrobial therapy was modified in four patients with the rapid SF results. While the number of positive samples was low in this single-site study, the ability to impact patient therapy was a significant finding.

Finally, Dark et al. (9) performed a systematic review and meta-analysis of diagnostic accuracy studies of SF versus blood cultures in the setting of suspected sepsis. Data were analyzed from 41 phase III diagnostic studies, with a total of 10,493 SF assays. Methodologic assessment was performed using the QUADAS tool (6). Analysis indicated that the overall study quality was variable with deficiencies that included representative sample size, selection criteria for inclusion, disease progression avoided, reference test applied equally, index test described sufficiently, reference standard described sufficiently, reference test blinded, index test blinded, uninterpretable results tests reported, discrepant analysis applied, and withdrawals explained. Despite these limitations, the following were calculated: the overall sensitivity was 68% (95% CI, 63 to 73%), and the overall specificity was 86% (95% CI, 84 to 89%). They conclude that it is difficult to make a firm recommendation of the use of SF in the setting of suspected sepsis. Note that although meta-analysis evaluation of data is useful, it is critical to remember that pooling data results in the heterogeneity of results because of a number of uncontrolled variables including the variety of sample types, clinical settings, patient populations, and study designs.

SepsiTest

Another system is the SepsiTest (ST) from Molzym (Bremen, Germany), which is commercially available (CE-IVD, non-FDA cleared) for direct identification of organisms in blood. ST uses broad-range PCR reactions that target the 16S and 18S rRNA genes with subsequent identification of positives by DNA sequence analysis. The assay requires 1 ml of whole blood (with an adaptive 10-ml modification). Human DNA is selectively degraded before isolation of microbial DNA. The sample is centrifuged and treated with reagents to hydrolyze the cell walls of bacteria and fungi.

Resulting DNA is then bound, washed, and eluted into 100-μl aliquots. PCR is performed with subsequent gel electrophoresis resolution, generating a positive or negative result within ~4 h. Positive samples are then subjected to DNA sequencing and data interpretation via an online BLAST tool (SepsiTest BLAST) to identify the microorganisms, which can detect >345 bacterial and fungal pathogens. Potential PCR inhibition in patient specimens, leading to false-negative results, is evaluated using an internal control. Limited evaluation is available at the time of this writing. Please see the package insert for additional information (http://www .goffinmoleculartechnologies.com/wp-content/uploads/2014/01/SepsiTest_ V3-0_IVD_CE.pdf, accessed December 26, 2016).

In a multicenter study by Nieman et al. (10), the authors evaluated the ST relative to blood culture with 236 samples from 166 patients with suspected sepsis. Results showed that, among 36 clinically relevant results, 11 bloodstream infections were detected by both ST and blood culture, while ST alone detected 15 and blood culture alone detected 10. The overall sensitivity and specificity for the assay were 66.7% and 94.4%, respectively. The authors noted that the added detection of organisms by ST could augment blood culture results. The authors commented that from a technical perspective, performance of ST in the clinical laboratory would be improved with automation and additional improvements to test methodology (e.g., melt curve analysis instead of gel electrophoresis for product detection).

In another report, Wellinghausen et al. (11) performed a prospective, multicenter study with 342 blood samples from 187 patients with ST compared with blood cultures. Thirty-four positive blood culture patients were detected. The diagnostic sensitivity and specificity of ST were 87.0% and 85.8%, respectively. Thirty-one patients were ST positive but negative by blood cultures, of which 25 were deemed as possibly or probably clinically significant. Six patients were blood culture positive, but ST negative. The authors concluded that ST can serve as an adjunctive to blood cultures, and recommended additional studies to assess the impact on patient outcome and costs.

VYOO Assay

Another CE-IVD, non-FDA-cleared system is the VYOO assay from Analytikjena (Jena, Germany), which is a multiplex PCR assay with microarray analysis to detect the most commonly isolated organisms in sepsis. Up to 5 ml of blood is used in the assay. The VYOO system utilizes a proprietary cell lysis method and automated sample preparation on magnetic beads to isolate and enrich for microbial DNA. Multiplex PCR plus micro-array analysis is then performed with an automated readout of results. An internal control is included with specimens to detect inhibition of PCR amplification. The assay includes 34 bacteria, seven fungi, and five antibiotic resistance mechanisms, as listed in Table 2. Limited studies are reported on utilization of VYOO.

Bloos et al. (12) evaluated the VYOO system compared with blood culture in critically ill patients with evidence of infection. They included patients either with severe sepsis (sepsis group) or systemic inflammatory response syndrome without evidence of infection (control group). Thirty-six samples were collected from septic patients (n = 24), and 32 samples were collected from control patients (n = 22) for blood culture and VYOO analysis. In the control group, the VYOO results were negative, whereas five blood cultures (15.6%) were positive. In the sepsis group, five blood cultures (13.4%) were positive, while 14 VYOO results (38.9%) were positive. While no clinical data are given to assess the significance of these data, positive PCR results were associated with higher serum procalcitonin levels. Note that since this study, significant steps in automation are now part of the VYOO system.

In another study by Schreiber et al. (13), the authors compared three commercial PCR assays for the detection of pathogens in critically ill sepsis patients. This single-center study compared blood cultures to ST (Molzym, Bremen, Germany), VYOO (Analytikjena, Jena, Germany), and SF (Roche, Mannheim, Germany). Fifty patients were included: 36 (72%) were pre-treated with antibiotics, and blood cultures were positive in 13 cases (26%), of which eight (16%) were deemed clinically significant. Two of the eight were detected in all three systems. In 32 cases (64%) there were concordant negative results. The detection rate for all three molecular-based assays was less than that of blood cultures. ST detected organisms in six specimens (12%), of which three were also detected in blood cultures. Of the five remaining positive blood cultures deemed clinically significant, five had negative ST results, but two negative cultures were positive by the ST assay with clinically significant organisms. VYOO detected pathogens in five cases (10%), of which two were also detected in culture. For five positive blood cultures deemed clinically significant, the VYOO was negative, but two VYOO-positive results were deemed clinically significant in the absence of a positive blood culture. SF identified eight organisms in seven speci-mens, but only matched three clinically significant blood culture results. Two clinically significant organisms were only detected in the SF system but failed to grow in blood cultures. While these numbers are low, a consistent trend indicates the need for culture, with the molecular assays as an add-on test. All systems suffer from the low volume of blood tested in the molecular-based assays, and the study has a major limitation of low specimen numbers tested.

IRIDICA BAC BSI Assay

The IRIDICA BAC BSI assay (IRIDICA) from Abbott Molecular (Des Plaines, IL) is a CE-IVD, non-FDA-cleared test for direct pathogen detection from blood specimens. The system uses an innovative new technology that combines PCR with electrospray ionization mass spectrometry (ESI-MS) to identify a variety of bacteria, fungi, viruses, and antimicrobial resistance markers directly from clinical specimens, including blood. Specifically, the system can detect 780 bacteria, *Candida* spp., and four antibiotic resistance markers (*mecA*, *vanA*, *vanB*, *bla*$_{KPC}$), as well as 200+ fungi and 13 viral reporting groups. The IRIDICA system contains several automated units to process up to 5 ml of whole blood from cell lysis by bead beating, to nucleic acid extraction, amplification, and purification, and finally ESI-MS analysis and data interpretation.

In a single-center study by Bacconi et al. (14), the authors evaluated IRIDICA and blood cultures in 331 specimens from patients suspected of BSI. Limit of detection (LOD) studies were performed by inoculating blood with known microbial concentrations, indicating that the LOD ranged from 16 CFU/ml to 4 CFU/ml for the bacterial and yeast pathogens tested. Thirty-five specimens (10.6%) were positive by IRIDICA, while there were only 18 (5.4%) positive blood cultures. Compared with culture, the sensitivity and specificity of IRIDICA were 83% and 94%, respectively. Additionally, the authors used replicate IRIDICA testing as a comparator for identifying true-positive results in IRIDICA-positive but blood culture-negative specimens. Based on these results, they reported a sensitivity and specificity of 91% and 99%, respectively.

In another single-center study, Jordana-Lluch et al. (15) evaluated the IRIDICA system for direct diagnosis from 410 whole-blood specimens. When compared with blood culture results, the positive and negative percent agreement for the IRIDICA system was 74.8% and 78.6%, respectively. Taking clinical information into account, the positive and negative agreement increased to 76.9% and 87.2%, respectively. IRIDICA detected 80 organisms that did not grow in culture: 41 (51.2%) were deemed clinically significant; seven (8.9%) were not supported as significant by clinical parameters; and 32 (40%) were considered to be contaminants (i.e., skin and environmental organisms).

T2Candida Panel

The T2Candida Panel (T2C) from T2 Biosystems (Lexington, MA) is a CE-IVD, FDA-cleared assay that uses T2 magnetic resonance (T2MR)-based technology to detect five *Candida* spp. directly from ~3 ml of whole blood. T2MR technology has been used to detect other analytes beside *Candida* spp., including cells, proteins, and hemostasis markers, with all these targets detected directly from patient specimens (16). *Candida* spp. detection occurs via supraparamagnetic particles that are attached to DNA probes, which when bound to a target, cluster, and change the T2MR signal, resulting in target detection.

The T2C is run on the T2DxInstrument, which is a random access analyzer with six modules and requires minimal hands-on time (<5 min) for specimen loading. Once a specimen is loaded on the T2DxInstrument, the instrument performs all processing and analysis steps. First, the host cells are lysed by detergent, and any yeast cells present along with cell debris are concentrated by centrifugation. Yeast cells are then lysed by bead beating, releasing DNA for PCR amplification of the *intervening transcribed space 2* (*ITS2*) region of the ribosomal DNA operon, of which there are 50 to 100 copies per genome. Amplified products are then detected using T2MR, and then the specimen is decontaminated with bleach. Total run time on the T2DxInstrument is between 3 and 5 h. A synthetic DNA marker serves as an internal control for each processed specimen. The *Candida* spp. detected by the T2C assay are listed in Table 2. Results are reported as negative or positive for *Candida albicans*/*Candida tropicalis*, *Candida glabrata*/*Candida krusei*, and/or *Candida parapsilosis*.

Based on controlled spiked sample testing, the LOD of the T2C assay is 3 CFU/ml for *C. albicans* and *C. tropicalis*, 2 CFU/ml for *C. krusei* and *C. glabrata*, and 1 CFU/ml for *C. parapsilosis* (17). Two separate studies evaluated the T2C assay relative to seeded BACTEC (Becton Dickinson and Company, Franklin Lakes, NJ) blood culture bottles (17, 18). In the study by Beyda et al. (18), growth occurred in all seeded bottles by 5 days, except that all *C. glabrata*-inoculated bottles (n = 20) failed to flag positive, but terminal subcultures showed that all contained viable *C. glabrata* cells. The T2C assay demonstrated a 100% detection rate for all seeded cultures (n = 91), reported all negative control bottles (n = 10) as negative, but did call out four false-positive results from the seeded blood cultures. In a second study using seeded blood culture bottles, the T2C assay demonstrated a 98% positive agreement (88/90) and 100% negative agreement (n = 43) with conventional cultures (17).

In the multicenter study by Mylonakis et al. (19), a total of 1,801 patient specimens were tested, of which 1,501 had concurrent blood cultures (i.e., prospective arm of the study), 50 specimens were collected as negative controls, and 250 separate specimens were spiked with *Candida* spp. at a range of clinically relevant concentrations (<1 to 100 CFU/ml). The last group served as a contrived control to increase the number of *Candida* spp.- positive specimens, because of the small number of *Candida* spp.-positive blood cultures (n = 6) in the prospective arm. Within the contrived arm, T2C detected *Candida* spp. in 70% (n = 35) of the specimens inoculated with <1 CFU/ml. Of the six culture-positive specimens, two were negative by the T2C assay, with both cultures positive for *C. albicans*. The overall sensitivity and specificity for all specimens tested were 91.1% (95% CI, 86.9 to 94.2%) and 99.4% (95% CI, 99.1 to 99.6%), respectively.

Summary

The assays highlighted in the chapter represent the forefront of rapid diagnostics for sepsis management, but methodologies for detecting infection directly from blood specimens are still an area of diagnostics in its infancy. Compared with traditional blood culture results, the specificity of these tests remains relatively high (>85%), but the sensitivity is more varied (50 to 91%). In addition, the clinical significance of blood-culture-negative but molecular-test-positive specimens is an area in need of additional investigation. Similar to the conundrum of blood cultures positive with skin contaminants, the results from molecular tests will need to be analyzed in the appropriate clinical context.

Despite the advancements offered by these direct-from-blood assays, there remain several important issues that laboratorians and clinicians need to consider with such testing. Importantly, such testing in its current and near-future iterations can be a supplement but not a substitute for traditional blood-culturing methods. Importantly, the targeted direct methods (e.g., SeptiFast, VYOO, and T2Candida) only identify pathogens for which they are designed to detect, thus missing all off-panel targets and/or genetic variants of target organisms. Cultured isolates are still needed to provide antimicrobial susceptibility results, and for epidemiologic studies of public health importance. The supplemental use of such tests is complicated in the pediatric population, because the available blood volume for testing can be severely limited in neonates and small children.

From a laboratory workflow standpoint, the complexity of performing direct-from-blood testing is an important factor to consider. It is important to note that the turnaround times noted in Table 1 likely represent average to minimal times, and may not always reflect real-world results. The SeptiFast and SepsiTest require more hands-on time relative to sample-to-answer system (e.g., T2Candida assay). The most efficient performance of such laborious tests would be batch testing, which in part negates the advantages of quicker turnaround times relative to blood cultures. Finally, these molecular methods come at an increased cost to laboratories and hospital systems. In the ever increasingly cost-conscious environment of medicine, studies are needed to justify the effectiveness of such methods from an economic and health outcomes perspective. Such data may indicate specific patient populations that would benefit most from such testing and provide support for purchasing and performing these assays.

References
1. Buehler SS, Madison B, Snyder SR, Derzon JH, Cornish NE, Saubolle MA, Weissfeld AS, Weinstein MP, Liebow EB, Wolk DM. 2016. Effectiveness of practices to increase timeliness of providing targeted therapy for inpatients with bloodstream infections: a laboratory medicine best practices systematic review and meta-analysis. *Clin Microbiol Rev* 29:59–103.
2. Hall MM, Ilstrup DM, Washington JA II. 1976. Effect of volume of blood cultured on detection of bacteremia. *J Clin Microbiol* 3:643–645.
3. Tenney JH, Reller LB, Mirrett S, Wang WL, Weinstein MP. 1982. Controlled evaluation of the volume of blood cultured in detection of bacteremia and fungemia. *J Clin Microbiol* 15:558–561.
4. Kaditis AG, O'Marcaigh AS, Rhodes KH, Weaver AL, Henry NK. 1996. Yield of positive blood cultures in pediatric oncology patients by a new method of blood culture collection. *Pediatr Infect Dis J* 15:615–620.
5. Chang SS, Hsieh WH, Liu TS, Lee SH, Wang CH, Chou HC, Yeo YH, Tseng CP, Lee CC. 2013. Multiplex PCR system for rapid detection of pathogens in patients with presumed sepsis - a systemic review and meta-analysis. *PLoS One* 8:e62323.
6. Whiting P, Rutjes AW, Reitsma JB, Bossuyt PM, Kleijnen J. 2003. The development of QUADAS: a tool for the quality assessment of studies of diagnostic accuracy included in systematic reviews. *BMC Med Res Methodol* 3:25.
7. Warhurst G, Maddi S, Dunn G, Ghrew M, Chadwick P, Alexander P, Bentley A, Moore J, Sharman M, Carlson GL, Young D, Dark P. 2015. Diagnostic accuracy of SeptiFast multi-pathogen real-time PCR in the setting of suspected healthcare-associated bloodstream infection. *Intensive Care Med* 41:86–93.

8. Markota A, Seme K, Golle A, Poljak M, Sinkovič A. 2014. SeptiFast real-time PCR for detection of bloodborne pathogens in patients with severe sepsis or septic shock. *Coll Antropol* 38:829–833.

9. Dark P, Blackwood B, Gates S, McAuley D, Perkins GD, McMullan R, Wilson C, Graham D, Timms K, Warhurst G. 2015. Accuracy of LightCycler(®) SeptiFast for the detection and identification of pathogens in the blood of patients with suspected sepsis: a systematic review and meta-analysis. *Intensive Care Med* 41:21–33.

10. Nieman AE, Savelkoul PH, Beishuizen A, Henrich B, Lamik B, MacKenzie CR, Kindgen-Milles D, Helmers A, Diaz C, Sakka SG, Schade RP. 2016. A prospective multicenter evaluation of direct molecular detection of blood stream infection from a clinical perspective. *BMC Infect Dis* 16:314.

11. Wellinghausen N, Kochem AJ, Disqué C, Mühl H, Gebert S, Winter J, Matten J, Sakka SG. 2009. Diagnosis of bacteremia in whole-blood samples by use of a commercial universal 16S rRNA gene-based PCR and sequence analysis. *J Clin Microbiol* 47:2759–2765.

12. Bloos F, Sachse S, Schmidt K-H, Lehmann M, Schmitz R, Russwurm S, Straube E, Reinhart K. 2008. Nucleic acid amplification-based pathogen detection in the blood of severe sepsis patients. *Critical Care* 12(Suppl 5):P43.

13. Schreiber J, Nierhaus A, Braune SA, de Heer G, Kluge S. 2013. Comparison of three different commercial PCR assays for the detection of pathogens in critically ill sepsis patients. *Med Klin Intensivmed Notf Med* 108:311–318.

14. Bacconi A, Richmond GS, Baroldi MA, Laffler TG, Blyn LB, Carolan HE, Frinder MR, Toleno DM, Metzgar D, Gutierrez JR, Massire C, Rounds M, Kennel NJ, Rothman RE, Peterson S, Carroll KC, Wakefield T, Ecker DJ, Sampath R. 2014. Improved sensitivity for molecular detection of bacterial and *Candida* infections in blood. *J Clin Microbiol* 52:3164–3174.

15. Jordana-Lluch E, Giménez M, Quesada MD, Rivaya B, Marcó C, Domínguez MJ, Arméstar F, Martró E, Ausina V. 2015. Evaluation of the broad-range PCR/ESI-MS technology in blood specimens for the molecular diagnosis of bloodstream infections. *PLoS One* 10:e0140865.

16. Pfaller MA, Wolk DM, Lowery TJ. 2016. T2MR and T2Candida: novel technology for the rapid diagnosis of candidemia and invasive candidiasis. *Future Microbiol* 11:103–117.

17. Neely LA, Audeh M, Phung NA, Min M, Suchocki A, Plourde D, Blanco M, Demas V, Skewis LR, Anagnostou T, Coleman JJ, Wellman P, Mylonakis E, Lowery TJ. 2013. T2 magnetic resonance enables nanoparticle-mediated rapid detection of candidemia in whole blood. *Sci Transl Med* 5:182ra54.

18. Beyda ND, Alam MJ, Garey KW. 2013. Comparison of the T2Dx instrument with T2Candida assay and automated blood culture in the detection of *Candida* species using seeded blood samples. *Diagn Microbiol Infect Dis* 77:324–326.

19. Mylonakis E, Clancy CJ, Ostrosky-Zeichner L, Garey KW, Alangaden GJ, Vazquez JA, Groeger JS, Judson MA, Vinagre YM, Heard SO, Zervou FN, Zacharioudakis IM, Kontoyiannis DP, Pappas PG. 2015. T2 magnetic resonance assay for the rapid diagnosis of candidemia in whole blood: a clinical trial. *Clin Infect Dis* 60:892–899.

The Dark Art of Blood Cultures
Edited by Wm. Michael Dunne, Jr. and Carey-Ann D. Burnham
© 2018 American Society for Microbiology, Washington, DC
doi:10.1128/9781555819811.ch8

Pediatric Blood Cultures

8

Paula Revell[1] and Christopher Doern[2]

Introduction

In pediatrics as in adult medicine, the clinical microbiology laboratory plays an integral role in providing accurate and timely data to aid in the diagnosis, treatment, and monitoring of various infectious diseases. Because of the associated morbidity and mortality with bloodstream infection (BSI), blood cultures are among the most critical diagnostic tests in pediatric laboratory medicine. Despite the critical nature of the pediatric blood culture, there remains a great deal of myth and misunderstanding surrounding these cultures. The unique challenges associated with pediatric blood cultures include the wide range of patient blood volumes making one standard recommended culture volume impossible, an ever evolving epidemiology of sepsis due in large part to the availability of various vaccines, and a diverse range of clinical presentations due to the dynamic patient population, ranging from neonates through the late teenage years. This chapter focuses on these uniquely pediatric challenges.

Epidemiology of Pediatric Bacteremia

The epidemiology of bacteremia in pediatrics is ever evolving and varies significantly by patient population. Factors that influence the epidemiology include, but are not limited to, patient age, corrected gestational age, birth weight, vaccination status, immune status, and presence or absence of an indwelling venous access line. The first several months of life are a high-risk

[1]Departments of Pathology and Pediatrics, Baylor College of Medicine, Houston, TX 77030
[2]Department of Pathology, Virginia Commonwealth University Health System, Richmond, VA 23298

period for sepsis for all newborns. As such, neonatal sepsis is an important focus of pediatric blood culture diagnosis. Neonatal sepsis can be divided into three defined age ranges, and the etiologic agents vary between these groups. Early-onset sepsis (EOS) occurs from birth to day 6 of life; late-onset sepsis (LOS) occurs from 7 to 30 days of life, and late, late-onset sepsis (LLOS) occurs from 30 days of life to 3 months.

The epidemiology of pediatric BSI has changed dramatically over the past several decades. In the 1970s, *Streptococcus agalactiae* was the primary cause of EOS in the United States, with case fatality rates as high as 50%. Maternal colonization with *S. agalactiae* was shown to be the primary risk factor. The epidemiology of EOS began to change with the recommendation for universal screening of all pregnant women at 35 to 37 weeks of gestation (1). Prior to the introduction of the *Haemophilus influenzae* type b (Hib) vaccines, one in 200 children less than 5 years of age experienced invasive Hib disease, and, as such, Hib was a leading cause of pediatric BSI. Greater than 60% of cases occurred in patients less than 15 months of age (2). Following the introduction of the Hib conjugate vaccine, the epidemiology of pediatric BSI shifted enormously with the dramatic reduction and near-elimination of Hib disease. After the implementation of the Hib vaccine, the next early childhood vaccine to significantly alter the epidemiology of pediatric BSI was the pneumococcal conjugate vaccine (PCV). In the post-Hib and -PCV era the agents associated with pediatric BSI vary directly based on the age of sepsis onset and the preexisting conditions of the patient.

Several studies have shown that, in previously healthy infants, the overall rate of BSI has decreased and the associated microorganisms have changed as well (3, 4). Mischler et al. demonstrated in a multicenter retrospective review of previously well, febrile infants ≤90 days old in the United States, that *Escherichia coli* was the primary bacterial pathogen isolated, followed by *S. agalactiae* (5). A retrospective analysis of 4,255 blood cultures from previously well, febrile patients ≤90 days old in a single geographical region of the United States showed similar findings, with *E. coli* being the most common pathogen isolated followed by *S. agalactiae* and *Staphylococcus aureus* (6, 7).

The focus of the above-mentioned studies was the febrile, previously healthy, term infant, but the epidemiology of sepsis in neonates cared for in the intensive care unit setting has been shown to be quite different. Two reports published from the longest-running, single-center database of neonatal sepsis show a striking increase in BSIs caused by commensal organisms, namely coagulase-negative *Staphylococcus* (CoNS). Of 755 episodes of sepsis,

29% were caused by CoNS, followed by *E. coli* (12%), *S. agalactiae* (10%), and *S. aureus* (8%) (8).

In the post-Hib and -PCV era, the rate of BSI in children older than 90 days is quite low, and, in many clinical scenarios, a positive blood culture is more likely to represent a contaminant than a true pathogen. In the cases where a pathogen is isolated, the leading etiologies are different from the epidemiology of infant BSIs, with *Streptococcus pneumoniae* and *S. aureus* being the primary pathogens isolated (9, 10).

The changing epidemiology not only impacts empiric therapy for patients but also affects the diagnostic sensitivity of the blood culture itself. Historically, there has been a long-held belief that the concentration of bacteria in the blood is typically higher in pediatric patients than in adult patients (11). This concept was likely due in part to the common pathogens isolated in the prevaccination era. Unfortunately, despite many studies that have shown this not to be the case in the majority of cases of pediatric BSI, this myth is perhaps the most widely held misconception surrounding pediatric blood cultures.

Specimen Collection

There are many factors that influence the practice of blood culture collection. However, in pediatrics as in adults one truth is constant: the amount of blood cultured is the primary factor influencing the sensitivity of detection (12, 13). Culturing larger volumes of blood increases the sensitivity of pathogen detection and also decreases the time to detection (14). Despite the misconception that children have higher concentrations of bacteria in the bloodstream compared with adults, several studies have definitively demonstrated that pediatric patients often have low-level bacteremia (≤10 colony-forming units of bacteria per milliliter of blood). Kellogg et al. showed that, in infants from birth to 2 months of age, in the post-Hib and -PCV era, nearly two-thirds of patients from whom a pathogen was recovered had low-level bacteremia (12). In a subsequent study, Kellogg et al. showed similar frequency of low-level bacteremia in patients up to 15 years of age (13).

In addition to the improved sensitivity of pathogen detection achieved through increased volume of blood cultured, the specificity of the positive blood culture is also influenced by the volume of blood submitted. Studies have shown an inverse correlation between the volume of blood drawn and the likelihood of isolating a contaminant. In other words, not only is a blood culture more likely to be positive if more blood volume is cultured, but also a positive culture is more likely to be a true pathogen (15, 16).

Contaminated blood cultures can confound diagnosis and lead to unnecessary hospitalization and antimicrobial therapy. The most commonly
isolated contaminants are components of skin flora such as CoNS, viridans
group streptococci, and coryneform bacteria. In order to decrease the likelihood of contamination, not only should adequate blood volume be drawn,
but appropriate skin antisepsis must also be performed. In pediatrics, as in
adults, chlorhexidine gluconate has been shown to be superior to povidone-
iodine in reducing central line-associated bloodstream infections and in
decreasing blood culture contamination rates (17). Importantly, however,
chlorhexidine is not used in children less than 2 months of age because
of possible associated safety risks, and alcohol should be used in this age
group.

Given the fact that blood volume obtained correlates with the sensitivity
and specificity of pathogen detection, the question remains, what is an
"adequate" volume of blood to detect pediatric bacteremia? Unlike in adults,
no one volume can be recommended because of the range of blood volumes
in pediatric patients. Two primary approaches have been used to guide
appropriate practice in terms of drawing adequate blood volumes, weight-
and age-based guidelines (Fig. 1). Both of these approaches address the issue
that, as a child grows, the volume of blood that can be safely drawn increases
as well.

OPTIMAL BLOOD CULTURE VOLUME

Volume by Patient's Weight

Weight in Kilograms (kg)	Total Recommended Volume (ml) over 24 hrs	Total Volume per Bottle (ml)	Total # of Bottles
≤ 3	2	2	1
> 3-5	3	3	1
> 5-7	5	5	1
> 7-12	10	5	2
> 12-20	15	5	3
> 20-30	30	10	3
> 30-45	40	10	4
> 45	60	10	6

Volume by Patient's Age

Age (years)	Total Volume per Bottle (ml)
< 1	1-3*
1-4	3-4*
5-9	6-8*
≥10	10**

*Include anaerobic bottle for at-risk patients.
**Include anaerobic bottle for all patients.

Write the volume of blood on each bottle!

Figure 1 Examples of weight- and age-based blood volume recommendations for pediatric
blood cultures.

When adequate blood volume is cultured, the time it takes for the culture to flag as positive is influenced by the nature of the organism and whether or not the culture contains a pathogen or contaminant. Studies have shown that, in patients with or without indwelling central venous catheters, blood cultures containing significant pathogens take less time to become positive than blood cultures containing contaminants. A study of 10,200 blood cultures obtained at a large tertiary care pediatric hospital showed that the mean time to positivity for cultures of true pathogens was 18.41 h compared to 32.77 h for cultures that grew contaminants (18). Gram-negative organisms on average take less time to signal positive than Gram-positive organisms, and nearly all true pathogens are detected within 36 h of incubation.

Yet another myth surrounding pediatric blood cultures is one that is shared with adults, i.e., the concept that drawing a blood culture as near as possible to the onset of fever will optimize pathogen detection. This assumption has been shown to be untrue. In a large multicenter study in the United States, nearly 1,500 patient charts were retrospectively reviewed to assess whether the timing of culture draw with onset of fever optimized pathogen detection. This adult study concluded that there was no association between fever and the likelihood of a culture being positive, and recommended that specimens be collected based on convenience and the likelihood of obtaining maximum volume using aseptic technique rather than association with fever (19). In a smaller study of exclusively pediatric patients, the authors drew the same conclusion, that the timing of blood culture collection in relation to fever is not important (20).

Blood Culture Media
Media Options
The current state of diagnosing bacterial BSI includes the incubation of blood on a continuously monitored blood culture system. Some manufacturers of these systems provide both high-volume (up to 10 ml of blood) bottles as well as low-volume (up to 3 to 4 ml of blood), or as some manufacturers designate, the pediatric bottles. As discussed in the specimen collection section, it is often difficult to obtain high volumes of blood from children; low-volume bottles are designed to accommodate these lower blood volumes. The rationale for these bottles is based on the dilution of the blood culture medium that occurs when blood volume is added to the bottle. In theory, low blood volume added to bottles designed to accommodate up to 10 ml of blood may lead to a suboptimal concentration of certain reagents. The low-volume bottles are adjusted accordingly and claim to be optimized

for the lower volumes typically drawn from children. In addition, many believe that these bottles optimize time to detection for low blood volume cultures.

While studies have shown that these low-volume blood culture bottles perform with high sensitivity (21), few studies have compared their performance directly with that of high-volume blood cultures. As a result, it is unclear whether the low-volume blood culture bottles are really necessary to optimize organism recovery from pediatric patients. A popular argument against the use of low-volume blood culture bottles is that you "can't drown bacteria," meaning that organisms will readily grow, regardless of the volume of blood culture medium. However, a counterargument would submit that the low-volume blood culture bottles are superior in media types that contain sodium polyanetholesulfonate (SPS, a commonly used anticoagulant supplement) because the bottles contain a lower concentration of this agent. SPS is well known to inhibit the isolation of some organisms if present at elevated concentrations. Examples include *Neisseria gonorrhoeae, Neisseria meningitidis*, anaerobic cocci, and *Streptobacillus* (22–24). However, most commonly isolated organisms are not affected by SPS, even at high concentrations (25). In addition, while SPS is present in most (but not all) currently manufactured blood culture systems, no studies have been performed to confirm the initial findings referenced above regarding the effects of SPS on organism growth. As a result, it is unclear whether the higher SPS concentrations present in the high-volume blood culture bottles would result in suboptimal recovery of some organisms.

Antibiotic Absorbing Substances

Many contemporary blood culture bottles contain reagents or substances that are designed to absorb antibiotics present in the specimens of patients receiving therapy. By absorbing and inactivating the antibiotics, the likelihood of a falsely negative blood culture result is reduced. There are limited data demonstrating the efficacy of these bottles to improve yield in pediatric patients receiving antibiotic therapy. However, one pediatric-focused study compared the yield of a charcoal-containing medium with a resin-containing medium and found that the resin medium identified significantly more pathogens from patients receiving antimicrobial therapy (21).

Anaerobic Blood Culture Media

In children, it is often not safe to draw the same volume of blood required to optimize blood culture sensitivity in adult patients. This reality necessitates that the limited blood volume be used as judiciously as possible and has led practitioners to question whether anaerobic blood culture media are warranted in all cases. As was discussed above, the majority of pediatric BSI is caused by aerobically growing organisms that are readily isolated from aerobic blood culture media. In addition, some organisms, such as *Pseudomonas aeruginosa* and *Candida* spp. are obligate aerobes and are almost never isolated from anaerobic blood culture media (26). However, some facultative anaerobes, such as *S. pneumoniae*, may be isolated preferentially from anaerobic blood culture media. So the question, ultimately, is which strategy (all blood into aerobic bottles or blood divided between aerobic and anaerobic bottles) will yield the greatest number of positives. A study by Dunne et al. attempted to answer this question in a multicenter trial that compared the yield of these strategies and found that the aerobic bottle-only strategy detected more episodes of bacteremia than the aerobic/anaerobic bottle strategy (27). While an aerobic bottle-only strategy may lead to higher yield in some patient populations (i.e., otherwise healthy children), the fact that some facultative anaerobes, such as *S. pneumoniac, S. aureus*, and the *Enterobacteriaceae*, are occasionally isolated only in anaerobic media should be considered. In addition, some patient populations are at greater risk for anaerobic bacteremia and may benefit from inclusion of an anaerobic bottle. Patients at risk for anaerobic bacteremia include those with abdominal signs and symptoms, patients with sacral decubitus ulcers, neutropenic patients, patients with bacteremia following human bite wounds, and patients who have experienced crush trauma, to name a few examples (28). In the final analysis, it should be appreciated that, in children, true anaerobic bacteremia is exceedingly rare and probably represents less than 1% of all bloodstream infections (28). However, there are few data conclusively showing that it is or is not appropriate to eliminate anaerobic blood cultures.

As such, no recommendation can be made as to whether or not an anaerobic bottle should be added to routine blood culture collection in pediatrics. However, if the volume of blood drawn is limited (e.g., less than or equal to 1 ml), the recommendation is to inoculate the entire volume into an aerobic bottle.

Fungal Blood Cultures

Fungal blood cultures are typically performed by collecting blood specimens in a tube (i.e., Wampole Isolator Tubes) that facilitates the direct plating of specimen onto fungal media. These tubes are available in 10-ml and 1.5-ml volumes and contain anticoagulants such as SPS, as well as reagents that lyse red and white blood cells. If the 10-ml tube is used, a centrifugation step is included in the processing to concentrate the specimen. Following centrifugation, the supernatant is withdrawn and discarded, leaving the microbial concentrate to be pipetted onto agar plates. If the 1.5-ml tube is used, there is no centrifugation, and the specimen is simply plated directly onto the fungal agar plates.

The advantage of this culture method is that it permits the direct plating of blood onto fungal media, in lieu of inoculating blood into bottles for continuously monitored blood culture systems that are not optimized for the isolation of filamentous fungi. The disadvantage of this system is that it is prone to contamination because of the increased handling required to process the cultures.

An important consideration when ordering fungal blood cultures is the relative risk for a given patient population for developing disseminated fungal infection. Filamentous fungal bloodstream infection is very rare in pediatric patients, even in at-risk patients, such as those with hematologic malignancies, or other immunocompromised states. A recent 10-year, multicenter review of 9,442 pediatric fungal blood cultures identified only nine clinically significant episodes of filamentous or dimorphic fungal bloodstream infection (29). Importantly, the majority of molds isolated from blood cultures over this time were considered to be contaminants. The nine true infections identified in this study were caused by *Histoplasma capsulatum*, *Coccidioides immitis/posadasii*, *Fusarium oxysporum*, *Aspergillus* spp., and *Bipolaris* spp.

Last, fungal blood cultures are capable of isolating yeast in candidemic patients. However, *Candida* spp. are readily identified by continuously monitored blood culture systems, and the manual fungal blood culture offers little advantage in diagnosing candidemia. Although most yeast will grow from a routine blood culture, an important exception is *Malassezia furfur*. This organism requires nutritional supplementation and can only be isolated from cultures in which sterile olive oil has been added to the fungal media. This supplement is not present in routine blood culture bottles, and *M. furfur* will not be isolated from routine cultures. Most clinical microbiology laboratories do not routinely supplement their fungal blood cultures with olive oil and require a specific request to do so. Considering that many physicians may not be aware of the unique growth requirements of *M. furfur*, ordering may be best facilitated by having a specific test order for the isolation of this organism. Patients at particular risk for *M. furfur* may be those receiving total parenteral nutrition (30).

Sterile Body Fluid Infections

In microbiology laboratories, it is relatively common practice to inject sterile body fluid (SBF) specimens directly into blood culture bottles, which are then incubated on continuously monitored blood culture systems. Some SBF specimens that may be injected into blood culture bottles include peritoneal dialysis fluid, ascites fluid from patients suspected of spontaneous bacterial peritonitis, prosthesis sonicate fluid, and joint fluid from patients suspected to have septic arthritis. The theoretical benefit of inoculating SBFs into blood culture bottles is that these bottles will increase the yield in low organism burden infections and that false-negative results in patients on antibiotic therapy will be reduced by the blood culture bottles. With the exception of joint fluid, these specimens are almost exclusively collected in adults; thus, the focus of this discussion will be on the utility of injecting joint fluid from children into blood culture bottles.

The epidemiology of septic arthritis in children varies significantly by age and patient population. Common pathogens isolated from the joint fluid of children include *S. aureus*, *S. pneumoniae*, *Streptococcus pyogenes*, *S. agalactiae*, *N. gonorrhoeae*, and *Kingella kingae* (31). *K. kingae* septic arthritis is almost exclusively a pediatric disease with most infections occurring in children <3 years of age (32). Blood culture medium is particularly important for isolating *K. kingae* from joint fluid specimens where it has been shown that solid medium fails to isolate the organism in a high percentage of cases (33). The reasons for this are not clear, but it is postulated that pus exerts an inhibitory effect on the organism and that growth is enhanced when the specimen is diluted in the blood culture bottle. This same principle may explain why other organisms, such as *S. aureus*, *Brucella melitensis*, and *S. pyogenes*, can occasionally be preferentially isolated from blood culture bottles (33).

Conclusion

It is clear that the practice of diagnosing bloodstream infections in children poses challenges not present in adults. The primary factor to be considered is the blood volume that can be drawn from the patient. There is good evidence that optimal blood culture yield is obtained when volume is maximized, but finding the balance between optimal yield and patient safety can be difficult, especially in young or undersized children. Unfortunately, we know that the blood culture practices used in young children are erroneously extrapolated to older children from whom optimal blood cultures can be safely drawn. Last, it is well documented that contamination rates are higher from pediatric, rather than adult, patients. This reality is complicated by the fact that many practitioners only draw a single blood culture, which makes interpreting the clinical significance of common contaminants very difficult. These issues, as well as those discussed above, should be addressed by bringing awareness to the health care providers through educational and feedback programs.

References

1. Verani JR, McGee L, Schrag SJ, Division of Bacterial Diseases, National Center for Immunization and Respiratory Diseases, Centers for Disease Control and Prevention (CDC). 2010. Prevention of perinatal group B streptococcal disease–revised guidelines from CDC, 2010. *MMWR Recomm Rep* **59**(RR-10):1–36.
2. Anonymous. 1991. Haemophilus b conjugate vaccines for prevention of *Haemophilus influenzae* type b disease among infants and children two months of age and older. Recommendations of the immunization practices advisory committee (ACIP). *MMWR Recomm Rep* **40**(RR-1):1–7.
3. Cantey JB, Farris AC, McCormick SM. 2016. Bacteremia in early infancy: etiology and management. *Curr Infect Dis Rep* **18**:1.
4. Biondi E, Evans R, Mischler M, Bendel-Stenzel M, Horstmann S, Lee V, Aldag J, Gigliotti F. 2013. Epidemiology of bacteremia in febrile infants in the United States. *Pediatrics* **132**:990–996.
5. Mischler M, Ryan MS, Leyenaar JK, Markowsky A, Seppa M, Wood K, Ren J, Asche C, Gigliotti F, Biondi E. 2015. Epidemiology of bacteremia in previously healthy febrile infants: a follow-up study. *Hosp Pediatr* **5**:293–300.
6. Greenhow TL, Hung YY, Herz AM. 2012. Changing epidemiology of bacteremia in infants aged 1 week to 3 months. *Pediatrics* **129**:e590–e596.
7. Greenhow TL, Hung YY, Herz AM, Losada E, Pantell RH. 2014. The changing epidemiology of serious bacterial infections in young infants. *Pediatr Infect Dis J* **33**:595–599.
8. Bizzarro MJ, Raskind C, Baltimore RS, Gallagher PG. 2005. Seventy-five years of neonatal sepsis at Yale: 1928-2003. *Pediatrics* **116**:595–602.
9. Gomez B, Hernandez-Bou S, Garcia-Garcia JJ, Mintegi S, Bacteraemia Study Working Group from the Infectious Diseases Working Group, Spanish Society of Pediatric Emergencies (SEUP). 2015. Bacteremia in previously healthy children in emergency departments: clinical and microbiological characteristics and outcome. *Eur J Clin Microbiol Infect Dis* **34**:453–460.
10. Sard B, Bailey MC, Vinci R. 2006. An analysis of pediatric blood cultures in the postpneumococcal conjugate vaccine era in a community hospital emergency department. *Pediatr Emerg Care* **22**:295–300.
11. Campos JM. 1989. Detection of bloodstream infections in children. *Eur J Clin Microbiol Infect Dis* **8**:815–824.
12. Kellogg JA, Ferrentino FL, Goodstein MH, Liss J, Shapiro SL, Bankert DA. 1997. Frequency of low level bacteremia in infants from birth to two months of age. *Pediatr Infect Dis J* **16**:381–385.
13. Kellogg JA, Manzella JP, Bankert DA. 2000. Frequency of low-level bacteremia in children from birth to fifteen years of age. *J Clin Microbiol* **38**:2181–2185.

14. Isaacman DJ, Karasic RB, Reynolds EA, Kost SI. 1996. Effect of number of blood cultures and volume of blood on detection of bacteremia in children. *J Pediatr* 128:190–195.

15. Connell TG, Rele M, Cowley D, Buttery JP, Curtis N. 2007. How reliable is a negative blood culture result? Volume of blood submitted for culture in routine practice in a children's hospital. *Pediatrics* 119:891–896.

16. Gonsalves WI, Cornish N, Moore M, Chen A, Varman M. 2009. Effects of volume and site of blood draw on blood culture results. *J Clin Microbiol* 47:3482–3485.

17. Marlowe L, Mistry RD, Coffin S, Leckerman KH, McGowan KL, Dai D, Bell LM, Zaoutis T. 2010. Blood culture contamination rates after skin antisepsis with chlorhexidine gluconate versus povidone-iodine in a pediatric emergency department. *Infect Control Hosp Epidemiol* 31:171–176.

18. McGowan KL, Foster JA, Coffin SE. 2000. Outpatient pediatric blood cultures: time to positivity. *Pediatrics* 106:251–255.

19. Riedel S, Bourbeau P, Swartz B, Brecher S, Carroll KC, Stamper PD, Dunne WM, McCardle T, Walk N, Fiebelkorn K, Sewell D, Richter SS, Beekmann S, Doern GV. 2008. Timing of specimen collection for blood cultures from febrile patients with bacteremia. *J Clin Microbiol* 46:1381–1385.

20. Kee PP, Chinnappan M, Nair A, Yeak D, Chen A, Starr M, Daley AJ, Cheng AC, Burgner D. 2016. Diagnostic yield of timing blood culture collection relative to fever. *Pediatr Infect Dis J* 35:846–850.

21. Doern CD, Mirrett S, Halstead D, Abid J, Okada P, Reller LB. 2014. Controlled clinical comparison of new pediatric medium with adsorbent polymeric beads (PF Plus) versus charcoal-containing PF medium in the BacT/alert blood culture system. *J Clin Microbiol* 52:1898–1900.

22. Staneck JL, Vincent S. 1981. Inhibition of *Neisseria gonorrhoeae* by sodium polyanetholesulfonate. *J Clin Microbiol* 13:463–467.

23. Rintala L, Pollock HM. 1978. Effects of two blood culture anticoagulants on growth of *Neisseria meningitidis*. *J Clin Microbiol* 7:332–336.

24. Wilkins TD, West SE. 1976. Medium-dependent inhibition of *Peptostreptococcus anaerobius* by sodium polyanetholsulfonate in blood culture media. *J Clin Microbiol* 3:393–396.

25. Rosner R. 1975. Comparison of recovery rates of various organisms from clinical hypertonic blood cultures by using various concentrations of sodium polyanethol sulfonate. *J Clin Microbiol* 1:129–131.

26. Freedman SB, Roosevelt GE. 2004. Utility of anaerobic blood cultures in a pediatric emergency department. *Pediatr Emerg Care* 20:433–436.

27. Dunne WM Jr, Tillman J, Havens PL. 1994. Assessing the need for anaerobic medium for the recovery of clinically significant blood culture isolates in children. *Pediatr Infect Dis J* 13:203–206.

28. Zaidi AK, Knaut AL, Mirrett S, Reller LB. 1995. Value of routine anaerobic blood cultures for pediatric patients. *J Pediatr* 127:263–268.

29. Campigotto A, Richardson SE, Sebert M, McElvania TeKippe E, Chakravarty A, Doern CD. 2016. Low utility of pediatric isolator blood culture system for detection of fungemia in children: a 10-year review. *J Clin Microbiol* 54:2284–2287.

30. Dankner WM, Spector SA, Fierer J, Davis CE. 1987. *Malassezia* fungemia in neonates and adults: complication of hyperalimentation. *Rev Infect Dis* 9:743–753.

31. **Carter K, Doern C, Jo CH, Copley LA.** 2016. The clinical usefulness of polymerase chain reaction as a supplemental diagnostic tool in the evaluation and the treatment of children with septic arthritis. *J Pediatr Orthop* **36:**167–172.
32. **Yagupsky P.** 2004. *Kingella kingae*: from medical rarity to an emerging paediatric pathogen. *Lancet Infect Dis* **4:**358–367.
33. **Yagupsky P, Dagan R, Howard CW, Einhorn M, Kassis I, Simu A.** 1992. High prevalence of *Kingella kingae* in joint fluid from children with septic arthritis revealed by the BACTEC blood culture system. *J Clin Microbiol* **30:**1278–1281.

The Dark Art of Blood Cultures
Edited by Wm. Michael Dunne, Jr. and Carey-Ann D. Burnham
© 2018 American Society for Microbiology, Washington, DC
doi:10.1128/9781555819811.ch9

Epidemiology of Bloodstream Infections

9

Allison R. McMullen,[1] Craig B. Wilen,[2] and Carey-Ann D. Burnham[2]

The detection of microorganisms in the setting of bloodstream infection is one of the most important functions of the clinical microbiology laboratory. A number of advances and practice changes in health care, including hematopoietic stem cell transplantation (HSCT) and solid organ transplantation (SOT) and resulting immunosuppressive regimens, as well as the aging population, emergence of antimicrobial resistance, and increased use of invasive procedures in health care settings (as well as improvements in blood culture methods), have resulted in changing epidemiology of bloodstream infections over the past 4 decades. This chapter will discuss trends in the epidemiology of positive blood cultures.

Bacteria

Over the past 40 years, the most commonly recovered microorganisms from blood cultures have been aerobic and facultative anaerobic bacteria, with *Escherichia coli* and *Staphylococcus aureus* being the most common species in almost all of the comprehensive studies to date (Figs. 1 and 2) (1–6). Other frequently recovered Gram-negative bacteria include *Pseudomonas aeruginosa*, *Klebsiella* spp., *Enterobacter* spp., and *Proteus* spp. Other Gram-positive bacteria commonly recovered in blood cultures include *Enterococcus* spp. and *Streptococcus pyogenes*. Overall, the incidence of *Streptococcus pneumoniae* has decreased and is no longer in the top 10 in studies evaluated during the 21st century. This decrease in invasive pneumococcal disease can

---

[1]Medical College of Georgia at Augusta University, Augusta, GA 30912
[2]Washington University School of Medicine, St. Louis, MO 63110

> **BACTERIA MOST COMMONLY**
> **ASSOCIATED WITH BLOODSTREAM**
> **INFECTIONS**
>
> | | |
> |---|---|
> | *Staphylococcus aureus* | *Klebsiella* spp. |
> | *Escherichia coli* | *Pseudomonas aeruginosa* |
> | *Enterococcus* spp. | *Enterobacter* spp. |

Figure 1 Overview of bacteria most commonly associated with bloodstream infections.

be attributed to the implementation of the pneumococcal conjugate vaccine; first PCV7 (available in the United States in 2000), which covers seven serotypes, and later PCV13 (available in the United States in 2010), which adds six additional serotypes (7). Although these vaccines are commonly given to children, they appear to have reduced the incidence of disease in nonvaccinated populations (7). Coagulase-negative staphylococci (CoNS) were also frequently recovered in multiple studies; the recovery of this organism can be difficult to interpret and may represent true infection or contamination of the blood culture specimen. This will be discussed later in the chapter.

Anaerobes account for 2 to 13% of all positive blood cultures. The most commonly recovered anaerobes include *Bacteroides fragilis* group, *Clostridium* spp. (*Clostridium perfringens, Clostridium septicum, Clostridium ramosum,* and others), *Fusobacterium* spp., *Prevotella* spp., *Porphyromonas* spp., and Gram-positive anaerobic cocci including *Peptostreptococcus* spp., *Parvimonas* spp., *Finegoldia magna,* and *Peptoniphilus* spp. (1, 3, 8, 9). Risk factors for anaerobic bloodstream infections include liver failure, diabetes mellitus, malignancy, and hematologic disease (10) and may be secondary to an infectious process occurring in or related to the alimentary tract, female genital tract, or skin and soft tissue infection (11). Mortality rates from anaerobic bloodstream infections have been reported to range from 1 to 60% (8, 11).

The necessity of anaerobic blood cultures has been a topic for great debate for several decades. Some studies have reported a decrease in the incidence of anaerobes in positive blood cultures (12–16), while others have shown this rate to remain steady or increase (8, 10). One study in a large hospital (1,750 to 2,500 beds) in Spain evaluating the incidence of anaerobic bacteremia over 22 years (1985 to 2006) demonstrated that the rate of anaerobes recovered from blood cultures was constant (4.0%), while rates of Gram-positive and Gram-negative microorganisms increased (17, 18).

Rank	1975-1977 (1)	1984-1992 (2)	1992-1993 (3)	1995-2002 (4)	1997-2002 (5)	2004 (6)	2014-2015 (This chapter)
1	E. coli	S. aureus	S. aureus	CoNS	S. aureus	S. aureus	CoNS
2	S. aureus	E. coli	E. coli	S. aureus	E. coli	E. coli	S. aureus
3	S. pneumoniae	C. albicans	CoNS	Enterococcus spp.	CoNS	Enterococcus spp.	E. coli
4	K. pneumoniae	CoNS	K. pneumoniae	Candida spp.	Enterococcus spp.	K. pneumoniae	Enterococcus spp.
5	P. aeruginosa	P. aeruginosa	Enterococcus spp.	E. coli	Klebsiella spp.	CoNS	Klebsiella spp.
6	Bacteroides fragilis	Enterococcus faecalis	P. aeruginosa	Klebsiella spp.	VGS	P. aeruginosa	VGS
7	Enterococcus spp.	K. pneumoniae	S. pneumoniae	P. aeruginosa	S. pneumoniae	C. albicans	Pseudomonas spp.
8	Streptococcus pyogenes	S. pneumoniae	VGS	Enterobacter spp.	P. aeruginosa	E. cloacae	Corynebacterium spp.
9	C. albicans	VGS	C. albicans	Serratia spp.	Enterobacter spp.	Serratia marcescens	Bacillus spp. not B. anthracis
10	Proteus mirabilis	E. cloacae	E. cloacae	Acinetobacter baumannii	Serratia spp.	Bacteroides spp.	Enterobacter spp.

Figure 2 The organisms most frequently recovered from blood cultures, 1975 to 2015. (1) Weinstein et al., 1983; (2) Cockerill et al., 1997; (3) Weinstein et al., 1997; (4) Wisplinghoff et al., 2004; (5) Biedenbach et al., 2004; (6) Pien et al., 2010.

The variation in the detection of anaerobes in blood cultures reported in the literature can be explained by numerous factors, including individual laboratory practices or protocols for including anaerobic media routinely during blood culture collection, and improvements in anaerobe media and blood culture systems. Because of the potential severity of anaerobic bacteremia and the need for appropriate antimicrobial therapy, especially in patients with underlying comorbidities, there is abundant evidence to support the practice of including anaerobic medium in blood culture sets. Furthermore, some facultative anaerobes, including *S. pneumoniae*, nutrient variant staphylococci, and enterococci, may be recovered more efficiently in anaerobic blood culture bottles (2).

Multidrug-Resistant Organisms

Beginning in the mid-1990s, antimicrobial-resistant organisms, including methicillin-resistant *S. aureus* (MRSA), vancomycin-resistant enterococci (VRE), and extended-spectrum β-lactamases (ESBL) *Enterobacteriaceae*, began to emerge as a major cause of bloodstream infections. In a large study from Spain, fewer than 1% of *E. coli* producing ESBLs were recovered each year until 2003 when the numbers increased steadily each year to almost 10% of the *E. coli* isolates recovered in 2006 (18). Additionally, resistance to ciprofloxacin among *E. coli* isolates increased from 3% in 1991 to 32% in 2006 in the same study (17, 18). A small proportion of *P. aeruginosa* isolates were resistant to piperacillin (11%), imipenem (14%), and ceftazidime (16%), with ceftazidime resistance increasing from 12 to 29% from 1995 to 2001 (4). Also during this time, antimicrobial resistance was also developing in Gram-positive microorganisms. The SCOPE study, which collected data from across the United States, demonstrated that methicillin resistance among *S. aureus* isolates increased from 22% (1995) to 57% (2001). Additionally, 75% of CoNS isolates were resistant to methicillin. Vancomycin resistance was detected in 60% of *Enterococcus faecium* and 2% of *Enterococcus faecalis* isolates (4, 19). Another study, over a similar time period, also showed increasing prevalence of MRSA in blood cultures from 22% of *S. aureus* isolates in 1997 to almost 40% in 2002 (5). Rates of VRE also increased over the same time period, although at a lower rate of change (13 to 18%) (5). While resistance in Gram-positive bacteria increased from 1997 to 2002, rates of resistance in Gram-negative bacteria including *Klebsiella* spp. and *P. aeruginosa* remained steady. Rates of resistant *Klebsiella* spp. and *P. aeruginosa* were much lower in North America than in Latin America and Europe (5).

Blood Culture-Negative Endocarditis

It is estimated that blood culture-negative endocarditis (BCNE) represents 5 to 70% of all cases of endocarditis (20). This may be a result of initiation of antibiotic treatment prior to the collection of blood cultures, fastidious organisms including *Brucella* spp., *Legionella* spp., mycobacteria, *Candida* spp., and intracellular organisms including *Coxiella burnetii, Tropheryma whipplei,* and *Bartonella* spp., as well as noninfectious causes of endocarditis (20, 21). Studies have shown that automated blood culture systems are able to support the growth of many organisms previously considered to be attributed to BCNE, such as nutritionally deficient streptococci (e.g., *Abiotrophia* spp. and *Granulicatella* spp.) and HACEK organisms (*Haemophilus, Aggregatibacter, Cardiobacterium, Eikenella, Kingella*), and that these organisms are readily detected within the routine incubation period of 5 days (22, 23).

Epidemiology of Bloodstream Infection in Children

There are few multicenter studies examining the epidemiology of bloodstream infections in children. One study examining 181 cases of bacteremia in infants (<90 days old) from six hospital systems from 2006 to 2012 in the United States showed that the most common pathogen isolated was *E. coli* (42%) followed by *Streptococcus agalactiae* (group B streptococcus) (23%). *S. pneumoniae, S. aureus,* and *Klebsiella* spp. were found in less than 10% of the cases each (24). A second study examining blood cultures from infants from 17 hospitals from throughout the United States from 2006 to 2013 had similar findings, with *E. coli* causing 44% of all infections, followed by *S. agalactiae* (22%), viridans group streptococci (8%), *S. aureus* (6%), and *S. pneumoniae* (5%) (25). These studies excluded infants who were in an intensive care unit. In both studies, *E. coli* bacteremia was frequently associated (90 to 92%) with a concurrent urinary tract infection and 20 to 27% of the group B streptococci cases were associated with meningitis (24, 25). Neither of these studies identified any cases of *Listeria monocytogenes* bacteremia (24, 25). A meta-analysis of 16 studies examining the rates of *L. monocytogenes* bacteremia (1998 to 2014) in infants was only 0.03% (26). Rates of *S. pneumoniae* bacteremia in children have decreased since the introduction of PCV-7 vaccination (7).

Polymicrobial bloodstream infections in pediatric populations are rare. One study examining cultures from 1998 to 2004 from the United States identified 18 patients with 29 episodes of polymicrobial infections. The primary organisms isolated from these cases include *Enterococcus* spp., coagulase-negative staphylococci, and *Candida* spp. (27).

Fungal Bloodstream Infections

Immunosuppressive agents including chemotherapy and biologics have created a large population of patients at risk for bloodstream infections with fungi. Over the past 3 decades, a dramatic increase in the number of fungal bloodstream infections has been reported (28–30). In addition, the use of broad-spectrum antimicrobials and routine use of fluconazole prophylaxis have contributed to the changing epidemiology of fungal bloodstream infections (28, 31, 32). The fungi most commonly recovered in blood cultures are shown in Fig. 3.

Yeast

Candida spp. are the most frequent cause of fungal bloodstream infections, with the most commonly implicated species being *C. albicans*, *C. glabrata*, and *C. parapsilosis* complex (*C. parapsilosis*, *C. orthopsilosis*, *C. metapsilosis*) (28–30, 33–35). *C. glabrata* is more often associated with infection in older adults, compared with *C. parapsilosis* complex infections, which occur more frequently in neonates and other pediatric patients. *C. parapsilosis* colonization has been demonstrated on the hands of health care workers, and this is thought to be an important risk factor in transmission and nosocomial infection (36). The mortality rate attributed to *C. glabrata* fungemia is higher than other *Candida* spp. (37). The other *Candida* spp. associated with bloodstream infection include *C. krusei* and C. *tropicalis* (28, 33, 38). With the emergence of *C. auris* worldwide, it is possible that this species may be noted more frequently in future epidemiological studies of *Candida* spp. bloodstream infections (39–41). A recent report from the SENTRY program reported that of 1,354 instances of candidemia, 655 (48.4%) were *C. albicans*, 247 (18.2%) were *C. glabrata*, 232 (17.1%) were *C. parapsilosis*, 143 (10.6%) were *C. tropicalis*, 27 (2.0%) were *C. krusei*, and 50 (3.7%) were miscellaneous species, including *C. dubliniensis*, *C. guilliermondii*, *C. famata*, *C. rugosa*, *C. kefyr*, and others (42).

Figure 3 Overview of fungi most commonly associated with bloodstream infections.

FUNGI MOST COMMONLY RECOVERED IN BLOOD CULTURES

YEAST	MOLD
Candida albicans	Fusarium spp.
Candida glabrata	Scedosporium spp.
Candida parapsilopsis	Mucorales
Candida tropicalis	
Candida krusei	

In many studies, candidemia is the fourth most common hospital-acquired infection. Invasive candidiasis is a leading cause of mycosis-associated mortality in developed nations (33). In the SENTRY study mentioned above, 37% of candidemia episodes were community associated and 64% were nosocomial; the frequency of candidemia was higher in North America (51%) than in Europe (22%) or Latin America (28%) (42); this is consistent with other investigations reporting on the increasing rate of candidemia in North America (30, 43, 44). It is thought that mucous membrane colonization with *Candida* spp. typically precedes infection and is the major risk factor associated with infection, especially in those with indwelling intravascular devices, but exogenous acquisition has also been reported, most commonly associated with parenteral nutrition (45).

These yeasts are generally detected by continuously monitored blood culture systems (i.e., "routine" blood cultures); specialized "fungal" blood cultures are not usually required for detection of *Candida* spp. Non-culture-based diagnostics are emerging to improve the rate and speed of detection of *Candida* bloodstream infections; these are discussed in detail in other chapters (46–49) (please see chapters 7, 11, and 12).

Most episodes of candidemia are monomicrobial, but polymicrobial infections do occur, especially in patients with underlying gastrointestinal disease, indwelling catheters, and urinary tract infections (50, 51); the reported rate of polymicrobial infections is 1 to 6% (50, 51). The mixed infections might be coinfection with another *Candida* spp. or a concomitant bacterial infection; staphylococci and *P. aeruginosa* are the bacterial pathogens most associated with these coinfections (50–52). Mortality with polymicrobial *Candida* spp. bloodstream infections has been reported to be similar to monomicrobial infections.

Although *Candida* spp. are the most common yeasts causing bloodstream infection, there are other important genera to consider. *Cryptococcus neoformans* is an important cause of bloodstream infection in individuals with poorly controlled HIV, and other non-*neoformans Cryptococcus* can also cause bloodstream infection in immunocompromised individuals (32, 53). *Malassezia furfur* is associated with bloodstream infection in those receiving total parenteral nutrition and/or lipid supplementation (53). *Trichosporon* spp. are emerging as an important cause of catheter-associated bloodstream infections in immunosuppressed individuals (54). Other yeasts associated with bloodstream infection include *Saccharomyces cerevisiae*, *Rhodotorula* spp., *Pseudozyma* spp., and *Geotrichum* spp. (32, 36, 53, 55, 56).

Invasive Mold Infections

The incidence of invasive mold infections is increasing, largely attributed to the increasing number of HSCT and SOT patients. Other risk factors include neutropenia, prolonged courses of broad-spectrum antimicrobials, corticosteroid therapy, other immunosuppressive conditions, and traumatic inoculation (36, 57). The most common taxa associated with invasive mold infection are *Aspergillus* spp., the *Mucorales*, *Fusarium* spp., and *Scedosporium* spp. (34, 58, 59). Although the incidence of invasive infection with filamentous mold is increasing, it remains relatively uncommon to isolate filamentous fungi in blood cultures. *Fusarium* spp. and *Scedosporium* spp. are the most commonly recovered molds in blood cultures, but it is very unusual to recover *Aspergillus* or the *Mucorales* in blood culture specimens.

Fusarium spp. are found in the soil and other organic substrates. Although there are many species in this genus, most human infections are attributed to *Fusarium solani* and *Fusarium oxysporum*. The prognosis for *Fusarium* spp. bloodstream infection is usually poor (36, 60). Similar to *Fusarium* spp., *Scedosporium* spp. are commonly found in soil and other organic matter (34). Disseminated *Scedosporium* infection is reported most frequently in lung transplant patients, but other forms of immunosuppression are also a risk factor. The prognosis for *Scedosporium* spp. bloodstream infection is not favorable; this is usually attributed to the high level of antifungal resistance and the extreme level of immunosuppression in the patients that are most commonly affected.

The *Aspergillus* spp. associated most frequently with invasive infection are *A. fumigatus*, followed by *A. flavus*, *A. terreus*, and *A. niger* (36). It can be very challenging to determine if cases of invasive aspergillosis are community associated or hospital associated; air, soil, food, water, and decaying plant matter can be important point sources for *Aspergillus* spp. (36, 57).

The incidence of invasive zygomycosis is increasing worldwide, especially in the HSCT population; other risk factors include intravenous drug use, neutropenia, and poorly controlled diabetes mellitus (36, 57). Disseminated infection may follow colonization of the sinus cavity or respiratory tract or may be secondary to traumatic inoculation. Less common modes of infection include dissemination from the gastrointestinal tract, burns, and peritoneal dialysis. The genera most commonly associated with disseminated zygomycoses are *Rhizopus*, *Mucor*, and *Rhizomucor*.

The agents of endemic mycosis are occasionally recovered in blood cultures, especially in patients with HIV, SOT, and other forms of immunosuppression (61). *Histoplasma* spp. are seen in peripheral blood films, bone marrow biopsies, and blood cultures most frequently; it is much less common to recover *Blastomyces* spp. or *Coccidioides* spp. in blood cultures (62–67).

Mycobacterial Bloodstream Infections

Although mycobacterial bloodstream infections are far less common than bacterial and fungal causes, the prevalence is rising concomitant with increases in immunocompromised patients and the use of indwelling catheters and medical devices (68). Mycobacteria are classified as either rapid or slow growers depending on whether they form colonies when subcultured in less or more than 7 days. Among mycobacteria, members of the *Mycobacterium tuberculosis* complex are of particular clinical and public health importance. In regions of nontuberculosis endemicity, the most frequently identified mycobacteria species from blood cultures are rapid-growing mycobacteria and the slow-growing *Mycobacterium avium-intracellulare* complex (MAI).

Rapid-growing mycobacteria are ubiquitous environmental organisms and frequent opportunistic pathogens in susceptible hosts. When rapid-growing mycobacteria are found as a cause of bloodstream infection, it is usually associated with a chronic indwelling catheter in both pediatric and adult settings (69–71). This is likely due to the ability of rapid-growing mycobacteria to establish biofilms on catheters and implanted medical devices (72). The most frequently identified rapid-growing mycobacteria species are *Mycobacterium fortuitum* complex, *Mycobacterium abscessus*, and *Mycobacterium mucogenicum* (68, 70, 71). Patient outcomes are generally favorable upon catheter or device removal and antimicrobial therapy (69–71).

In severely immunocompromised individuals, especially those with poorly controlled HIV infection, the most common mycobacteria isolates identified in the bloodstream are MAI followed by *M. tuberculosis* (73, 74). Disseminated MAI disease, which is diagnosed by culture of MAI from the bloodstream, is an AIDS-defining illness and heralds a poor prognosis if not adequately treated. For this reason, MAI prophylaxis is administered to HIV-infected individuals with CD4 counts below 100 cells/mm^3 (75).

Recently, a prolonged global outbreak of *Mycobacterium chimaera* associated with heater-cooler units used in cardiopulmonary bypass has been identified (76–80). The outbreak investigation revealed that the devices were contaminated with *M. chimaera* during the manufacturing process. Although the contaminated water in the heater-cooler unit does not come into physical contact with the patient, the fan on the heater-cooler unit aerosolizes the organism, leading to direct contamination of the surgical wound, resulting in surgical site infections and/or endocarditis. *M. chimaera* has been recovered from mycobacterial blood cultures of some of the infected patients. Because the time to diagnosis is frequently 4 years (or longer) postinfection, it is likely that clinical laboratories will continue to recover this organism in mycobacterial blood cultures for many years to come (76–80).

Unlike other mycobacteria that cause bloodstream infections, *M. tuberculosis* is an obligate human pathogen and identification of such requires targeted therapy, patient isolation, and public health intervention. While identification of *M. tuberculosis* is rare in blood cultures from regions of nontuberculosis endemicity, in settings where tuberculosis is endemic, the prevalence has been reported as 13% for adults and 1% for children (81). Although blood culture is not the preferred diagnostic modality, *M. tuberculosis* bacteremia is associated with poor clinical outcomes (82).

While bloodstream infection due to mycobacteria is infrequent relative to other Gram-positive and -negative bacteria and fungi, it is a critical problem in certain populations, particularly those who are immunocompromised or have long-term indwelling catheters. In regions of nontuberculosis endemicity, rapid-growing mycobacteria and MAI are the predominant organisms isolated while in regions of tuberculosis endemicity, *M. tuberculosis* represents a substantial minority of isolates with significant public health implications.

Recovery of Contaminants in Blood Culture Specimens

The contamination of blood cultures typically occurs during specimen collection or processing and involves microbes commonly found on the patient's skin or environment; these contaminants are not the cause of the patient's infection (83, 84). Although ideally contamination of blood culture specimens should be kept to a minimum, this can be difficult; as a result, laboratories have a benchmark of maintaining contamination rates below <3% (85). Studies have demonstrated that actual rates range from <1% to over 6%, with higher rates in emergency departments, in pediatric patients, and in settings where blood cultures are not collected by a centralized phlebotomy service (83, 84). Contaminated blood cultures lead to increased costs for hospitals with increased length of stay and unnecessary use of antibiotics. The differentiation of contaminants in blood cultures is determined by using organism identity, number of positive blood culture sets, time to positivity, and source of culture (83, 86). The most common organisms reported as blood culture contaminants include coagulase-negative staphylococci, coryneforms/diphtheroids (including *Corynebacterium* spp.), *Bacillus* spp. (other than *B. anthracis*), *Propionibacterium* spp., and viridans group streptococci (3, 83, 86, 87). In certain cases, including patients with indwelling devices or venous catheters or who are immunocompromised, these organisms may also represent true infection, therefore making it difficult to interpret blood culture results and definitively define blood culture contamination. Studies have shown that coagulase-negative staphylococci are frequently the most common cause of contamination, but may also represent between 10 and 26% of cases of true bacteremia (3, 83).

Contemporary Epidemiology of Positive Blood Cultures at a Tertiary Care Academic Medical Center

At our institution, a 1,350-bed tertiary care hospital in Saint Louis, Missouri, we examined the epidemiology of positive blood cultures over a 2-year period (2014 to 2015). There were a total of 8,699 positive blood cultures; only the first positive culture from each patient from each visit was included for a total of 4,896 positive cultures. The top 10 most frequently recovered organisms are listed in Fig. 2 and were similar to previous studies with CoNS, *S. aureus*, *E. coli*, *Enterococcus* spp., and *Klebsiella* spp. representing the most frequently identified organisms. Our data included *Corynebacterium* spp. and *Bacillus* spp. as frequently recovered, but like CoNS, may represent contaminants of unknown clinical significance. Table 1 lists all bacteria that were recovered at least 10 times and all fungi and mycobacteria recovered from blood cultures during the 2-year period at our medical center. Of the 19 instances of mycobacteria bloodstream infections occurring during this time period, eight (42%) were caused by a *M. avium-intracellulare* complex, four were caused by rapidly growing mycobacteria, and four cases of *Mycobacterium xenopi* infection. Of the filamentous fungi recovered, 54% likely represent contaminants (*Cladosporium* spp., *Epicoccum* spp., and *Penicillium* spp.), 36% of the isolates were *Histoplasma capsulatum*, and one case of *Scedosporium* spp. was documented. The three yeast species most commonly recovered (*C. albicans*, *C. glabrata*, and *C. parapsilosis*) parallel the findings of other studies. Overall, the epidemiology of positive blood cultures at our medical center is similar to findings from studies published during the previous 40 years, with a few notable exceptions including the decline in *S. pneumoniae* and increases in the recovery of coagulase-negative staphylococci. Differences in patient populations and geographical locations may account for some of the small differences among studies.

Table 1 Microorganisms isolated from positive blood cultures at a tertiary care academic medical center, 2014 to 2015

Organism(s)	No. (%) detected
All detected	4,896
Bacteria (≥10 isolates)	
Coagulase-negative staphylococci	1,740 (35.5)
Staphylococcus aureus	559 (11.4)
Escherichia coli	341 (6.9)
Klebsiella pneumoniae	188 (3.8)
Pseudomonas aeruginosa	171 (3.5)
Corynebacterium species	168 (3.4)
Enterococcus faecalis	158 (3.2)
Enterococcus faecium	129 (2.6)
Bacillus species, not *B. anthracis*	116 (2.4)
Viridans group streptococci	103 (2.1)
Micrococcus species	93 (1.9)
Enterobacter cloacae complex	79 (1.6)
Streptococcus mitis group	70 (1.4)
Streptococcus agalactiae (group B beta-hemolytic streptococci)	63 (1.3)
Streptococcus pneumoniae	55 (1.1)
Bacteroides fragilis group	53 (1.1)
Proteus mirabilis	40 (0.8)
Klebsiella oxytoca	34 (0.7)
Propionibacterium species	33 (0.7)
Stenotrophomonas maltophilia	30 (0.6)
Lactobacillus species	28 (0.6)
Serratia marcescens	24 (0.5)
Streptococcus anginosus group	21 (0.4)
Streptococcus pyogenes (group A beta-hemolytic streptococci)	19 (0.4)
Acinetobacter species	18 (0.4)
Enterobacter aerogenes	17 (0.3)
Peptostreptococcus species	17 (0.3)
Haemophilus influenzae	16 (0.3)
Granulicatella species	14 (0.3)
Streptococcus dysgalactiae	13 (0.3)
Citrobacter species	13 (0.3)
Clostridium perfringens	12 (0.2)
Enterococcus species	11 (0.2)
Rothia species	11 (0.2)
Pseudomonas species, not *Pseudomonas aeruginosa*	10 (0.2)
Prevotella species	10 (0.2)
Mycobacterium	
Mycobacterium avium–intracellulare complex	8 (0.2)
Mycobacterium xenopi	4 (<0.1)
Mycobacterium chelonae	2 (<0.1)
Mycobacterium fortuitum	1 (<0.1)
Mycobacterium mucogenicum	1 (<0.1)
Mycobacterium porcinum	1 (<0.1)

(*continued on next page*)

Table 1 (*continued*)

Organism(s)	No. (%) detected
Mycobacterium terrae complex	1 (<0.1)
Mycobacterium spp.	1(<0.1)
Fungi	
Mold	
Cladosporium species	13 (0.3)
Histoplasma capsulatum	10 (0.2)
Aspergillus species, not *A. fumigatus* or *A. flavus*	1 (<0.1)
Aspergillus terreus	1 (<0.1)
Epicoccum species	1 (<0.1)
Penicillium species	1 (<0.1)
Scedosporium species	1 (<0.1)
Yeast	
Candida albicans	75 (1.5)
Candida glabrata	42 (0.9)
Candida parapsilosis	28 (0.6)
Candida tropicalis	21 (0.4)
Candida dubliniensis	8 (0.2)
Candida krusei	6 (0.1)
Cryptococcus neoformans	6 (0.1)
Candida guilliermondii	4 (<0.1)
Candida lusitaniae	2 (<0.1)
Candida kefyr	1 (<0.1)
Candida species	1 (<0.1)
Saccharomyces cerevisiae	1 (<0.1)
Trichosporon species	1 (<0.1)

Summary/Conclusion

The identification of microbes in blood culture specimens continues to be an important function of the clinical microbiology laboratory. Bacteria continue to be the most frequently recovered organisms, but fungi, especially yeast, are being recovered with increasing frequency.

References

1. Weinstein MP, Reller LB, Murphy JR, Lichtenstein KA, Laboratory and Epidemiologic Observations. 1983. The clinical significance of positive blood cultures: a comprehensive analysis of 500 episodes of bacteremia and fungemia in adults. I. Laboratory and epidemiologic observations. *Rev Infect Dis* 5:35–53.
2. Cockerill FR III, Hughes JG, Vetter EA, Mueller RA, Weaver AL, Ilstrup DM, Rosenblatt JE, Wilson WR. 1997. Analysis of 281,797 consecutive blood cultures performed over an eight-year period: trends in microorganisms isolated and the value of anaerobic culture of blood. *Clin Infect Dis* 24:403–418.
3. Weinstein MP, Towns ML, Quartey SM, Mirrett S, Reimer LG, Parmigiani G, Reller LB. 1997. The clinical significance of positive blood cultures in the 1990s: a

prospective comprehensive evaluation of the microbiology, epidemiology, and outcome of bacteremia and fungemia in adults. *Clin Infect Dis* 24:584–602.

4. **Wisplinghoff H, Bischoff T, Tallent SM, Seifert H, Wenzel RP, Edmond MB.** 2004. Nosocomial bloodstream infections in US hospitals: analysis of 24,179 cases from a prospective nationwide surveillance study. *Clin Infect Dis* 39:309–317.

5. **Biedenbach DJ, Moet GJ, Jones RN.** 2004. Occurrence and antimicrobial resistance pattern comparisons among bloodstream infection isolates from the SENTRY Antimicrobial Surveillance Program (1997-2002). *Diagn Microbiol Infect Dis* 50:59–69.

6. **Pien BC, Sundaram P, Raoof N, Costa SF, Mirrett S, Woods CW, Reller LB, Weinstein MP.** 2010. The clinical and prognostic importance of positive blood cultures in adults. *Am J Med* 123:819–828.

7. **Myint TT, Madhava H, Balmer P, Christopoulou D, Attal S, Menegas D, Sprenger R, Bonnet E.** 2013. The impact of 7-valent pneumococcal conjugate vaccine on invasive pneumococcal disease: a literature review. *Adv Ther* 30:127–151.

8. **Vena A, Muñoz P, Alcalá L, Fernandez-Cruz A, Sanchez C, Valerio M, Bouza E.** 2015. Are incidence and epidemiology of anaerobic bacteremia really changing? *Eur J Clin Microbiol Infect Dis* 34:1621–1629.

9. **Ng LS, Kwang LL, Rao S, Tan TY.** 2015. Anaerobic bacteraemia revisited: species and susceptibilities. *Ann Acad Med Singapore* 44:13–18.

10. **Blairon L, De Gheldre Y, Delaere B, Sonet A, Bosly A, Glupczynski Y.** 2006. A 62-month retrospective epidemiological survey of anaerobic bacteraemia in a university hospital. *Clin Microbiol Infect* 12:527–532.

11. **De Keukeleire S, Wybo I, Naessens A, Echahidi F, Van der Beken M, Vandoorslaer K, Vermeulen S, Piérard D.** 2016. Anaerobic bacteraemia: a 10-year retrospective epidemiological survey. *Anaerobe* 39:54–59.

12. **Fenner L, Widmer AF, Straub C, Frei R.** 2008. Is the incidence of anaerobic bacteremia decreasing? Analysis of 114,000 blood cultures over a ten-year period. *J Clin Microbiol* 46:2432–2434.

13. **Dorsher CW, Rosenblatt JE, Wilson WR, Ilstrup DM.** 1991. Anaerobic bacteremia: decreasing rate over a 15-year period. *Rev Infect Dis* 13:633–636.

14. **Lombardi DP, Engleberg NC.** 1992. Anaerobic bacteremia: incidence, patient characteristics, and clinical significance. *Am J Med* 92:53–60.

15. **Murray PR, Traynor P, Hopson D.** 1992. Critical assessment of blood culture techniques: analysis of recovery of obligate and facultative anaerobes, strict aerobic bacteria, and fungi in aerobic and anaerobic blood culture bottles. *J Clin Microbiol* 30:1462–1468.

16. **Goldstein EJ.** 1996. Anaerobic bacteremia. *Clin Infect Dis* 23(Suppl 1):S97–S101.

17. **Muñoz P, Cruz AF, Rodríguez-Créixems M, Bouza E.** 2008. Gram-negative bloodstream infections. *Int J Antimicrob Agents* 32(Suppl 1):S10–S14.

18. **Rodríguez-Créixems M, Alcalá L, Muñoz P, Cercenado E, Vicente T, Bouza E.** 2008. Bloodstream infections: evolution and trends in the microbiology workload, incidence, and etiology, 1985-2006. *Medicine (Baltimore)* 87:234–249.

19. **Karchmer AW.** 2009. Bloodstream infections: the problem and the challenge. *Int J Antimicrob Agents* 34(Suppl 4):S2–S4.

20. **Lamas CC, Fournier PE, Zappa M, Brandão TJ, Januário-da-Silva CA, Correia MG, Barbosa GI, Golebiovski WF, Weksler C, Lepidi H, Raoult D.** 2016. Diagnosis of

blood culture-negative endocarditis and clinical comparison between blood culture-negative and blood culture-positive cases. *Infection* **44**:459–466.

21. Tattevin P, Watt G, Revest M, Arvieux C, Fournier PE. 2015. Update on blood culture-negative endocarditis. *Med Mal Infect* **45**:1–8.

22. Baron EJ, Miller JM, Weinstein MP, Richter SS, Gilligan PH, Thomson RB Jr, Bourbeau P, Carroll KC, Kehl SC, Dunne WM, Robinson-Dunn B, Schwartzman JD, Chapin KC, Snyder JW, Forbes BA, Patel R, Rosenblatt JE, Pritt BS. 2013. Executive summary: a guide to utilization of the microbiology laboratory for diagnosis of infectious diseases: 2013 recommendations by the Infectious Diseases Society of America (IDSA) and the American Society for Microbiology (ASM)(a). *Clin Infect Dis* **57**:485–488.

23. Weinstein MP, Mirrett S, Wilson ML, Reimer LG, Reller LB. 1994. Controlled evaluation of 5 versus 10 milliliters of blood cultured in aerobic BacT/Alert blood culture bottles. *J Clin Microbiol* **32**:2103–2106.

24. Biondi E, Evans R, Mischler M, Bendel-Stenzel M, Horstmann S, Lee V, Aldag J, Gigliotti F. 2013. Epidemiology of bacteremia in febrile infants in the United States. *Pediatrics* **132**:990–996.

25. Mischler M, Ryan MS, Leyenaar JK, Markowsky A, Seppa M, Wood K, Ren J, Asche C, Gigliotti F, Biondi E. 2015. Epidemiology of bacteremia in previously healthy febrile infants: a follow-up study. *Hosp Pediatr* **5**:293–300.

26. Leazer R, Perkins AM, Shomaker K, Fine B. 2016. A meta-analysis of the rates of *Listeria monocytogenes* and *Enterococcus* in febrile infants. *Hosp Pediatr* **6**:187–195.

27. Sutter D, Stagliano D, Braun L, Williams F, Arnold J, Ottolini M, Epstein J. 2008. Polymicrobial bloodstream infection in pediatric patients: risk factors, microbiology, and antimicrobial management. *Pediatr Infect Dis J* **27**:400–405.

28. Swinne D, Nolard N, Van Rooij P, Detandt M. 2009. Bloodstream yeast infections: a 15-month survey. *Epidemiol Infect* **137**:1037–1040.

29. Lagrou K, Verhaegen J, Peetermans WE, De Rijdt T, Maertens J, Van Wijngaerden E. 2007. Fungemia at a tertiary care hospital: incidence, therapy, and distribution and antifungal susceptibility of causative species. *Eur J Clin Microbiol Infect Dis* **26**:541–547.

30. Shorr AF, Gupta V, Sun X, Johannes RS, Spalding J, Tabak YP. 2009. Burden of early-onset candidemia: analysis of culture-positive bloodstream infections from a large U.S. database. *Crit Care Med* **37**:2519–2526, quiz 2535.

31. Geha DJ, Roberts GD. 1994. Laboratory detection of fungemia. *Clin Lab Med* **14**:83–97.

32. Miceli MH, Díaz JA, Lee SA. 2011. Emerging opportunistic yeast infections. *Lancet Infect Dis* **11**:142–151.

33. Pfaller MA, Diekema DJ. 2007. Epidemiology of invasive candidiasis: a persistent public health problem. *Clin Microbiol Rev* **20**:133–163.

34. Slavin MA, Australian Mycology Interest Group. 2002. The epidemiology of candidaemia and mould infections in Australia. *J Antimicrob Chemother* **49**(Suppl 1):3–6.

35. Bonfietti LX, Martins MA, Szeszs MW, Pukiskas SB, Purisco SU, Pimentel FC, Pereira GH, Silva DC, Oliveira L, Melhem MS. 2012. Prevalence, distribution and antifungal susceptibility profiles of *Candida parapsilosis*, *Candida orthopsilosis* and *Candida metapsilosis* bloodstream isolates. *J Med Microbiol* **61**:1003–1008.

36. Richardson M, Lass-Flörl C. 2008. Changing epidemiology of systemic fungal infections. *Clin Microbiol Infect* **14**(Suppl 4):5–24.

37. Gupta A, Gupta A, Varma A. 2015. Candida glabrata candidemia: an emerging threat in critically ill patients. *Indian J Crit Care Med* **19**:151–154.

38. Fernández-Ruiz M, Puig-Asensio M, Guinea J, Almirante B, Padilla B, Almela M, Díaz-Martín A, Rodríguez-Baño J, Cuenca-Estrella M, Aguado JM, CANDIPOP Project, GEIH-GEMICOMED (SEIMC), REIPI. 2015. Candida tropicalis bloodstream infection: incidence, risk factors and outcome in a population-based surveillance. *J Infect* **71**:385–394.

39. Borman AM, Szekely A, Johnson EM. 16 February 2017. Isolates of the emerging pathogen *Candida auris* present in the UK have several geographic origins. *Med Mycol* doi:10.1093/mmy/myw147.

40. Lockhart SR, Etienne KA, Vallabhaneni S, Farooqi J, Chowdhary A, Govender NP, Colombo AL, Calvo B, Cuomo CA, Desjardins CA, Berkow EL, Castanheira M, Magobo RE, Jabeen K, Asghar RJ, Meis JF, Jackson B, Chiller T, Litvintseva AP. 2017. Simultaneous emergence of multidrug-resistant *Candida auris* on 3 continents confirmed by whole-genome sequencing and epidemiological analyses. *Clin Infect Dis* **64**:134–140.

41. Vallabhaneni S, Kallen A, Tsay S, Chow N, Welsh R, Kerins J, Kemble SK, Pacilli M, Black SR, Landon E, Ridgway J, Palmore TN, Zelzany A, Adams EH, Quinn M, Chaturvedi S, Greenko J, Fernandez R, Southwick K, Furuya EY, Calfee DP, Hamula C, Patel G, Barrett P, MSD, Lafaro P, Berkow EL, Moulton-Meissner H, Noble-Wang J, Fagan RP, Jackson BR, Lockhart SR, Litvintseva AP, Chiller TM. 2016. Investigation of the first seven reported cases of *Candida auris*, a globally emerging invasive, multidrug-resistant fungus - United States, May 2013-August 2016. *MMWR Morb Mortal Wkly Rep* **65**:1234–1237.

42. Pfaller MA, Moet GJ, Messer SA, Jones RN, Castanheira M. 2011. Candida bloodstream infections: comparison of species distributions and antifungal resistance patterns in community-onset and nosocomial isolates in the SENTRY Antimicrobial Surveillance Program, 2008-2009. *Antimicrob Agents Chemother* **55**:561–566.

43. Zilberberg MD, Shorr AF, Kollef MH. 2008. Secular trends in candidemia-related hospitalization in the United States, 2000-2005. *Infect Control Hosp Epidemiol* **29**:978–980.

44. Gulia J, Aryal S, Saadlla H, Shorr AF. 2010. Health care-associated candidemia–a distinct entity? *J Hosp Med* **5**:298–301.

45. Tortorano AM, Kibbler C, Peman J, Bernhardt H, Klingspor L, Grillot R. 2006. Candidaemia in Europe: epidemiology and resistance. *Int J Antimicrob Agents* **27**:359–366.

46. Hamula CL, Hughes K, Fisher BT, Zaoutis TE, Singh IR, Velegraki A. 2016. T2Candida provides rapid and accurate species identification in pediatric cases of candidemia. *Am J Clin Pathol* **145**:858–861.

47. Pfaller MA, Wolk DM, Lowery TJ. 2016. T2MR and T2Candida: novel technology for the rapid diagnosis of candidemia and invasive candidiasis. *Future Microbiol* **11**:103–117.

48. Mylonakis E, Clancy CJ, Ostrosky-Zeichner L, Garey KW, Alangaden GJ, Vazquez JA, Groeger JS, Judson MA, Vinagre YM, Heard SO, Zervou FN, Zacharioudakis IM, Kontoyiannis DP, Pappas PG. 2015. T2 magnetic resonance assay for the rapid diagnosis of candidemia in whole blood: a clinical trial. *Clin Infect Dis* **60**:892–899.

49. Schuetz AN. 2013. Invasive fungal infections: biomarkers and molecular approaches to diagnosis. *Clin Lab Med* **33**:505–525.

50. Pulimood S, Ganesan L, Alangaden G, Chandrasekar P. 2002. Polymicrobial candidemia. *Diagn Microbiol Infect Dis* 44:353–357.
51. Guerra-Romero L, Telenti A, Thompson RL, Roberts GD. 1989. Polymicrobial fungemia: microbiology, clinical features, and significance. *Rev Infect Dis* 11:208–212.
52. Klotz SA, Chasin BS, Powell B, Gaur NK, Lipke PN. 2007. Polymicrobial bloodstream infections involving Candida species: analysis of patients and review of the literature. *Diagn Microbiol Infect Dis* 59:401–406.
53. Arendrup MC, Boekhout T, Akova M, Meis JF, Cornely OA, Lortholary O, European Society of Clinical Microbiology and Infectious Diseases Fungal Infection Study Group, European Confederation of Medical Mycology. 2014. ESCMID and ECMM joint clinical guidelines for the diagnosis and management of rare invasive yeast infections. *Clin Microbiol Infect* 20(Suppl 3):76–98.
54. Liao Y, Lu X, Yang S, Luo Y, Chen Q, Yang R. 2015. Epidemiology and outcome of trichosporon fungemia: a review of 185 reported cases from 1975 to 2014. *Open Forum Infect Dis* 2:ofv141.
55. Siddiqui W, Ahmed Y, Albrecht H, Weissman S. 12 December 2014. *Pseudozyma* spp catheter-associated blood stream infection, an emerging pathogen and brief literature review. *BMJ Case Rep* 2014. doi:10.1136/bcr-2014-206369.
56. Pande A, Non LR, Romee R, Santos CA. 18 January 2017. *Pseudozyma* and other non-*Candida* opportunistic yeast bloodstream infections in a large stem cell transplant center. *Transpl Infect Dis* doi:10.1111/tid.12664.
57. Sanz Alonso MA, Jarque Ramos I, Salavert Lletí M, Pemán J. 2006. Epidemiology of invasive fungal infections due to *Aspergillus* spp. and Zygomycetes. *Clin Microbiol Infect* 12:2–6.
58. Pagano L, Caira M, Candoni A, Offidani M, Fianchi L, Martino B, Pastore D, Picardi M, Bonini A, Chierichini A, Fanci R, Caramatti C, Invernizzi R, Mattei D, Mitra ME, Melillo L, Aversa F, Van Lint MT, Falcucci P, Valentini CG, Girmenia C, Nosari A. 2006. The epidemiology of fungal infections in patients with hematologic malignancies: the SEIFEM-2004 study. *Haematologica* 91:1068–1075.
59. Park BJ, Pappas PG, Wannemuehler KA, Alexander BD, Anaissie EJ, Andes DR, Baddley JW, Brown JM, Brumble LM, Freifeld AG, Hadley S, Herwaldt L, Ito JI, Kauffman CA, Lyon GM, Marr KA, Morrison VA, Papanicolaou G, Patterson TF, Perl TM, Schuster MG, Walker R, Wingard JR, Walsh TJ, Kontoyiannis DP. 2011. Invasive non-*Aspergillus* mold infections in transplant recipients, United States, 2001-2006. *Emerg Infect Dis* 17:1855–1864.
60. Dabas Y, Bakhshi S, Xess I. 2016. Fatal cases of bloodstream infection by *Fusarium solani* and review of published literature. *Mycopathologia* 181:291–296.
61. Campigotto A, Richardson SE, Sebert M, McElvania TeKippe E, Chakravarty A, Doern CD. 2016. Low utility of pediatric isolator blood culture system for detection of fungemia in children: a 10-year review. *J Clin Microbiol* 54:2284–2287.
62. Kauffman CA. 2007. Histoplasmosis: a clinical and laboratory update. *Clin Microbiol Rev* 20:115–132.
63. Saccente M, Woods GL. 2010. Clinical and laboratory update on blastomycosis. *Clin Microbiol Rev* 23:367–381.
64. Roberts GD, Washington JA II. 1975. Detection of fungi in blood cultures. *J Clin Microbiol* 1:309–310.

65. Graybill JR. 1988. Histoplasmosis and AIDS. *J Infect Dis* **158**:623–626.
66. Paya CV, Roberts GD, Cockerill FR III. 1987. Laboratory methods for the diagnosis of disseminated histoplasmosis: clinical importance of the lysis-centrifugation blood culture technique. *Mayo Clin Proc* **62**:480–485.
67. Ampel NM, Ryan KJ, Carry PJ, Wieden MA, Schifman RB. 1986. Fungemia due to *Coccidioides immitis*. An analysis of 16 episodes in 15 patients and a review of the literature. *Medicine (Baltimore)* **65**:312–321.
68. El Helou G, Viola GM, Hachem R, Han XY, Raad II. 2013. Rapidly growing mycobacterial bloodstream infections. *Lancet Infect Dis* **13**:166–174.
69. Al Yazidi LS, Marais BJ, Hazelton B, Outhred A, Kesson A. 2017. Nontuberculous mycobacteria in children - a focus on bloodstream infections. *Pediatr Infect Dis J* **36**:374–378.
70. Hawkins C, Qi C, Warren J, Stosor V. 2008. Catheter-related bloodstream infections caused by rapidly growing nontuberculous mycobacteria: a case series including rare species. *Diagn Microbiol Infect Dis* **61**:187–191.
71. van Duin D, Goldfarb J, Schmitt SK, Tomford JW, Tuohy MJ, Hall GS. 2010. Nontuberculous mycobacterial blood stream and cardiac infections in patients without HIV infection. *Diagn Microbiol Infect Dis* **67**:286–290.
72. Zambrano MM, Kolter R. 2005. Mycobacterial biofilms: a greasy way to hold it together. *Cell* **123**:762–764.
73. Oplustil CP, Leite OH, Oliveira MS, Sinto SI, Uip DE, Boulos M, Mendes CF. 2001. Detection of mycobacteria in the bloodstream of patients with acquired immunodeficiency syndrome in a university hospital in Brazil. *Braz J Infect Dis* **5**:252–259.
74. Pedro-Botet ML, Mòdol JM, Vallés X, Romeu J, Sopena N, Giménez M, Tor J, Clotet B, Sabrià M. 2002. Changes in bloodstream infections in HIV-positive patients in a university hospital in Spain (1995-1997). *Int J Infect Dis* **6**:17–22.
75. Pierce M, Crampton S, Henry D, Heifets L, LaMarca A, Montecalvo M, Wormser GP, Jablonowski H, Jemsek J, Cynamon M, Yangco BG, Notario G, Craft JC. 1996. A randomized trial of clarithromycin as prophylaxis against disseminated *Mycobacterium avium* complex infection in patients with advanced acquired immunodeficiency syndrome. *N Engl J Med* **335**:384–391.
76. Sommerstein R, Schreiber PW, Diekema DJ, Edmond MB, Hasse B, Marschall J, Sax H. 2017. *Mycobacterium chimaera* outbreak associated with heater-cooler devices: piecing the puzzle together. *Infect Control Hosp Epidemiol* **38**:103–108.
77. Kohler P, Kuster SP, Bloemberg G, Schulthess B, Frank M, Tanner FC, Rössle M, Böni C, Falk V, Wilhelm MJ, Sommerstein R, Achermann Y, Ten Oever J, Debast SB, Wolfhagen MJ, Brandon Bravo Bruinsma GJ, Vos MC, Bogers A, Serr A, Beyersdorf F, Sax H, Böttger EC, Weber R, van Ingen J, Wagner D, Hasse B. 2015. Healthcare-associated prosthetic heart valve, aortic vascular graft, and disseminated Mycobacterium chimaera infections subsequent to open heart surgery. *Eur Heart J* **36**:2745–2753.
78. Sax H, Bloemberg G, Hasse B, Sommerstein R, Kohler P, Achermann Y, Rössle M, Falk V, Kuster SP, Böttger EC, Weber R. 2015. Prolonged outbreak of *Mycobacterium chimaera* infection after open-chest heart surgery. *Clin Infect Dis* **61**:67–75.
79. Williamson D, Howden B, Stinear T. 2017. *Mycobacterium chimaera* spread from heating and cooling units in heart surgery. *N Engl J Med* **376**:600–602.

80. Svensson E, Jensen ET, Rasmussen EM, Folkvardsen DB, Norman A, Lillebaek T. 2017. *Mycobacterium chimaera* in heater-cooler units in Denmark related to isolates from the United States and United Kingdom. *Emerg Infect Dis* 23:507–509.

81. Pavlinac PB, Lokken EM, Walson JL, Richardson BA, Crump JA, John-Stewart GC. 2016. *Mycobacterium tuberculosis* bacteremia in adults and children: a systematic review and meta-analysis. *Int J Tuberc Lung Dis* 20:895–902.

82. Jacob ST, Pavlinac PB, Nakiyingi L, Banura P, Baeten JM, Morgan K, Magaret A, Manabe Y, Reynolds SJ, Liles WC, Wald A, Joloba ML, Mayanja-Kizza H, Scheld WM. 2013. Mycobacterium tuberculosis bacteremia in a cohort of hiv-infected patients hospitalized with severe sepsis in uganda–high frequency, low clinical suspicion [corrected] and derivation of a clinical prediction score. *PLoS One* 8:e70305.

83. Hall KK, Lyman JA. 2006. Updated review of blood culture contamination. *Clin Microbiol Rev* 19:788–802.

84. Dawson S. 2014. Blood culture contaminants. *J Hosp Infect* 87:1–10.

85. CLSI. 2007. *Principles and Procedures for Blood Cultures; Approved Guideline.*, CLSI document M47-A ed. CLSI, Wayne, PA.

86. Weinstein MP. 2003. Blood culture contamination: persisting problems and partial progress. *J Clin Microbiol* 41:2275–2278.

87. Schifman RB, Strand CL, Meier FA, Howanitz PJ. 1998. Blood culture contamination: a College of American Pathologists Q-probes study involving 640 institutions and 497134 specimens from adult patients. *Arch Pathol Lab Med* 122:216–221.

The Dark Art of Blood Cultures
Edited by Wm. Michael Dunne, Jr. and Carey-Ann D. Burnham
© 2018 American Society for Microbiology, Washington, DC
doi:10.1128/9781555819811.ch10

Best Practices in Blood Cultures 10

Robert J. Tibbetts[1] and Barbara Robinson-Dunn[2]

Rapid and accurate detection of sepsis is critical, yet errors in collection lead to unnecessary testing, use of antimicrobial agents, and prolonged hospitalizations. Strict attention to the various components that compose the blood culture collection process can help to reduce factors leading to rising costs in health care as well as inaccurate test results.

The single most important factor contributing to successful isolation of an infectious agent in a blood culture is the volume of blood placed into culture. Blood should be collected by venipuncture and (if at all possible) prior to administration of antimicrobial therapy. For detection of bacteremia/fungemia in patients who weigh at least 80 lbs (36.3 kg), at least two sets of blood cultures (each consisting of both an aerobic and an anaerobic bottle) should be obtained. These two bottles constitute one set of blood cultures. For patients with a vascular access device, one set of blood cultures should be obtained by venipuncture and the other may be obtained through the device for comparison. These cultures should be labeled to indicate the source of the blood (venipuncture or vascular access device).

In general, blood for cultures may be collected as rapidly as venipuncture sites can be adequately disinfected and accessed as long as the blood is obtained from different sites. No more than three sets of blood cultures should be obtained within a 24-h period (1). Several studies have attempted to determine the optimal time to obtain blood for culture. Although in the past it was frequently stated that blood should be obtained at 30- to 60-min

[1]Henry Ford Health System, Detroit MI 48202
[2]Beaumont Health System, Royal Oak, MI 48073

intervals, there are few data to support this practice. Multiple studies (2–4) have shown no significant differences in recovery of isolates when blood was obtained at spaced intervals or when it was obtained in concordance with fever spikes. If labels are printed prior to collection every effort should be made to include the exact time and site of draw on the label as well as in the laboratory information system.

As the volume of blood placed into culture increases, the likelihood of detecting the causative agent of bacteremia also increases. Ideally, a total of 20 to 30 ml of blood is obtained from persons weighing more than 80 lbs, and half of this amount is placed aseptically into each of two bottles. Realistically, this may be problematic because the vacuum in the bottles continues to aspirate the sample, so that one bottle may be overfilled with the other bottle being underfilled. The yield of blood cultures in adults increases approximately 3% per milliliter of blood cultured (5). Therefore, clinical microbiology laboratories should strive to obtain the optimal amount of blood for cultures. It should be noted that both Cockerill et al. (3) and Lee et al. (6) showed that more than three sets of blood cultures were necessary to reach 99% sensitivity of the culture system.

If endocarditis is suspected, at least three sets of blood cultures should be obtained from different venipuncture sites with the first and last samples drawn at least 1 h apart (7). If the acuity of the patient's condition is such that antimicrobial agents must be immediately administered (meningitis, acute sepsis, etc.), obtain two blood cultures of maximum volume from different sites consecutively before starting therapy.

Usually blood is inhibitory to the growth of microbial pathogens because blood contains substances such as antibodies, complement, lysozyme, and white blood cells capable of phagocytizing foreign substances. Additionally, the patient might have received antimicrobial agents prior to the veni-puncture. Therefore, to minimize the inhibitory activity of these factors, blood must be diluted into the blood culture media at a ratio of 1:5 to 1:10. Blood cultures may be falsely negative if the blood is not properly diluted at this ratio into the blood culture media (8). For both adult and pediatric patients, the time to detection inversely correlates with volume of blood cultured (9). For these patients, the recovery of pathogens increases as larger amounts of blood are placed into culture, since children frequently have lower levels of bacteremia than were previously thought to occur (10, 11). Guidelines published in 2013 recommended that smaller volumes of blood be placed into culture for pediatric patients or other patients who weigh less than 80 lbs (36.3 kg), Table 1 (see also chapter 8).

Table 1 Recommended pediatric blood culture volume[a]

Weight in kg (lb)	Venipuncture	Culture set[b]	Culture set[c]	Total blood volume
≤1 (≤2.2 lbs)	1 site	2 ml	–	2 ml
1.1–2 (2.4–5 lbs)	2 sites	2 ml	2 ml	4 ml
2.1–12.7 (5–28 lbs)	2 sites	4 ml	2 ml	6 ml
12.8–36.3 (28–80 lbs)	2 sites	5 ml	5 ml	10 ml
>36.3 (>80 lbs)		Treat as an adult		

[a]Adapted from reference 43.
[b]Aerobic bottle/pediatric bottle (if available).
[c]Aerobic, aerobic resin, or anaerobic bottle.

Pediatric blood culture bottles have been specifically designed to support the needs of these patients. As such, they have a smaller volume and better detection of fastidious organisms, thus optimizing the blood-to-broth ratio and time to detection when small volumes of blood are cultured. The media in these bottles have been reformulated to support the growth of known fastidious pediatric pathogens such as *Streptococcus pneumoniae*, *Haemophilus influenzae*, and *Neisseria meningitidis*. Despite these improvements over conventional blood culture bottles, it is debatable whether pediatric formulations provide any advantage over conventional blood culture bottles for small-volume samples (12).

Modern blood culture instruments are continuously monitored systems and indicate when cultures need to be examined for growth. Microscopic examination of a positive blood culture using a Gram stain is the most important and rapid factor influencing appropriate therapy. Barenfanger and colleagues (13) looked at the value of timely Gram stains and whether the results could improve patient outcomes. They documented a statistically significant increase in the mortality rate for patients who had blood cultures processed ≥1 h after being detected as positive. Of the 112 patients whose Gram stain reports were delayed, 21 patients (18.8%) died versus 8 of 86 patients (9%) whose Gram stains were read in less than 1 h ($P = 0.0624$). These results indicate that delay in obtaining Gram stain results was associated with significantly higher rates of mortality in septic patients. Possible solutions include periodic education and regular monitoring of turnaround times (TATs) for critical results and ensuring that time to detection is minimized by loading bottles into the instrument as soon as possible, as well as mandating the priority of reporting blood culture (and other sterile site) results.

Blood Cultures and Contamination

Contaminated blood cultures occur for a variety of reasons. They are responsible for increased health care costs and can lead to increased length of stay in hospitals, increased use of antimicrobial agents, and additional diagnostic testing. Although blood culture contamination rates vary between institutions, numerous studies have shown that blood obtained from indwelling vascular access devices has a much higher probability of being contaminated, particularly if the device has been in use longer than 48 h (14). When attempting to determine whether organisms isolated from a blood culture are significant or a contaminant, the following factors should be considered:

1. Was the isolate recovered from just one set of blood cultures or from two or more sets?
2. Was the isolate recovered from blood obtained by venipuncture or from an intravascular access device? If it was from an intravascular access device, was the same isolate recovered from venipuncture and from how many sets of blood cultures?
3. If any of the following organisms are recovered, they should only be considered significant if present in more than one set of blood cultures collected within a 24-h period:
   a. A single species of coagulase-negative staphylococci (excluding *Staphylococcus lugdunensis*)
   b. *Bacillus* species (excluding *B. anthracis*)
   c. *Corynebacterium* species
   d. *Propionibacterium* species
   e. Viridans group streptococci (excluding *Streptococcus bovis* group/ *gallolyticus*)
   f. *Lactobacillus* species
   g. *Micrococcus* species
4. Positive cultures may be excluded as contaminants if they are recovered from more than one blood culture in a series, provided that the isolates are of the same species and the antibiograms are identical or similar.

Since most blood for culture is obtained by venipuncture, skin antisepsis is critical to minimize the risk of contamination of blood cultures with skin flora. Although many skin disinfectants have been recommended for use, most laboratories/guidelines recommend the use of either chlorhexidine gluconate, tincture of iodine, or povidone-iodine. A randomized cross-over trial was performed to determine the effect of these skin disinfectants on blood culture contamination rates when blood was collected by trained phlebotomy teams (15, 16). In this study, all phlebotomy carts were kept stocked with supplies and all blood was obtained by venipuncture. A total of 12,904 sets of blood cultures were obtained. Of these, 735 sets of cultures (5.7%) were positive. There were also 98 contaminated cultures (13.3% of all positive cultures). Thus, the overall blood culture contamination rate was 0.76%. Importantly, rates of contaminated blood cultures were not significantly different among the three disinfectants. Other studies have shown that chlorhexidine gluconate was superior to povidone-iodine when blood was obtained by students, residents, or nurses in adult or pediatric emergency departments (17, 18). Povidone-iodine may be the best disinfectant based on price, but, when drying time is factored in, as well as the need to first clean the site with alcohol, phlebotomy costs increase.

As mentioned above, many factors are responsible for the increased cost of contaminated blood cultures to the health care system. Gilligan (15) described this eloquently in the following example: If a hospital performs 20,000 blood cultures annually and has a 2.5% contamination rate, while another hospital runs 30,000 blood cultures annually and has a 1% contamination rate, the cost of a contaminated blood culture at each hospital is approximately $5,000. The annual expense of contaminated blood cultures to the first hospital is $2,500,000 while the cost to the second hospital is $1,500,000. Additionally, in the first hospital, there would be more than 200 more days when a bed is unnecessarily occupied compared with the second hospital because of an increased length of stay of just 1 day per contamination event, typical of the effect on hospital stay of a contaminated blood culture.

Gilligan also described other negative effects of contaminated blood cultures. Patients are likely to receive antimicrobials that they do not need (15) and that may put them at risk for other complications such as allergic reactions, increased rates of colonization with vancomycin-resistant *Enterococcus* spp., methicillin-resistant *Staphylococcus aureus*, other multidrug-resistant organisms, and disease due to *Clostridium difficile*.

Each laboratory should maintain a monthly determination of the blood culture contamination rate. It is determined by dividing the number of cultures containing recognized contaminants by the total number of blood cultures. Separate blood culture contamination rates can be calculated for phlebotomy staff, nonlaboratory personnel who obtain blood cultures (physicians and nurses), separate collection locations, etc. With this information, additional training can be directed to those groups of persons involved in the collection of blood for culture but whose contamination rate exceeds 3% (although lower rates of contamination are admirable and achievable). In addition to having a well-trained phlebotomy team obtain blood for cultures, several studies have reported other factors that led to lower blood culture contamination rates, i.e., having phlebotomy supplies readily available on well-stocked carts and excellent adherence to aseptic techniques (16, 19–21).

Reducing blood culture contamination takes vigilance. All three skin disinfectants (chlorhexidine gluconate, tincture of iodine, povidone-iodine) are highly effective if used properly (16). Fewer contaminated blood cultures occur when dedicated phlebotomy teams perform the venipuncture compared with other medical personnel. If at all possible, avoid obtaining blood for culture from intravascular devices. If this is not possible, one blood culture should be obtained by venipuncture at the same time that blood is obtained from intravascular devices for comparison. Do not allow the collection of a single blood culture set, since it is impossible to determine if organisms such as viridans group streptococci and coagulase-negative staphylococci are contaminants or are significant. Finally, by following the contamination rate and tracking personnel who obtained those specimens, it is possible to reeducate and retrain so that there will be improved outcomes.

Verification and Validation of Blood Culture Systems

The most important qualities of an *in vitro* diagnostic (IVD) laboratory test are its ability to produce accurate, precise, and reproducible results over time. Two very important evaluations, verification and validation, are designed for this purpose. Automated blood culture instruments are considered to be IVDs and are, therefore, under the regulatory control of the FDA and the Centers for Medicare and Medicaid Services (CMS). As such, these systems require full verification prior to implementation (22). Designing appropriate test verification and validation plans can be confusing. The purpose of this section is to clarify the various regulatory requirements and discuss the various processes and procedures that can be used to fulfill these requirements (23).

In 1976, the Medical Device Amendments to the existing Food, Drug, and Cosmetic Act sought to expand the role of the FDA in the regulation of medical devices and further the Safe Medical Devices Act of 1990. A major revision of the 1976 amendments added additional provisions to better ensure that devices entering the market were safe and effective (22). This oversight confirms that there is appropriate and adequate scientific evidence supporting the claims of the manufacturers. In addition, as required by law outlined in the Federal Register 21 CFR 809.10: Labeling for *in vitro* diagnostic products, the FDA critically ensures the components of the package insert including intended use, specimen collection, transport, and storage recommendations; warnings and limitations; expected values; validation of cutoff; results and their interpretation; quality control recommendations; and specific performance characteristics (22).

All microbiology products that undergo this scientific evaluation of performance (verification) are expected by the FDA to maintain that performance throughout the life of the product (validation) and failure to maintain that expected performance could result in compliance or regulatory action. Oversight of the requirements for verification and validation is achieved through regulations contained within the Clinical Laboratory Improvement Amendments (CLIA) and enforcement through the College of American Pathology (CAP) and/or other regulatory bodies (22). According to Federal document 42 CFR 493.1253 Standard: Establishment and verification of performance specifications, each laboratory that introduces an unmodified, FDA-cleared test system must do the following before reporting patient test results: (i) Demonstrate that it can obtain performance specifications comparable to those established by the manufacturer for the following performance characteristics: (a) accuracy, (b) precision, (c) reportable range of test results for the test system. (ii) Verify that the manufacturer's reference intervals (normal values) are appropriate for the laboratory's patient population. In addition, all reagents, controls, and associated protocols included in the product insert must be followed exactly; this includes the FDA-approved specimens, collection devices, and transport conditions (22, 24). Therefore, verification is a one-time process to determine the performance characteristics of the test as claimed by the manufacturer (22). Verification must be able to demonstrate that the laboratory can obtain performance specifications comparable to those established by the manufacturer. The extent of this verification process, i.e., the number of positive and negative specimens, and required performance characteristics, is dependent on the FDA IVD class level and CLIA-defined complexity. Verification can range from a rather simple comparison between two systems to a much more complex analysis.

In addition to initial verification requirements, document 42 CFR 493.1701 Standard: Medicare, Medicaid and CLIA programs; laboratory requirements relating to quality systems and certain personnel qualifications; final rule, continued analysis of a test performance is required. This process, known as validation, is ongoing to monitor and ensure that the test continues to perform as expected and is typically achieved through the laboratory's quality assurance plan (22).

Deviations from FDA-approved protocols can occur, but they must first be put through a more rigorous verification process similar to that for laboratory-developed tests (LDTs); for more information on LDTs, please see Cumitech 31A (22). A deviation for a blood culture instrument might include any body fluids not initially approved by the FDA, such as peritoneal, synovial, or bile, or other specimens such as bone marrow. In addition to specimen type, any new media, i.e., antimicrobial neutralization media, need to be verified prior to implementing in the clinical microbiology laboratory. While there are no official guidelines on which and how many antimicrobials are tested in the new media, there are several published studies outlining some options. In one case, the authors chose to test the most frequently used antimicrobials overall in their particular health system (25), while others chose those antimicrobials that were typically used to empirically treat sepsis (26, 27). Therefore, the choice of which and how many antimicrobial agents to test in the new system and/or media is left to the laboratory director; however, the choice of agents should, at the very least, be those antimicrobials that are used to empirically treat sepsis and/or acute illness and should cross over several families of antimicrobials.

Federal Regulation: The Role of the FDA

The FDA divides medical devices into four main classes (exempt, class I, class II, or class III) based on two primary factors: (i) the level of quality control necessary to ensure the safety and effectiveness of the device. For example, class II devices may require additional, specialized controls, including special labeling requirements, mandatory performance standards, and development of patient registries, and (ii) devices may include a requirement for postmarket surveillance (22, 24) depending on the level of risk of causing harm to a patient associated with their use, for example, whether the device is a tongue depressor (class I) or replacement heart valves (class III) (22). Not only do these classifications define the level of quality control (QC) needed, they also dictate one of two processes the manufacturer must complete to obtain FDA clearance or approval to market their product, namely, premarket notification [510(k)] or premarket approval (PMA). Most devices are cleared for commercial distribution in the United States by the premarket notification, also known as a [510(k)] process (22). Premarket notifications are generally associated with class I, class II, and some class III devices, whereby there are existing devices currently FDA approved and in use in the United States. If the FDA analysis of a premarket notification submission determines that it is significantly comparable to a currently approved and marketed device, the device is cleared and the manufacturer is free to market it in the United States (22). However, a premarket approval is a much more stringent and rigorous process required by the FDA for class III devices where there are no currently FDA-approved devices in use. For approval, submission must contain sufficient valid scientific evidence that provides reasonable assurance that the device is safe and effective for its intended use (22). There are some minor exclusions to these classifications, for example, some class I devices may require a premarket notification [510(k)] based on their stated or purported use. These devices are referred to as "reserved" class I devices, and blood culture systems are an example (22, 28).

Blood Culture Systems and Media: Verification of Automated Systems

The ability to detect agents of bacteremia and fungemia with speed and precision remains one of the most important roles of the clinical microbiology laboratory because their ascribable mortality can be as high as 12% (29). Furthermore, rapid and accurate detection and identification of the infecting agent are crucial for the implementation of appropriate antimicrobial therapy (30). Consequently, a well-designed, meaningful verification of a new blood culture system can be one of the most difficult tasks facing the clinical microbiologist. There are two primary methods of performing a blood culture system verification: a prospective, parallel-draw blood culture comparison and a seeded blood culture analysis of performance. While the choice of performing a parallel-draw, prospective study may seem like the best option over a seeded study, parallel-draw testing requires collection of additional blood from each patient, which may not be possible in some patient populations or institutions. Furthermore, this type of study would require an institutional review board-approved procedure to obtain patient consent for the extra blood draw. Because of the low level of positivity for clinical pathogens (usually in the range of 8 to 14%) (31), most of the specimens collected will be of little value in the comparison, with the exception of assay specificity. In addition, the incidence of contamination (usually 1 to 3%) and predominance of a limited number of pathogens may result in an evaluation skewed toward only a few of the potentially clinically significant organisms. Because of this, a French working group had made the recommendation of evaluating at least 1,000 blood culture sets where both positive and negative cultures were to be subsequently subcultured to determine sensitivity and specificity versus culture as the gold standard (32). Seeded blood culture studies are considerably less difficult and require fewer sets to reach a similar goal, as is outlined in more detail below and in Appendix B.

Blood Culture Systems

There are three primary FDA-cleared, automated blood culture detection systems currently available using a variety of different media types, antimicrobial inhibitor solutions and concentrations, and detection methods (28, 33). Depending on the patient population, primarily pediatric versus adult and/or organisms targeted (fungal, bacterial, acid fast), the choice of instrument and media type and the subsequent verification study can vary.

All automated blood cultures systems detect growth as a measure of CO_2 production during bacterial growth; however, there are two primary mechanisms to monitor CO_2 production. Both the BD Bactec system (Becton Dickinson, Sparks, MD) and the various BacT/Alert systems (bioMérieux, Durham, NC) use colorimetric or fluorometric detection of CO_2 over time (33). In contrast, the VersaTREK system (TREK Diagnostics, Cleveland, OH) measures the CO_2 pressure in the headspace of the bottles (33). These systems monitor the CO_2 production anywhere from 10 to 24 times per minute. Computer algorithms then analyze the data to determine whether the CO_2 is increasing or remains stable and, if the appropriate criteria are met, flag the bottles as positive for removal and subsequent culture (33). For a detailed review of all blood culture systems and available detection technologies, see subsequent chapters in this text, the CLSI M47-A (8), or Cumitech 1C (34). In addition to variation in detection methods, there are a number of different types of media that can be used. Some of these are designed for low-volume application such as the BD Bactec Peds Plus/F medium bottles and the BacT/Alert PF bottles; media designed for specific organisms such as the Bactec Lytic bottles for anaerobes or those media containing compounds designed to inhibit antimicrobials in the blood, such as the BacT/Alert FAN and FAN Plus bottles and the Bactec Plus aerobic bottles. To this end, there may be differences in the time to positivity that is dependent on both detection method and type of media bottles used (35). Therefore, blood culture system verification studies should be designed to answer the following fundamental questions:

- Will the instrument detect, in a timely fashion, the majority of pathogenic organisms from blood cultures that contain these microorganisms?
- Will the media used by the system support the growth of organisms (including yeasts, anaerobes, and fastidious organisms, where appropriate) commonly seen in the user's patient population?

There are two approaches for verification of blood culture systems, which are discussed below. As indicated previously, while performing a prospective, parallel-draw study would truly demonstrate the system's ability to detect bacteremia or fungemia in an actual patient population, the number of cultures and time required would be prohibitive in comparison with a seeded study. However, laboratories can choose to combine these approaches to take advantage of the strong points of each; for example, the laboratory could perform prospective parallel studies to assess the ability of the system to detect commonly isolated organisms and use seeded blood cultures to assess less common pathogens (22).

As blood culture instruments evolve, there may be circumstances in which the laboratory is implementing a newer version of its existing system. Depending on the nature of the changes to the new system version, a verification study may not be necessary. This is particularly true if the primary differences are limited to the blood culture instrument (e.g., hardware and software), and the blood culture bottles and/or media types did not change (22). If this is the case, then an instrument function check by the vendor's technical representative to verify that incubation and optical systems and software are operating per manufacturer's specifications is sufficient to verify the performance of the entire blood culture system (22).

Seeded Blood Culture Studies

Seeded blood culture studies are considerably faster and less expensive than a parallel-draw study. In addition, the laboratory can select any combination of true pathogens and typical contaminating bacterial species typically seen in its health system. Furthermore, a seeded study allows for the laboratory to use organisms that are rare but do cause very severe and often fatal infections, such as such as *N. meningitidis* and *Brucella* species (with appropriate biosafety!). Human blood contains a variety of compounds, enzymes, and antibodies, not to mention white blood cells, that may have an effect on microbial growth (33). Therefore, the primary downside to performing a seeded culture study is obtaining human blood for the study (see Appendix A). To have a robust verification study, a minimum of 20 representatives of blood culture isolates normally seen in the institution should be used. These organisms should include both Gram-positive and Gram-negative bacteria and yeasts, as appropriate for the health system and, whenever possible, use actual patient isolates previously cultured and stored at −20°C rather than stock strains (22). To challenge the system, the amount of blood to be used for the study would have to be greater than or equal to the minimum volume suggested or required by the manufacturer. The concentration of organisms placed in each bottle should also approximate those found in cases of septicemia (which can be less than 0.1 CFU per ml of blood) (31). This is done by making serial dilutions of the organisms prior to inoculation to achieve approximately 5 to 30 CFU per bottle (22). An example of how to prepare the organism suspension and seed human blood for this type of study is outlined in Appendix B.

There are no well-documented definitive requirements to guide acceptance of the results obtained from seeded blood culture system verification studies. However, Cumitech 31A does suggest at least 90% accuracy when performing verifications in general (22). It would be expected that, if one were to seed a blood culture with a specific organism with sufficient aseptic technique, the same organism would be recovered 100% of the time. The time to positivity (TTP) between the two systems or new units of the same system must be consistent with the literature for given organisms (22) and should not be significantly different among the seeded cultures. Typically, as few as 3 days may be sufficient to recover at least 95% of clinically relevant bacteria and yeasts (8), but, again, there are no guidelines that define "significant" in these settings. There are several very good papers that describe seeded studies and the acceptability criteria for time to positivity, etc., used therein (25, 36–39). As such, it is the clinical laboratory director's responsibility to determine the acceptability of any particular study design. Last, because the bottles are seeded with viable organisms, as confirmed with plate counts of organism suspensions, any problems with detection should be investigated by repeating the tests with the same strains. If detection is still not obtained, analysis of the root cause and corrective action must be taken by the user and/or the manufacturer prior to introducing use of the system in the laboratory. Overall, the method is considered verified if all isolates are detected within timeframes specified by the user.

Parallel Blood Culture Studies

Performance of parallel blood cultures allows the laboratory to evaluate all aspects of the new system under actual patient and laboratory conditions. When a laboratory chooses to perform parallel studies of commercially available systems, duplicate sets of blood cultures inoculated with equivalent blood volumes should be obtained until a minimum of 20 positive blood cultures (not to include contaminants [8]) representative of the blood culture isolates normally seen in the institution are evaluated (8). As with seeded studies, there is scant literature on the acceptability criteria for the study; however, as suggested in Cumitech 31A, the new method is considered verified if the sensitivity is at least 95%, relative to the reference method, and times to positivity are not significantly different (22). Since blood culture bottles from a parallel study are inoculated simultaneously, any discrepant results, i.e., growth in one and not the other, obtained between the two systems should be critically analyzed via chart review to determine contamination versus true pathogens.

A note on TTP: It is important to note that it is up to the laboratory director's discretion to define what difference in TTP is "significant" because there are no available guidelines; however, there is good evidence that delays in TTP, for whatever reason, can have significant effects on patient outcomes. For example, Kumar et al. (40) determined that for every hour of delay in TTP resulting in a delay in the administration of appropriate antimicrobial agents resulted in an increase in mortality or timely and effective deescalation of empiric therapy (1). Further, it has been shown that delays in TTP may result in delays in performing and reporting Gram stain results. In one study by Barenfanger et al., it was reported that delays of ≥ 1 h in processing positive blood cultures resulted in a significant increase in crude patient mortality (10.1 and 19.2%, respectively, $P = 0.389$) (13). Therefore, it would be reasonable to deduce that delays in TTP will result in delays in processing blood cultures and reporting Gram stain results. To that end, it is recommended herein that differences in TTP should be within ≤ 2 h of each instrument and/or media type used for aerobic/facultative anaerobic organisms and within 5 hours for anaerobes and yeast. For health systems that use core microbiology laboratories where blood cultures are delivered to the laboratory from outside locations, it is also important that the verification includes a simulated delay in receiving the bottles and placing on the instruments to determine sensitivity of the system. Several early studies noted that delayed blood culture incubation does lead to an increase in time to detect growth and, in some cases, false negatives (35, 41). More recently, Koh et al. demonstrated that in the case of microbiology laboratories that do not have an evening shift, delaying loading of the bottles on the instruments, preincubation of the bottles at 37°C still results in an earlier TTP (42). Therefore, in performing a study such as this, it may become apparent that logistics require the laboratory to place instruments at the outside locations or prepare to incubate the bottles during transport to the core laboratory.

Conclusion

In conclusion, the ability to detect agents of bacteremia and fungemia with speed and precision remains one of the most important roles of the clinical microbiology laboratory because their ascribable mortality can be as high as 12% (29). Conversely, errors in collection resulting in poor sensitivity associated with low blood volumes and improper handling of the blood draw leading to contaminants may result in unnecessary testing, use of antimicrobial agents, and lengthier hospitalization. Therefore, it is critical for the clinical microbiology laboratory to determine which automated blood system and media combination works best for the local health system. Unfortunately, a meaningful verification of a new blood culture system can be one of the most difficult tasks facing the clinical microbiologist. While there are no definitive guidelines for verification acceptance of blood culture systems specifically, the minimum recommendations here are for at least 90% accuracy if performing a seeded verification and at least 95% accuracy criteria for parallel-draw verifications. Measurement of accuracy should include the standard deviation of time to positivity between different systems and/or similar units of the same system and organism identification.

Acknowledgments

The authors would like to thank Dr. Linoj Samuel for the use of some of the information contained in the verification example in Appendix A and Appendix B.

References

1. Dellinger RP, Levy MM, Rhodes A, Annane D, Gerlach H, Opal SM, Sevransky JE, Sprung CL, Douglas IS, Jaeschke R, Osborn TM, Nunnally ME, Townsend SR, Reinhart K, Kleinpell RM, Angus DC, Deutschman CS, Machado FR, Rubenfeld GD, Webb SA, Beale RJ, Vincent JL, Moreno R, Surviving Sepsis Campaign Guidelines Committee including the Pediatric Subgroup. 2013. Surviving sepsis campaign: international guidelines for management of severe sepsis and septic shock: 2012. *Crit Care Med* **41**:580–637.
2. Jaimes F, Arango C, Ruiz G, Cuervo J, Botero J, Vélez G, Upegui N, Machado F. 2004. Predicting bacteremia at the bedside. *Clin Infect Dis* **38**:357–362.
3. Lee A, Mirrett S, Reller LB, Weinstein MP. 2007. Detection of bloodstream infections in adults: how many blood cultures are needed? *J Clin Microbiol* **45**:3546–3548.
4. Riedel S, Bourbeau P, Swartz B, Brecher S, Carroll KC, Stamper PD, Dunne WM, McCardle T, Walk N, Fiebelkorn K, Sewell D, Richter SS, Beekmann S, Doern GV. 2008. Timing of specimen collection for blood cultures from febrile patients with bacteremia. *J Clin Microbiol* **46**:1381–1385.
5. Mermel LA, Maki DG. 1993. Detection of bacteremia in adults: consequences of culturing an inadequate volume of blood. *Ann Intern Med* **119**:270–272.
6. Cockerill FR III, Wilson JW, Vetter EA, Goodman KM, Torgerson CA, Harmsen WS, Schleck CD, Ilstrup DM, Washington JA II, Wilson WR. 2004. Optimal testing parameters for blood cultures. *Clin Infect Dis* **38**:1724–1730.

7. Baddour LM, Wilson WR, Bayer AS, Fowler VG Jr, Tleyjeh IM, Tybak MJ, Barsic B, Lockhart PB, Gewitz MH, Levison ME, Bolger AF, Steckelberg JM, Baltimore RS, Fink AM, O'Gara P, Taubert KA; American Heart Association Committee on Rheumatic Fever, Endocarditis, and Kawasaki Disease of the Council on Cardiovascular Disease in the Young, Council of Clinical Cardiology, Council on Cardiovascular Surgery and Anesthesia, and Stroke Council. 2015. Infective endocarditis in adults: diagnosis, antimicrobial therapy, and management of complications: a scientific statement for healthcare professionals from the American Heart Association. *Circulation* 132:1435–1486.

8. CLSI. 2007. Principles and Procedures for Blood Cultures; Approved Guideline. CLSI Document M47-A. CLSI, Wayne, PA.

9. Isaacman DJ, Karasic RB, Reynolds EA, Kost SI. 1996. Effect of number of blood cultures and volume of blood on detection of bacteremia in children. *J Pediatr* 128:190–195.

10. Kellogg JA, Manzella JP, Bankert DA. 2000. Frequency of low-level bacteremia in children from birth to fifteen years of age. *J Clin Microbiol* 38:2181–2185.

11. Schelonka RL, Chai MK, Yoder BA, Hensley D, Brockett RM, Ascher DP. 1996. Volume of blood required to detect common neonatal pathogens. *J Pediatr* 129:275–278.

12. Dien Bard J, McElvania TeKippe E. 2016. Diagnosis of bloodstream infections in children. *J Clin Microbiol* 54:1418–1424.

13. Barenfanger J, Graham DR, Kolluri L, Sangwan G, Lawhorn J, Drake CA, Verhulst SJ, Peterson R, Moja LB, Ertmoed MM, Moja AB, Shevlin DW, Vautrain R, Callahan CD. 2008. Decreased mortality associated with prompt Gram staining of blood cultures. *Am J Clin Pathol* 130:870–876.

14. Bryant JK, Strand CL. 1987. Reliability of blood cultures collected from intravascular catheter versus venipuncture. *Am J Clin Pathol* 88:113–116.

15. Gilligan PH. 2013. Blood culture contamination: a clinical and financial burden. *Infect Control Hosp Epidemiol* 34:22–23.

16. Washer LL, Chenoweth C, Kim HW, Rogers MA, Malani AN, Riddell J IV, Kuhn L, Noeyack B Jr, Neusius H, Newton DW, Saint S, Flanders SA. 2013. Blood culture contamination: a randomized trial evaluating the comparative effectiveness of 3 skin antiseptic interventions. *Infect Control Hosp Epidemiol* 34:15–21.

17. Marlowe L, Mistry RD, Coffin S, Leckerman KH, McGowan KL, Dai D, Bell LM, Zaoutis T. 2010. Blood culture contamination rates after skin antisepsis with chlorhexidine gluconate versus povidone-iodine in a pediatric emergency department. *Infect Control Hosp Epidemiol* 31:171–176.

18. Suwanpimolkul G, Pongkumpai M, Suankratay C. 2008. A randomized trial of 2% chlorhexidine tincture compared with 10% aqueous povidone-iodine for venipuncture site disinfection: effects on blood culture contamination rates. *J Infect* 56:354–359.

19. Bekeris LG, Tworek JA, Walsh MK, Valenstein PN. 2005. Trends in blood culture contamination: a College of American Pathologists Q-Tracks study of 356 institutions. *Arch Pathol Lab Med* 129:1222–1225.

20. Boyce JM, Nadeau J, Dumigan D, Miller D, Dubowsky C, Reilly L, Hannon CV. 2013. Obtaining blood cultures by venipuncture versus from central lines: impact on

blood culture contamination rates and potential effect on central line-associated bloodstream infection reporting. *Infect Control Hosp Epidemiol* 34:1042–1047.

21. **Weinstein MP.** 2003. Blood culture contamination: persisting problems and partial progress. *J Clin Microbiol* **41:**2275–2278.
22. **Clark RB, Lewinski MA, Loeffelholz MJ, Tibbetts RJ.** 2009. *Cumitech 31A, Verification and Validation of Procedures in the Clinical Microbiology Laboratory.* ASM Press, Washington, DC.
23. **Tibbetts R.** 2015. Verification and validation of tests used in the clinical microbiology laboratory. *Clin Microbiol Newsl* **37:**153–160.
24. **CDC, Centers for Medicare & Medicaid Services.** 2003. Medicare, Medicaid, and CLIA programs; laboratory requirements relating to quality systems and certain personnel qualifications; final rule. *Fed Regist* **68:**3639–3714.
25. **Flayhart D, Borek AP, Wakefield T, Dick J, Carroll KC.** 2007. Comparison of BACTEC PLUS blood culture media to BacT/Alert FA blood culture media for detection of bacterial pathogens in samples containing therapeutic levels of antibiotics. *J Clin Microbiol* **45:**816–821.
26. **Crepin O, Roussel-Delvallez M, Martin GR, Courcol RJ.** 1993. Effectiveness of resins in removing antibiotics from blood cultures. *J Clin Microbiol* **31:**734–735.
27. **Mitteregger D, Barousch W, Nehr M, Kundi M, Zeitlinger M, Makristathis A, Hirschl AM.** 2013. Neutralization of antimicrobial substances in new BacT/Alert FA and FN Plus blood culture bottles. *J Clin Microbiol* **51:**1534–1540.
28. **Truant AL.** 2002. *Manual of Commercial Methods in Clinical Microbiology.* ASM Press, Washington, DC.
29. **Pien BC, Sundaram P, Raoof N, Costa SF, Mirrett S, Woods CW, Reller LB, Weinstein MP.** 2010. The clinical and prognostic importance of positive blood cultures in adults. *Am J Med* **123:**819–828.
30. **Wilson ML, Weinstein MP, Reller LB.** 2007. Laboratory detection of bacteremia and fungemia, p 15–28. *In* Murray PR, Baron EJ, Jorgenson JH, Landry ML, Pfaller MA (ed), *Manual of Clinical Microbiology,* 9th ed. American Society for Microbiology, Washington, DC.
31. **Carroll KC, Weinstein MP.** 2007. Manual and automated systems for detection and identification of microorganisms, p 192–217. *In* Murray PR, Baron EJ, Jorgenson JH, Landry ML, Pfaller MA (ed), *Manual of Clinical Microbiology,* 9th ed. American Society for Microbiology, Washington, DC.
32. **Rohner P, Auckenthaler R.** 1999. Review on evaluations of currently available bloodculture systems. *Clin Microbiol Infect* **5:**513–529.
33. **Riedel S, Carroll KC.** 2010. Blood cultures: key elements for best practices and future directions. *J Infect Chemother* **16:**301–316.
34. **Baron EJ, Weinstein MP, Dunne WM Jr, Yagupsky P, Welch DF, Wilson DM.** 2005. *Cumitech 1C, Blood Cultures IV.* ASM Press, Washington, DC.
35. **Banerjee R, Özenci V, Patel R.** 2016. Individualized approaches are needed for optimized blood cultures. *Clin Infect Dis* **63:**1332–1339.
36. **Almuhayawi M, Altun O, Abdulmajeed AD, Ullberg M, Özenci V.** 2015. The performance of the four anaerobic blood culture bottles BacT/ALERT-FN, -FN Plus, BACTEC-Plus and -Lytic in detection of anaerobic bacteria and identification by direct MALDI-TOF MS. *PLoS One* **10:**e0142398.

37. Altun O, Almuhayawi M, Lüthje P, Taha R, Ullberg M, Özenci V. 2016. Controlled evaluation of the new BacT/Alert Virtuo blood culture system for detection and time to detection of bacteria and yeasts. *J Clin Microbiol* 54:1148–1151.
38. Ericson EL, Klingspor L, Ullberg M, Ozenci V. 2012. Clinical comparison of the Bactec Mycosis IC/F, BacT/Alert FA, and BacT/Alert FN blood culture vials for the detection of candidemia. *Diagn Microbiol Infect Dis* 73:153–156.
39. Marlowe EM, Gibson L, Hogan J, Kaplan S, Bruckner DA. 2003. Conventional and molecular methods for verification of results obtained with BacT/Alert Nonvent blood culture bottles. *J Clin Microbiol* 41:1266–1269.
40. Kumar A, Haery C, Paladugu B, Kumar A, Symeoneides S, Taiberg L, Osman J, Trenholme G, Opal SM, Goldfarb R, Parrillo JE. 2006. The duration of hypotension before the initiation of antibiotic treatment is a critical determinant of survival in a murine model of *Escherichia coli* septic shock: association with serum lactate and inflammatory cytokine levels. *J Infect Dis* 193:251–258.
41. Sautter RL, Bills AR, Lang DL, Ruschell G, Heiter BJ, Bourbeau PP. 2006. Effects of delayed-entry conditions on the recovery and detection of microorganisms from BacT/ALERT and BACTEC blood culture bottles. *J Clin Microbiol* 44:1245–1249.
42. Koh EH, Lee DH, Kim S. 2014. Effects of preincubating blood culture bottles at 37oC during the night shift and of collected blood volume on time to detection and days to final report. *Ann Clin Microbio* 17:14–19.
43. Baron EJ, Miller JM, Weinstein MP, Richter SS, Gilligan PH, Thomson RB Jr, Bourbeau P, Carroll KC, Kehl SC, Dunne WM, Robinson-Dunn B, Schwartzman JD, Chapin KC, Snyder JW, Forbes BA, Patel R, Rosenblatt JE, Pritt BS. 2013. A guide to utilization of the microbiology laboratory for diagnosis of infectious diseases: 2013 recommendations by the Infectious Diseases Society of America (IDSA) and the American Society for Microbiology (ASM)(a). *Clin Infect Dis* 57:e22–e121.

APPENDIX A EXAMPLE OF BLOOD CULTURE SYSTEM VERIFICATION

The laboratory in this example currently has five units of Blood Culture System-A (BCSA) and wishes to bring in three additional units because volume has increased. No changes in the bottle or media types will be necessary. The following example outlines a seeded verification study designed to compare three new units with units currently used in the laboratory. This blood culture system uses bottles with a 5-ml minimum fill requirement. While this example is comparing the same instruments, the same type of study design can be used to verify entirely new systems without comparison to an existing system or two different systems. Bacterial isolates were subcultured on standard media, and expired blood product from the department's blood bank was used as a matrix. Instructions for making the bacterial dilutions used to spike human blood specimens are found in Appendix B.

Materials and methods

At least 20 various bacterial isolates comprising typical blood pathogens and contaminants of aerobic and anaerobic, Gram-negative and Gram-positive bacilli, and Gram-positive cocci will be used to spike blood culture bottle sets (one aerobic and one anaerobic bottle) with the addition of expired whole blood. The bottle sets will be made in quadruplicate: one set will be placed in any of the five existing BCSA instruments to act as the "gold standard" for the study, and each of the remaining three sets will be placed in each of the three new BSCA instruments as the "comparator." Approximately 5 to 50 CFU of each bacterial isolate will used to spike each bottle of each set. In addition, 10 negative controls containing whole blood only will be included, spread across the three new instruments, which will be incubated a total of 5 days before removing from the units. Plate counts of the bacterial suspensions will be performed in triplicate to ensure proper bacterial density in each set and no growth in the negative control sets (also see Appendix B). Time to positivity (TTP) will be recorded for each positive bottle/set. The TTP average for positive bottles for each bacterial species from the three new instruments will be averaged and recorded. As the primary means to compare the new and old instruments, the standard deviation between the TTP of the positive bottles from the existing instruments and the new instruments will be determined and compared. All positive bottles will be Gram stained and plated. Colony and bacterial morphologies will be compared with what was used to inoculate them for accuracy. Whole-blood-only negative cultures that did not flag positive will be terminally plated after 5 days to ensure the sensitivity of the instruments.

Validation assumption

The standard deviation of the average TTP of the new instruments should not exceed 1 h when compared to the TTP of the same bacterial species from the existing instruments. In addition, there will be no positive signals from the whole-blood-only negative cultures nor will there be any growth from these bottles after terminal plating.

Results

In this example, bacterial plate counts ranged from 0.0 to 14.7 CFU per bottle. Overall, the range of TTP standard deviation was 0.0 to 0.8 h for aerobic bottles and 0.0 to 4.1 h for anaerobic bottles. However, three culture sets exceeded the 1-h standard deviation assumption. Upon review of the data, two of the replicates where the standard deviation exceeded 1 h were attributed to aerobic/facultative anaerobic bacteria grown anaerobically and in the other was an anaerobe grown anaerobically. No whole-blood-only negative control cultures went positive nor was there any growth after terminal plating. All Gram stain and colony morphology accuracy was 100%. However, three of the positive bacterial cultures contained the spiked organism and an additional bacterial species, i.e., contaminated. A critical review of the process indicated that the contaminating organism was carried over from the bacterial species used in the previous replicates. Since bacterial cultures can be contaminated in clinical practice, we do not feel that these results invalidate the verification.

Conclusion
Based on the data obtained during this verification of new units of the same blood culture system currently in use in the laboratory, it was concluded that the new units performed as expected and were comparable to the existing units in place. The new blood culture system units were verified and placed into use in the laboratory.

APPENDIX B BACTERIAL DILUTIONS AND PLATE COUNTS
Materials

- Pipettes
- Dilution tubes and racks
- Disposable spreaders
- Appropriate agar plates for each organism
  - Sheep blood agar (SBA) for most organisms to be incubated in CO_2 at 37°C
  - Chocolate agar (CHOC) for *Haemophilus* species to be incubated in CO_2 at 37°C
  - MacConkey (MAC) agar for *Proteus* species to be incubated in CO_2 37°C
  - Pre-reduced anaerobic blood agar plate for *Bacillus fragilis*, *Fusobacterium nucleatum*, and *Clostridium perfringens* to be incubated at 37°C in the anaerobic chamber
  - Campylobacter media for *Campylobacter* species to be incubated at 42°C in microaerophilic bag
- 1-ml, 100-μl, and 10-μl pipettes and tips
- Plastic test tube for dilution A
- 50-ml conical tube
- Manual pipette and bulb for 50-ml tube

Methods to perform serial 1:1,000-fold dilutions and final concentration plate counts. All work should be performed aseptically in the hood with proper personal protective equipment (PPE).

1. Appropriately label five tubes A through E and aliquot sterile saline into dilution tubes prior to starting.
    * Tube A = 3.0 ml
    * Tubes B and C = 990 µl
    * Tube D = 900 µl
    * Tube E = 4.0 ml
2. Prepare a 0.5 McFarland preparation of the organism in 3.0 ml saline; this is dilution A, and the bacterial density is 1.0×10^8 CFU/ml. Pipette up and down several times and vortex vigorously.
3. Transfer 10 µl of dilution A into 990 µl of saline; this is dilution B, and the bacterial density is 1.0×10^6 CFU/ml. Pipette up and down several times and vortex vigorously.
4. Transfer 10 µl of dilution B to 990 µl of saline; this is dilution C, and the bacterial density is 1.0×10^4 CFU/ml. Pipette up and down several times and vortex vigorously.
5. Transfer 100 µl of dilution C to 900 µl of saline; this is dilution D and the bacterial density is 1.0×10^3 CFU/ml. Pipette up and down several times and vortex vigorously.
6. Transfer 500 µl of dilution D to 4.5 ml of saline; this is dilution E and the bacterial density is 1.0×10^2 CFU/ml. Pipette up and down several times and vortex vigorously.
7. Transfer dilution E into a 50-ml conical tube for easy access in hood.
8. Plate 100 µl of dilution D to appropriate culture media for the organism being diluted in triplicate for colony counts; make sure to vortex suspension between each plate. Using a disposable spreader, spread the aliquot over the entire plate until evenly distributed and incubated at the appropriate temperature and air conditions for the bacterial species being used.
9. Following incubation, count the number of colonies and enter values into the data collection sheet (see Table 2).
    * If there is more than one colony type on these plates, please indicate in the comments section and keep the plates. If there is no contamination, the plates can be discarded.

Table 2 Example of a data collection sheet[a]

| | Time to positivity (TTP) | | | | | | | | | | | |
| | Existing Instrument | | Instrument F | | Instrument G | | Instrument H | | Average | | SD-Aer | SD-Ana | Comments |
	Aer	Ana	Aer	Ana	Aer	Ana	Aer	Ana	Aer	Ana			
Enterobacteriaceae													
Escherichia coli	10.3	11.1	10.3	11.9	9.7	10.7	10.3	11.1	10.1	11.2	0.1	0.1	
Klebsiella	10.3	11.9	10.5	11.5	10.1	11.1	10.1	11.5	10.2	11.4	0.0	0.4	
Enterobacter cloacae	10.8	11.9	10.9	11.9	10.3	11.9	10.9	11.9	10.7	11.9	0.1	0.0	
Salmonella	11.9	13.1	11.5	13.1	10.7	12.7	11.7	13.1	11.3	13.0	0.4	0.1	
Gram-positive cocci													
Staphylococcus aureus	12.9	15.1	12.9	ND	12.7	14.3	13.1	19.1	12.9	16.7	0.0	1.1	

[a]The same format can be used for plate counts, TTP, Gram stain, and colony morphology. Aer, aerobic; Ana, anaerobic; SD, standard deviation.

Preparation of four sets of blood culture bottles appropriately labeled for each organism. All work should be performed aseptically in the hood with proper PPE.

Materials

- Alcohol and iodine wipes
- 10- and 20-ml syringes
- 1-ml tuberculin syringes
- 18-gauge needles
- Gauze and tape
- Bags of expired blood from blood bank and wire basket to place the bag into
- One SBA plate (for blood bag purity)
- Waste containers

Methods

1. Label each set of cultures with a unique identifier for recording results, including which instrument, 1 through 7, they will be placed into.
2. Prior to inoculation of the bottles, carefully clean the rubber septum with alcohol wipe and allow to dry. Do not use the iodine on the septum, because residual iodine may inhibit the bacteria in the bottles.
3. For each bacterial suspension, setup one aerobic bottle, one anaerobic bottle, and one agar plate that is appropriate for the species of bacteria used for the suspension.
4. Use iodine wipes to clean the puncture site on the outside of the blood bag (do not go in through the port; puncture the side of the bag).
   - Intermittently invert the blood bag several times to mix.
   - As the blood volume decreases, multiple puncture sites will be necessary.
5. Using a single 10-ml syringe per set, draw up just over 8.0 ml of blood and dispense 4.0 ml into each bottle of the set one after another. Do not go back into the blood bag with the same needle.
6. Immediately place a drop or two of blood remaining in the syringe used to inoculate the bottles onto the agar plate.
7. Using a disposable spreader, spread the blood over the entire plate until evenly distributed and incubated at the appropriate temperature and air conditions for the bacterial species being used.

- If sufficient blood remains in the bag following inoculation of the day's blood culture sets, thoroughly clean the outside of the bag with iodine and tape gauze over the puncture site(s).

8. From dilution E above use a single tuberculin syringe per set to draw up 500 µl of the bacterial suspension and inoculate each bottle with 250 µl.

9. Repeat steps 1 through 8 for the whole-blood-only negative controls. Replace dilution E with sterile saline.

10. Load bottles into the various BCSA units as described above.

11. For positive blood culture bottles
    - Depending on the type of detection system used, print out either the pressure graph and/or record the TTP, label with bottle number and unit in the data collection sheet and retain.
    - Prepare a Gram stain of each positive set from both the aerobic and anaerobic bottles from each replicate and record Gram reaction, morphology, and arrangement in the data collection sheet.
    - Subculture each bottle onto the appropriate agar plates as needed and incubate appropriately overnight or longer for some anaerobic organisms. Keep all bottles until the end of the study.
    - Following overnight incubation, record the colony morphology on the data collection sheet.
    - If there are differences in colony morphology between either the aerobic and anaerobic bottles or from machine to machine, indicate this in the comments section.
    - Gram stain each distinct colony type and indicate in the comments section.

12. For negative blood culture bottles
    - After 5 days, remove the negative bottles, print out the growth charts for each and retain.
    - Terminally culture the blood from these sets and incubate appropriately. Gram stain and record any positive growth; however, after 5 days of incubation record the results as no-growth.
    - If any negative bottle signals positive, perform the steps outlined above for positive blood culture bottles.

The Dark Art of Blood Cultures
Edited by Wm. Michael Dunne, Jr. and Carey-Ann D. Burnham
© 2018 American Society for Microbiology, Washington, DC
doi:10.1128/9781555819811.ch11

Processing Positive Cultures   11

Matthew L. Faron[1] and Nathan A. Ledeboer[1]

Introduction

It can be said that the diagnosis of bloodstream infections is one of the most important roles of the clinical microbiology laboratory; the mortality rate associated with bloodstream infection ranges from 25 to 80% (1, 2). There are a number of factors that contribute to the mortality rate subsequent to bloodstream infection, with time to appropriate antimicrobial therapy frequently cited as one of the most important variables correlating with clinical outcome (3–5). Herein, we describe procedures for optimization of positive blood culture specimens and describe current and future methodologies to augment blood culture to diagnose bloodstream infection.

Laboratory Organization

Results of a positive blood culture can be delayed if bottles that have signaled positive by a continuously monitored blood culture instrument are left unattended. As such, optimizing the layout and organization of the laboratory can impact timely report of blood culture results and ultimately patient welfare. In an ideal laboratory, the optimal setup would locate the blood culture system next to the technologist responsible for blood culture workup to ensure minimum delay from bottle positivity to diagnostic testing. Automated blood culture systems have a large footprint, and space constraints may limit instrument locations. Another approach, although less than optimal, is to create a policy where the blood bench performs periodic checks of the automated systems to pull positive bottles. This system may still delay

[1]Medical College of Wisconsin, Milwaukee, WI 53226

results based on when the bottle signals positive in relation to when the technologist performs a check. For instance, if a technologist checks the instrument at 0800 h and a bottle flags positive at 0802 h, that bottle will not be removed until 1000 h when the technologist performs another check, resulting in a delay to results by 2 h. Finally, smaller facilities or those that want to reduce processing time can place continuously monitoring blood culture systems into wards for near-patient testing and then bring positive bottles to the laboratory. Transportation will greatly increase a delay in testing, which is dependent on scheduled pickup times and the distance between laboratories. Data demonstrate that sites that pick up specimens twice a day increase turnaround time (TAT) by 3 to 10 h (6). Extended delay in the time from bottle inoculation to the time entered into the blood culture system can affect pathogen recovery if delayed for >24 h at 4°C or >12 h at room temperature and so it may be necessary for satellite laboratories to perform off-system incubation (7). Extended delay to processing can also be an issue for laboratories that are not open 7 days a week or only work up bottles on first shift.

Staining Techniques and Subculture

The use of Gram stain to evaluate the contents of a positive blood culture bottle has become nearly universal. The interpretation of the Gram stain is used as an algorithm not only to decide what to do next in the workflow of the positive blood culture, but also to initiate (or not) appropriate patient therapy based on local antibiograms. In addition, Gram stains can aid in the detection of polymicrobial infections, which occur at a rate of 5 to 11% and often affect the accuracy of rapid diagnostic assays (8). The Gram stain is not without pitfalls; interpretation of the Gram stain can require experience and skill. Figure 1 combines multiple organisms in a blood matrix to highlight common objects observed through the microscope differentiating large erythrocyte (large pink) cells from the smaller bacteria or yeast. Misinterpretation of organisms such as reporting Gram-positive (GP) cocci in pairs could easily represent the Gram-negative (GN) organism *Acinetobacter baumannii* and lead to inappropriate antimicrobial therapy. The recognition of small, faintly staining GN coccobacilli should send up a red flag for experienced technologists indicating the possible presence of highly infective organisms such as *Francisella tularensis* or *Brucella* spp. requiring additional safety measures. Furthermore, identification of unique morphologies such as comma-shaped *Campylobacter* or *Vibrio* spp. may suggest the need for additional media or growth conditions to efficiently recover the organism. Figure 2 represents several common morphologies that can be observed.

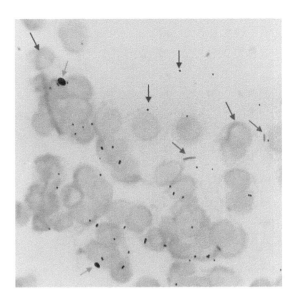

Figure 1 Example of blood culture Gram stains with multiple morphologies to illustrate size differences of various organisms. Image was acquired by adding cells from each organism with the contents of a negative blood culture. Based on size, large to small pink/brown erythrocytes can be observed throughout the Gram stain (red arrow). *Candida* cells are much larger than bacterial cells and stain GP (green arrow). Smaller bacteria are observed throughout the stain with *E. coli* GN rods (pink arrow) and *S. aureus* GPC (purple arrows).

Blood culture bottles that signal positive and are Gram stain negative can be difficult to interpret. False-positive rates vary from site to site and between continually monitoring blood culture systems, but range from 1 to 10% of all bottles entered (9–11). It should be noted that laboratories experiencing particularly high levels of false-positive bottles should evaluate bottle inoculation because overfilling can cause sensor positivity due to the increased number of leukocytes being added to the bottles (10). A conservative approach for these bottles is to perform acridine orange staining, blind subculture, and return the bottle to the blood culture system for further incubation. Acridine orange binds to nucleic acids and is more sensitive than a Gram stain. It may help detect yeast, which flag positive at a lower limit of detection (LOD) and can also detect organisms that stain faintly with a Gram stain such as *Helicobacter* spp. (12, 13). An alternative technique to interpreting bottles that are negative by acridine orange or subculturing is the use of 16S ribosomal DNA sequencing, although clinical utility is limited because studies have shown little to no bacterial presence in these bottles (10, 14).

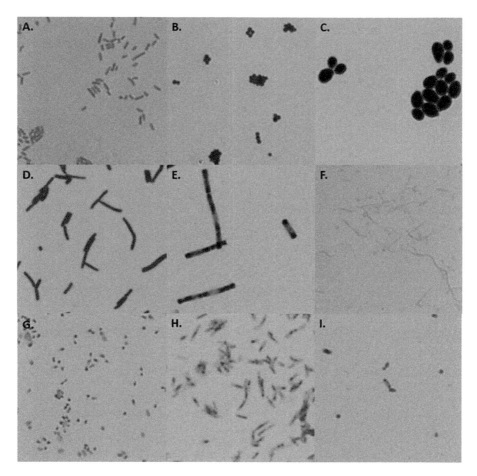

Figure 2 Representative image of several Gram stain morphologies that can be observed from blood culture. Most commonly observed are Gram-negative rods (GNR) and Gram-positive cocci (GPC) (**A**, *P. aeruginosa*; **B**, *S. aureus*). Larger budding yeasts are less common but may yield better growth when plated to Sabouraud agar (**C**, *C. albicans*). Gram-positive rods (GPR) are also less frequent and many not require unique agar to grow (**D**, *Lactobacillus* spp.), but boxy poor staining GPR may indicate *Clostridium* spp. which grow optimally at anaerobic conditions (**E**, *C. perfringens*). *Campylobacter* spp. are thin GN spirochetes often growing wavelike or "gull shaped" and may require growth at 42°C on specific agar depending upon the species (**F**, *C. jejuni*). Finally, morphologies that may require caution because of being highly infectious agents are small GN coccobacillus (**G**), beaded branching GP rods (**H**), or bipolar staining "safety pin" (**I**); however, many other organisms can be observed with these morphologies, and restrictions can be lifted after colony morphologies and testing rule out biological safety agents (morphology represented by **G**, *H. influenzae*; **H**, *M. fortuitum*; **I**, *K. pneumoniae*).

After the initial Gram stain, it is important to subculture each bottle even when laboratories use rapid identification methods. These assays can only detect organisms on the target panel above a certain threshold. Organisms not represented on the assay panel will not be detected. It is within the purview of each laboratory to select appropriate media for subculture, but, in general, positive bottles should be plated to sheep blood (BAP) agar, chocolate agar, and MacConkey agar (MAC) (some will also include Columbia colistin and nalidixic acid [CNA] agar for differentiation of GP organisms). If anaerobic bottles signal positive media that support anaerobic growth, such as anaerobic phenylethyl alcohol agar with vitamin K, CDC anaerobic blood agar, *Brucella* blood agar, or anaerobic laked blood kanamycin agar, these plates should be added and incubated in an anaerobic environment. Other media can be added, especially if unique Gram stain morphology was observed (e.g., *Campylobacter* or *Vibrio*). All plates should be held until the final report is issued and a frozen stock of the isolate should be saved for at least 2 years for epidemiological testing (15).

Rapid Diagnostics

Broad-spectrum empiric antimicrobial therapy commonly used for suspected bloodstream infections will typically provide coverage for approximately 85 to 90% of bloodstream infections (16, 17). A Gram stain can help guide deescalation of antimicrobial therapy (removal of opposite Gram stain coverage), but these data have limited utility in predicting resistance. Better predictions can be made once an organism is identified to genus and species level because known intrinsic resistance factors in combination with local antibiogram data can inform physicians of common response patterns. Traditionally, laboratories have relied on culture followed by biochemical analysis to identify bacteria, which can take up to 24 to 48 h. To improve patient care by reducing this TAT, several laboratory-developed tests (LDTs) and FDA-cleared assays have been introduced.

When developing diagnostic tests for blood cultures, several factors concerning the matrix need to be considered that can either benefit or decrease assay performance. As blood bottles are incubated for growth, the majority contain organisms at high bacterial loads ($\sim 10^7$ to 10^9 CFU/ml) by the time bottles are flagged positive (18). Polymicrobial cultures can also affect the performance of the assay because bottles may contain a ratio of organisms that can drop below the LOD of the assay, especially if nucleic acid amplification is not performed. In addition, blood cultures contain human cells and proteins that can inhibit amplification assays. Without purification prior to amplification, proteins such as immunoglobulin G and lactoferrin can bind to DNA polymerase or nucleic acids, inhibiting the assay's enzymes (19). Various approaches have been used in the development of assays that overcome these potential pitfalls such as matrix-assisted laser desorption ionization–time of flight mass spectrometry (MALDI-TOF MS), molecular methods both with and without amplification, sequencing, and a myriad of novel technologies to detect organism growth within the blood culture.

MALDI-TOF MS Detection from Positive Blood Cultures

MALDI-TOF MS has revolutionized bacterial identification by reducing the TAT for species identification compared with traditional biochemical methodologies. Specimen preparation for organisms recovered on subculture is simple, because a single colony can be added to a MALDI target plate, covered with matrix (a low-mass organic compound that facilitates ionization, often a derivative hydroxycinnamic or dihydroxybenzoic acid), followed by ionization of proteins, peptides, and other macromolecules using a high-power laser. As particles cross a detector, a spectrum based on the mass-to-charge ratio and amount of a particular molecule is generated. Identification is then deduced by matching it to a database of known organism spectra. An in-depth description of MALDI-TOF MS is beyond the scope of this chapter, but many excellent reviews on the subject can be found for greater detail (20, 21). The use of MALDI-TOF MS for direct identification from positive blood cultures is also possible as these specimens contain approximately 10^8 CFU/ml, well above the limit of detection for MALDI-TOF MS (approximately 10^4 to 10^5 CFU/ml) (22, 23). However, as MALDI-TOF MS detects proteins, the use of the technology requires specific processing to remove extraneous human cellular debris.

Specimen processing

To date, there are no FDA-cleared kits or protocols to perform bacterial identification using MALDI-TOF MS directly from positive blood bottles. Published protocols do share similar processing steps prior to plating. To remove larger cells such as erythrocytes and cellular debris, 1 to 1.5 ml of blood is often lysed with saponin or ammonium chloride and centrifuged at approximately 500 rpm for 5 to 15 min (24, 25). Protocols do differ with some adding detergents or using specific serum separator tubes to improve separation of the background matrix (26, 27). The supernatant containing the bacteria or yeast is then centrifuged, washed, and resuspended. Wash protocols and resuspension also differ, but common MALDI-TOF MS extraction chemicals are used such as formic acid, ethanol, or acetic acid to improve bacterial lysis prior to spotting to the MALDI target plate. One CE-marked kit does exist for automated processing of blood specimens, the Sepsityper kit (Bruker Daltonik GmbH, Bremen, Germany). The kit comes with a standardized protocol containing a lysis step along with several centrifugation steps to purify bacterial pellets and extract proteins. bioMérieux also offers a similar system: the VITEK MS Blood Culture Kit (bioMérieux Inc., Durham, NC), which uses a vacuum-filtered manifold that allows lysis and purification of positive blood cultures for MALDI-TOF MS identification. Finally, an alternative approach has been tested to remove the labor-intensive processing, which is to subculture blood to a BAP for several hours and perform testing on short incubation cultures (28, 29). These short incubation cultures allow for organism growth on the plate, which can be tested following normal MALDI-TOF MS procedures.

Performance

Comparing reported performances of direct MALDI-TOF MS identification of positive blood cultures is difficult because of the variability between laboratory-developed methods. Further, individual laboratory demographics can affect performance even when using the same protocol (A. Lau, personal communication, ASM Microbe 2016 presentation at session "Practical Considerations and Novel Application of MALDI-TOF MS in the Clinical Library"). In general, the sensitivity of MALDI-TOF MS direct from blood culture ranges from 56 to 98%, including both laboratory-developed and CE-marked *in vitro* diagnostic (IVD) kits (30, 31). The range in sensitivity is likely due to several contributing factors such as differences in protocols, reference methods, site variation, and the composition of specimens tested. Studies demonstrate that higher accuracy is achieved for GN organisms (usually approximately 90 to 95%) compared with GP (70 to 90%) and yeast (60 to 70%) (27, 32). Reduced accuracy for both yeast and GP organisms is likely attributable to a reduction in cell lysis, lowering recovery of proteins obtained while performing MALDI-TOF MS and a lower bacterial load for positive bottles, which also reduces protein concentration. Identification of yeast can be improved by adding wash steps with pure water and the addition of a detergent that leads to concordance as high as 91.3 to 100% compared with identification from colonies (33, 34). Viridans group streptococci appear to be especially difficult, because most studies fail to correctly identify these organisms and, in some cases, misidentify them as *Streptococcus pneumoniae* (26, 27). This issue is less common when using VITEK MS (bioMérieux, Inc., Durham, NC) due to the binning method utilized when assigning weight to the presence or absence of individual peaks (35). The use of short-term subculturing (plating and using small colonies after a few hours of growth) performs similarly to purification methods. Studies evaluating this method observed that correct identification (ID) was obtained for 81% of isolates after a short incubation with failure to identify organisms associated with anaerobes and yeast that may not contain sufficient growth for detection (28, 29).

A disadvantage of MALDI-TOF MS for identification of positive blood cultures is that mixed cultures tend to generate unacceptable or incorrect identifications (36). In one study, 15 polymicrobial specimens containing different species were tested by MALDI-TOF MS for direct identification from positive blood cultures. In 12 of 15 cultures, only one species was detected, while the other three resulted in no identification (26). Another study obtained similar results when testing 22 polymicrobial blood cultures of which 18 identified one of the two organisms, two resulted in no identification, and the remaining two had erroneous IDs reported (24). In cases where multiple organisms are observed in the Gram stain, subculture should be performed to reduce the risk of erroneous results.

The type of bottle used could affect MALDI-TOF MS results because of differences in growth medium composition. A meta-analysis of 21 studies using the Sepsityper kit did not observe any significant differences in the identification of organisms between Bactec (BD Diagnostic Systems, Sparks, MD) or the VersaTREK bottles (Thermo Fisher Scientific, Waltham, MA), although data using VersaTREK are limited because only two published papers were included in the analysis (32). The use of MALDI-TOF MS from anaerobic bottles was observed to be accurate in most studies; however, one article removed anaerobic bottles from their data analysis because of frequent errors (37–39).

Optimization

A challenge for MALDI-TOF MS is to reliably obtain acceptable identifications especially for both GP and yeast, which tend to have reduced accuracy. To improve the rate of identification, several studies have tested modifications to both methodology and result interpretation. A commonly studied approach to increase identifications, when using the Bruker biotyper CA system (Bruker Daltonics Inc., Billerica, MA), is to lower the acceptable criteria for species cutoff thresholds from ≥2.0 to ≥1.7 or even as low as ≥1.5

(40, 41). Lowering thresholds to ≥1.5 did not cause any incorrect identifications provided the top three potential organisms had the same genus and
species reported (40). By adjusting the acceptable criteria, one study found
that an additional 5.2% of specimens were able to be reported (26). The
VITEK MS system uses a percent probability score for identification purposes, and studies have suggested that a >95.0% identification score was
reliable to report results in comparison with culture, reaching 99.5% concordance (42). Lowering these criteria may increase identifications; however, to our knowledge, no studies have discussed the effect that lowering
acceptance criteria would have on performance.

Differences in extraction preparation also likely affect the performance of
MALDI-TOF MS identification from positive blood cultures. One study
compared four different procedures using the same specimens (27). All
specimens were treated the same for the removal of cellular debris, but the
final extracted supernatants were resuspended in different reagents: (i) 50 μl
of 30% formic acid, (ii) 50 μl of 30% acetic acid, or (iii) 50 μl of 100%
ethanol. The final method plated the pellet to BAP and incubated for 90 min
or 6 h when diphtheroids were observed via a Gram stain. The first three
methods performed equally for GN organisms (91% correct ID), and the
fourth method was 82% concordant with culture results. Differences were
detected when GP specimens were tested. Method 4 yielded the best results
with 94%, followed by methods 1 and 2 (89%) and method 3 (76%). Method
4 was able to correctly identify 2/5 viridans group streptococci organisms
tested, whereas methods 1 and 2 correctly identified one specimen, suggesting that validating separate methods based on the Gram stain result may
improve overall performance. A final study determined that detection of
yeast can be improved if additional wash steps were added prior to use of the
Sepsityper kit; however, only 42 specimens were tested with this method
(33).

Direct antimicrobial resistance testing

Performing resistance testing using MALDI-TOF MS directly from
positive blood culture uses the same principles as performing MALDI-TOF
MS antimicrobial susceptibility testing (AST) from colony growth. These
methods include detection of hydrolyzed product, methylation of ribosomes,
or detection of bacterial growth in the presence of an antibiotic based on
changes of peak intensity. Hrabák et al. discussed each of these methodologies in detail in a recent clinical microbiology review (43). Modifying
MALDI-TOF MS AST for positive blood cultures requires the user to

obtain a bacterial pellet, which was part of the identification process prior to extraction. A standardized McFarland solution can be created from the pellet to be used for AST.

Results using MALDI-TOF MS AST methods directly from a positive blood culture bottle show beneficial results to reduce time to result. In one study, detection of carbapenemases directly from positive blood cultures could be obtained within 4 h of incubation. Detection of several carbapenemases (OXA, KPC, IMP, GIM, and NDM) was 96% concordant with phenotypic antimicrobial susceptibility for most organisms tested with an exception for *A. baumannii* isolates where only 63% concordance was observed (44). With the use of isolates that grew from those bottles and following the same protocol, MALDI-TOF MS direct from colonies was concordant 98% with phenotypic results and 97% with *A. baumannii*, suggesting that MALDI-TOF MS AST direct from positive blood can be highly accurate. In the case of carbapenemases, these data aid in detecting resistance, but confirmation for susceptibility is still required because of the harboring of other resistance mechanisms. These methods can reduce the turnaround of AST results by 48 h; however, these methods are labor intensive and require validation as a LDT.

Molecular Detection from Positive Blood Cultures

In recent years, several molecular assays have come to market that reduce the TAT for positive blood cultures. Unlike MALDI-TOF MS, these assays are FDA cleared, allowing for easier introduction into routine laboratory practice. Most assays have greatly reduced hands-on time compared with standard biochemical procedures. Molecular detection can also target resistance markers to quickly identify specific drug resistance; however, these assays are costly compared with conventional methods. Deciding which assay to adopt can be difficult because there are several differences between assays such as number of targets, cost, and workflow (or labor intensity). A comparison of these assays can be found in Table 1.

Verigene BC-GN and BC-GP assay

The FDA-cleared Verigene system (Luminex, Austin, TX) is a sample-to-answer system that detects organisms through microarray technology. For the detection of positive blood cultures, two assays exist: the BC-GP and the BC-GN panels, which are used after an initial Gram stain. The complete list of targets is summarized in Table 1, but the BC-GN panel detects eight organisms (in addition to *Serratia marcescens* outside the United

States) and six resistance genes. The BC-GP panel detects 12 organisms (in addition to *Micrococcus* spp. outside the United States) and three resistance markers. Each test uses reagents for an onboard extraction, hybridization of purified nucleic acids, capture probes immobilized to a glass microarray slide, and finally hybridization of a conjugate nanoparticle detection probe. Each capture probe is present in triplicate to aid in removing background signal and to reduce false positives (FPs), and each test contains internal controls that confirm optimal extraction and binding. Setup takes approximately 2 min, and, after 2.5 h of extraction and hybridization, a technologist transfers the glass slide to the reader, which detects positive probe hybridization and reports the results within 1 min.

Performance of both assays has been measured by several laboratories, and, in general, these studies have observed a high concordance to reference testing (culture followed by biochemical identification) (45–48). Agreement for GN organisms ranged from 93 to 100% and genetic resistance detection correlated from 94 to 100% compared with PCR and bidirectional sequencing (46, 47). Studies evaluating the performance of the GP panel show similar high levels of performance, with sensitivity and specificity ranging from 93 to 100% and 99 to 100%, respectively (48). The target for *Klebsiella pneumoniae* was observed to be 93% concordant. Sequence analysis of these false-negative (FN) isolates demonstrated that 25 of 26 were actually *Klebsiella variicola* (47). Both species are known to be frequent causes of bloodstream infections, but recent studies have observed higher mortality rates from *K. variicola* infections than from *K. pneumoniae* (49). The lower sensitivity observed in the GP study was for detection of *Enterococcus faecium* and *Enterococcus faecalis*. The product insert notes that *Enterococcus avium* can cross-react with the *E. faecalis* probe.

The above evaluation of the Verigene assay only accounts for monomicrobial blood bottles. Concordance drops when polymicrobial bottles were included. In the study evaluating the BC-GP assay, a total of 95 polymicrobial specimens were enrolled for which 72% (68/95) of bottles detected all pathogens present in the specimen (48). *Staphylococcus epidermidis* was the most often missed organism, accounting for 60% of the missed polymicrobial isolates. The BC-GN panel found a similar decrease in performance, detecting all organisms in only 54% of polymicrobial cultures (47). It is unclear why certain organisms were not detected, but it may be because of differences in final organism load that affect analytics, because there is no amplification in the assay so that bacteria present at lower concentrations may be not detected.

Table 1 Comparison of rapid identification assays for blood culture

Assay	Methodology	Identification targets	Resistance targets	Turnaround time (h)	Refs
		Panels			
Verigene GP-BC	Nonamplified MicroArray	*Staphylococcus* spp., *S. aureus*, *S. epidermidis*, *S. lugdunensis*, *Streptococcus* spp., *Streptococcus anginosus* group, *S. agalactiae*, *S. pneumoniae*, *S. pyogenes*, *E. faecalis*, *E. faecium*, *Mirococcus* spp.,[a] *Listeria* spp.	*mecA, vanA, vanB*	2.5	45, 48
Verigene GN-BC	Nonamplified MicroArray	*E. coli*,[b] *K. pneumoniae, K. oxytoca, P. aeruginosa, S. marcescens*,[a] *Acinetobacter* spp., *Citrobacter* spp., *Enterobacter* spp., *Proteus* spp.	CTX-M, IMP, KPC, NDM, OXA, VIM	2.5	46, 47
iCubate	Amplified MicroArray	*S. aureus, S. epidermidis, S. pneumoniae, E. faecalis, E. faecium*	*mecA, vanA, vanB*	2.0	59
Biofire	Nested PCR	*Staphylococcus* spp., *S. aureus, Streptococcus* spp., *S. agalactiae, S. pyogenes, S. pneumoniae, Enterococcus* spp., *L. monocytogenes, Enterobacteriaceae* spp., *Enterobacter cloacae* complex, *E. coli, K. oxytoca, K. pneumoniae, Proteus* spp., *S. marcescens, A. baumannii, H. influenzae, N. meningitidis, P. aeruginosa, C. albicans, C. glabrata, C. krusei, C. parapsilosis, C. tropicalis*	*mecA, vanA, vanB*, KPC	1.0	53–55

Name	Method	Targets	Antimicrobial resistance	TAT (h)	References
HemoFISH	FISH[c]	*Staphylococcus* spp., *S. aureus*, *Streptococcus* spp., *S. pneumoniae*,[a] *S. agalactiae*,[a] *E. faecalis*,[a] *E. faecium*,[a] *Enterobacteriaceae* spp. *E. coli*, *K. pneumoniae*, *P. mirabilis*,[a] *P. aeruginosa*,[a] *Acinetobacter* spp.,[a] *S. maltophilia*[a]	None	0.5	N/A
Accelerate Pheno system	FISH + automated microscopy	*Staphylococcus* spp., *S. aureus*, *S. lugdunensis*, *E. faecalis*, *E. faecium*, *Streptococcus* spp.,[c] *S. pneumoniae*,[c] *S. agalactiae*,[c] *Enterobacter* spp., *E. coli*, *Klebsiella* spp., *Proteus* spp., *Citrobacter* spp., *S. marcescens*, *P. aeruginosa*, *A. baumannii*, *C. albicans*,[c] *C. glabrata*[c]	26 different drugs with various drug/bug combinations	1.0 (ID) 8.0 (ID+AST)	66, 67
AdvanDX	FISH[d]	Small panels: (i) *Staphylococcus* spp., *S. aureus*. (ii) *E. faecalis*, *E. faecium*, (iii) *E. coli*, *K. pneumoniae*, *P. aeruginosa*, (iv) *C. albicans/C. parapsilosis*;[e] *C. tropicalis*, *C. glabrata/C. krusei*[e]	None	0.5	60–62
MRSA specific					
Staph ID/R	PCR	*Staphylococcus* spp., *S. aureus*, *S. lugdunensis*	*mecA*	2.0	N/A
GeneOhm StaphSR	PCR	*S. aureus*	SCC*mec*	1.5	74, 75, 78
Xpert MRSA/SA BC	PCR	*S. aureus*	*mecA*, SCC*mec*	1.0	76–78
BinaxNOW	Immunochromatographic	*S. aureus*	PBP2a	0.5	80–82

[a]Target is not cleared within the United States.
[b]BC-GN does not distinguish *E. coli* from *Shigella* spp.
[c]ID only.
[d]Fluorescent *in situ* hybridization.
[e]Three fluorescent dyes are used and / indicates that targets will not be differentiated.

A study evaluating clinical impact was performed over a 6-month period before and after the implementation of the Verigene BC-GN panel (50). In this report, patient demographics, time to identification, and time to effective antimicrobial therapy were evaluated. No differences were observed in patient populations for comorbidities and sources of bacteremia. Organism identification was significantly faster, reducing TAT from an average of 37.9 h to 10.9 h ($P < 0.001$) (50). Improvement in TAT reduced overall length of stay and 30-day mortality with multidrug-resistant organisms, and resulted in a more rapid implementation of appropriate antibiotics when patients were infected with extended-spectrum beta-lactamase-producing (ESBL) organisms. However, this difference was not observed for all types of GN infections. These data demonstrate the effectiveness that rapid identification can have on patient care and outcomes.

FilmArray BCID panel

The FilmArray BCID panel (Biofire, Salt Lake City, UT) is an FDA-cleared sample to answer qualitative multiplexed nucleic acid assay able to detect 24 pathogens and three resistance genes (Table 1). The assay uses one consumable and setup is simple, consisting of a pouch that is placed into a loading station where two injection vials are used to hydrate lyophilized reagents and load the sample. The pouch is vacuum sealed, so insertion of the injector into the pouch automatically draws the appropriate volume needed for the assay. Once the assay is started, the specimen goes through nucleic acid purification using Boom extraction technology followed by an initial multiplex PCR to amplify nucleic acid (51). The multiplex PCR is then diluted and added to a hexagon-shaped array that contains targeted organism/resistance gene primers. A second nested PCR is performed in these wells, and a DNA-binding dye is incorporated into the amplification. Detection is then determined through a melt curve analysis through the loss of fluorescence as temperature is increased and the DNA denatures.

Several studies have evaluated the performance of the BCID assay, demonstrating good correlation between the assay and conventional blood culture (52–54). The largest study to date was a multicenter trial between eight centers and a total of 1,568 clinical specimens and 639 seeded specimens. The BCID assay results were compared with phenotypic identification (53). The authors found that, prior to discrepant resolution, sensitivity ranged from 92.2 to 100% with all but *Klebsiella oxytoca* obtaining sensitivity >96%. Specificity for all organisms ranged from 99 to 100%. Of the five discordant *K. oxytoca* specimens, four were misidentified by the phenotypic reference method and were determined to be *Raoultella ornithinolytica* based on 16S rRNA sequencing, which raises the postdiscrepant analysis sensitivity to 98.3%. Detection of resistance genes was also highly sensitive and specific as detection of *vanA/B* and bla$_{KPC}$ was 100% for both and *mecA* was 98.4% sensitive and 98.3% specific. Some studies have shown a lower sensitivity especially for staphylococci, with one study finding a sensitivity of 90.9% (54/60) (55). The BCID product insert reports that there is reduced sensitivity for five *Staphylococcus* species (*S. capitis, S. pasteuri, S. saprophyticus, S. simulans,* and *S. warneri*) and so it is possible that the reduced sensitivity observed in the cited study was attributed to an abnormally high number of coagulase-negative *Staphylococcus* (CoNS).

Polymicrobial cultures can be difficult to detect because the organisms at a lower concentration may have too low of a signal to be detected by the assay. This limitation can potentially be overcome by adding amplification steps, because this will increase the signal for both targets to allow detection of both organisms growing. The results from studies reporting the detection of polymicrobial cultures with the BCID suggest detection is possible, but with reduced sensitivity. One report observed polymicrobial sensitivity to be 78.6% (8/11), while others demonstrated that a high number of FP results were obtained from polymicrobial cultures (46% of FP) (53, 55). Another article reported a large number of FP due to detection of *Pseudomonas aeruginosa* that was not observed in culture. Upon further evaluation, these FP results were linked to the presence of nucleic acid from nonviable organisms in the bioMérieux BacT standard anaerobic bottles (BioMérieux Inc., Durham, NC) (56). These data suggest that polymicrobial cultures from amplification methods should be reviewed and correlated with the patient's clinical history.

Clinical outcomes studies have also been performed using the BCID panel comparing pre- and postimplementation of the assay. In a pediatric setting, the use of BCID with antimicrobial stewardship intervention showed that the average time to optimal therapy was significantly decreased from 60.2 h to 26.7 h ($P < 0.01$), with time to effective therapy reduced from 6.9 to 3.4 h ($P < 0.05$) (57). Overall, the study found that health care providers changed management of patients in 73% of all cases of bacteremia. These data are similar to the Verigene study discussed above, demonstrating significantly improved patient care management following implementation of molecular panels for positive blood culture evaluation. However, the contribution of the assay results on patient care may depend upon each hospital's prevalence of bacteremia caused by organisms that identification changes empirical treatment as another study found similar improvements of TAT, but only nine out of 173 patients had impact on antimicrobial prescribing when using either the Verigene or FilmArray BCID panels (58).

iCubate iC-GPC

The iCubate system (iCubate, Huntsville, AL) is another multiplex amplification assay that is composed of an iC-Processor that performs onboard extraction, amplification, and hybridization and an iC-Reader that scans the microarray to detect secondary binding of fluorescent probes to target sequences. The system uses a single-use, closed-system cartridge that is loaded by pipetting blood into a port on the cartridge. Each iC-Processor can hold up to four cartridges at once, and testing takes approximately 4 h per test with less than 5 min of hands-on time (59).

Currently, the platform only offers a GP panel that detects several bacterial targets and resistance markers (Table 1). Preliminary results evaluating the iC-GPC panel demonstrate that the assay has sensitivity and specificity similar to other multiplex platforms ranging from 93.8 to 100% and 98.9 to 100%, respectively, for each target when compared with culture-based standard of care (MALDI-TOF MS with routine biochemical tests) and disk diffusion tests for AST (59). A few limitations to this study were that only 203 total specimens were tested, less than 50 positives were tested for each target, and research used only reagents.

GenMark ePlex

Similar to the other platforms discussed above, the ePlex system (GenMark Diagnostics, Carlsbad, CA) is a single-cartridge multiplex system that performs onboard extraction, amplification, and detection in under 1.5 h. The system contains a touch screen monitor that connects to multiple processing bays that allow up to six random-access tests to be run at a time. The technology uses a process called electrowetting to move the sample sequentially from station to station within the consumable. Detection is performed using capture probes specific to several targets that are bound to gold electrodes. An electrochemical redox-dependent faradaic signal, which can only be generated when target DNA is bound to the probe, signifies the presence of pathogen in the sample. As of the writing of this chapter, blood culture panels were in development. The GP panel that is currently in development consists of 20 bacterial targets and four resistance genes and the GN panel consists of 24 bacterial targets and six resistance genes; the final product that is marketed may provide a different menu.

PNA-FISH

The use of peptide nucleic acid fluorescent *in situ* hybridization (PNA-FISH) for direct visualization of bacteria in positive blood cultures is an alternative approach that has gained some popularity over time. In these methods, specimen is fixed (heat or antibody immobilized) to a microscope slide and processed to allow for partial lysing of bacterial cells. This, in turn, allows for internalization of fluorescent PNA probes that target organism-specific RNA. Slides are then viewed on a fluorescent microscope to detect target organisms. Multiple probes can be utilized, allowing for small panels based on fluorescence wavelength. Currently, assays include both manual processing and detection, QuickFISH (AdvanDX, Woburn, MA) and HemoFISH (Miacom Diagnostics GmbH, Dusseldorf, Germany), and automated systems, Accelerate PhenoTest BC (Accelerate Diagnostics, Tucson, AZ).

Manual PNA-FISH

Both QuickFISH and HemoFISH require manual processing of the blood culture, requiring a technologist to perform the individual steps such as lysis, washes, and beacon hybridization. In general, these steps take approximately 20 to 30 min and can be performed individually or batched depending on the needs of the laboratory. The QuickFISH system contains multiple test kits that detect several organisms, including *Staphylococcus*, *Enterococcus*, GNs, and *Candida*, and a test for *mecA*. Each test only detects a single analyte and so a Gram stain would predict which assay is required (e.g., if *Staphylococcus aureus* was detected, the laboratory would then perform the *mecA* test on the specimen). The HemoFISH assay is a small panel manual FISH assay that utilizes a multispot slide containing eight wells and uses 14 probes to detect common blood pathogens (Table 1). After a dilution step, the sample is added to each well and heat fixed. The assay utilizes reagents that are best suited for a multichannel pipette so each well can be inoculated at the same time. Importantly, as beacons are placed into eight separate wells (two per well, green/red), they need to be loaded correctly, otherwise misidentification can occur. Currently, the system does not contain probes for any resistance markers such as *mecA* or *vanA/B*.

Both assays are FDA-cleared, although the HemoFISH is only cleared for the first half of the panel and detects *Staphylococcus* spp., *S. aureus*, *Streptococcus* spp., *Enterobacteriaceae*, *E. coli*, and *K. pneumoniae*. Evaluations of the QuickFISH assays demonstrate high sensitivity and specificity ranging from 96.5 to 98.6% and 96.8 to 100%, respectively, when compared with reference methods (60–62). No fluorescence was detected from targets not included in the assay, with the exception of one viridans group streptococcus, which was identified as a CoNS (60). In the same study, seven cultures containing CoNS were negative for the *S. aureus*/CoNS assay. To date, no results have been published on the HemoFISH assay, but posters presented at American Society for Microbiology (ASM) Microbe and at the European Congress of Clinical Microbiology and Infectious Diseases (ECCMID) demonstrate that positive percent agreement (PPA) and negative percent agreement (NPA) range from 96.8 to 100% and 99.8 to 100% depending on the target (63, 64).

Automated PNA-FISH

The Accelerate system removes the manual processing of PNA-FISH and reflects workflow similar to that of the FilmArray BCID and Verigene systems by pipetting a specific amount of the specimen into a bottle, which is then added to a cartridge and loaded into the instrument. Once testing is initialized, the instrument isolates bacteria through gel electrofiltration and transfers the specimen into multiple microscope flow cells that immobilize organisms using a low voltage to the transparent lower surface of the flow cell channel. PNA-FISH is then performed in several wells with each well using different beacons. A microscope housed within the instrument then detects fluorescence and performs quantitation, giving an identification in less than 2 h. Following identification, specific concentrations of antibiotics are placed into the remaining wells by using a universal probe that detects replicating, injured, and dead cells for bacteria visualization. Software interprets the growth of individual organisms with and without antibiotic and uses the changes in growth rates to report minimal inhibitory concentration (MIC) for several drugs testing within 4 to 5 h after identification.

The addition of MIC-based AST has some benefits for patient outcomes over genotypic testing. Genotypic testing informs physicians that a specific drug will not work, but does not provide data to inform the physician about which drugs will be effective. An assay that provides MIC data may lead to decreased time to optimal therapy and specifying appropriate antimicrobial therapy for multidrug-resistant organisms. In addition, genotypic data can be erroneous in cases where the gene is present but is functionally inactive because of mutations that are not within the primer binding sites. However, phenotypic resistance for certain classes of antibiotic resistance, such as ESBLs, can be falsely interpreted. One study showed that 4.8% of phenotypic ESBL-positive organisms identified between 2009 and 2012 and

29.5% in 2013 were genotypically negative for ESBL beta-lactamase genes using a combination of microarray and multiplex PCR assays (65).

At the time of writing this chapter, there were no published studies evaluating an FDA-cleared Accelerate platform. However, a few publications were generated during the development of the assay. In one such publication, *K. pneumoniae* susceptibility to ertapenem (ETP) and carbapenemases (KPC) was evaluated using a manually pipetted flow cell chamber. Of 47 isolates tested, the automated microscopy correctly reported susceptibilities to ertapenem for all, which include 24 ETP-S/23 ETP-R and 21 KPC+/26 KPC– organisms (66). Similar results were found for the identification and quantification of *S. aureus* and *P. aeruginosa* from remnant bronchoalveolar lavage specimens (n = 53) (67). In this study, all *S. aureus* (n = 9) and *P. aeruginosa* (n = 7) were correctly identified. Recent poster presentations at ECCMID demonstrated that the system had a 94% essential agreement and 94% categorical agreement compared to broth microdilution for *Enterobacteriaceae* using the CLSI breakpoints (68, 69). Blood cultures containing *A. baumannii* had an essential agreement of 99.4% and categorical agreement of 100% compared with broth microdilution. The ability of the assay to detect polymicrobial specimens has not been reported.

MRSA-Specific PCR Assays

The leading cause of bloodstream infections are *Staphylococcus* species, specifically *S. aureus* and *S. epidermidis*, and initial treatment is broad-spectrum antimicrobial agents until identification and antimicrobial susceptibility are reported (70). However, because many CoNS are contaminants, differentiating between *S. aureus* and CoNS and determining the status of methicillin resistance can greatly improve patient care and reduce hospital costs. One study reported a decrease in hospital stay of 6.2 days and a mean reduction of $21,387 per patient after switching to a rapid PCR for MRSA associated with reduced length of stay (71). Other studies have found similar results using rapid PCR assays. Using a PCR assay that differentiates *S. aureus* from CoNS and methicillin resistance from positive blood cultures concluded that 36% (21/57) of patients with methicillin-sensitive *S. aureus* would receive suboptimal care with traditional culture for up to 48 h (72). Reduction in vancomycin usage for methicillin-sensitive *S. aureus* infections has been observed by others at similar rates of 38% of treated patients (n = 65) (73). Because Gram-positive cocci in clusters (GPCCL) are the most common organisms identified in positive blood cultures, and determining methicillin resistance is a highly actionable result, some laboratories utilize molecular tests that detect MRSA alone because these tests are more cost-effective than the large panels described above.

Several FDA-cleared, MRSA-specific tests are available on the market such as Xpert MRSA/SA BC (Cepheid, Sunnyvale, CA), GeneOhm StaphSR (BD Diagnostics, Oakville, Canada), and the Staph ID/R Blood Culture Panel (Great Basin Scientific, Salt Lake City, UT). Primer design can differ among these assays compared with large panel options as the junction of the *mec* element (SCC*mec*) and *orfX* is targeted instead of *mecA* itself (Staph ID/R Blood Culture Panel uses *mecA* and detects *Staphylococcus lugdunensis*). The benefit of this approach is that the junction discriminates MRSA from methicillin-resistant CoNS in mixed cultures. However, the junction is more often subjected to genetic rearrangement or point mutations, which can increase the likelihood of false-negative (FN) results because there are currently 20 recognized junction types (74). The long-term effects of these mutations on assay performance can be observed by comparing the sensitivities of these assays over time. Initial evaluation of the GeneOhm and Xpert assays reported sensitivity and specificity of 98.3 to 100% and 98.4 to 99.4%, respectively (75, 76). Reevaluation of previously characterized isolates spiked into blood cultures has reported sensitivities of 50 to 92% and analysis demonstrates that missed specimens were due to variants in SCC*mec* types or genetic rearrangement/deletion in the SCC*mec* cassette (74, 77). These assays have been updated by the commercial vendors on a regular basis to detect variants. In a recent multicenter study comparing both the next-generation Xpert MRSA/SA BC assay and the GeneOhm StaphSR Assay versus routine culture determined sensitivity and specificity ranged from 96.4 to 100% and 89.2 to 100%, respectively, for *S. aureus* and 87.5 to 100% and 96.1 to 100%, respectively, for identifying MRSA at the eight study sites (78). To date, no reports have been published on the Staph ID/R Blood Culture Panel; however, it was recently cleared by the FDA.

Alternative Approaches

Besides MALDI-TOF MS and molecular assays, there are a few approaches that the laboratories can utilize to improve TAT for positive blood cultures. Some of these assays target MRSA specifically using immunochromatographic tests or shorten identification by directly plating to chromogenic agar. In general, these approaches may be less sensitive or require more time to identification than molecular methods, but are less expensive options for testing than traditional culture alone that can improve patient care.

Immunochromatographic assays

Many molecular tests require moderate- or high-complexity laboratories with well-trained laboratory professionals to ensure that contamination does not occur during the performance of the test. In addition, most molecular assays can significantly increase cost because they are generally more expensive than culture- and antigen-based testing. An alternative approach for the detection of *S. aureus* and methicillin resistance includes immunochromatographic assays such as the BinaxNOW *S. aureus* and the BinaxNOW PBP2a assay (Alere, Scarborough, ME). Both are antigen detection assays using a flow strip to transport sample over immobilized control and capture line antibodies. In response to the target antigen, a colorimetric line is produced indicating that the test is positive. The BinaxNOW *S. aureus* is used to detect for the presence of *S. aureus* from blood but cannot differentiate MRSA and methicillin-sensitive *S. aureus* nor can it detect other *Staphylococcus* species or detect mixed cultures. The BinaxNOW PBP2a assay detects penicillin-binding protein 2A (PBP2a), which is produced by *mecA* and has low affinity to beta-lactams causing resistance (79).

As both tests are sold separately, several studies have compared different testing algorithms to improve patient care and reduce the cost of reporting MRSA blood cultures. In one study, both BinaxNOW assays were used in combination with an initial BinaxNOW *S. aureus* followed by the PBP2a test for *S. aureus*-positive cultures, which resulted in a sensitivity and specificity of 94 and 87% (*S. aureus*) and 100% (PBP2a), respectively (80). Another article suggested the use of MALDI-TOF MS for the identification of *S. aureus* followed by PBP2a detection (81). In this study, the PBP2a assay was found to be 95% sensitive and 100% specific compared with a PCR assay for *mecA* (81). The authors did note that a common commercial PCR assay costs on average $30 compared with the PBP2a assay that costs $20 a test. However, this algorithm requires LDT verification of MALDI-TOF MS from positive blood bottles and increases hands-on time because of the identification processing. A final testing algorithm utilized the BinaxNOW *S. aureus* test in combination with the Xpert MRSA/SA assay (82). Blood identified as GPCCL was initially tested using the antigen test and upon a positive result was tested using the Xpert MRSA assay. Compared with phenotypic methods, the BinaxNOW assay was 92% sensitive and 99% specific (n = 581), and using the antigen test as a *S. aureus* screen reduced cost by 75% compared with testing all blood cultures with the Xpert assay (82). An additional benefit to this algorithm is that all assays are FDA cleared, allowing for easier validations for laboratories.

Direct plating to chromogenic agar

Another targeted approach to quickly identify high-impact targets such as MRSA or vancomycin-resistant *Enterococcus* (VRE) is to directly plate blood cultures to one of a variety of chromogenic agar plates. This method has several benefits such as simple workflow (adding a plate dependent on a Gram stain), lower cost than molecular, and no requirement for specialized training of technologists, which may benefit smaller laboratories with limited resources. Studies evaluating the use of MRSA chromogenic agar demonstrate high sensitivity and specificity ($\geq$98%) and showed a reduction of TAT for MRSA detection by approximately 24 h because initial 18 to 24 h growth was not needed prior to AST testing (83). It is possible to report MRSA earlier using chromogenic plates because colonies can be observed as early as 10 h postincubation (84). However, this method does increase TAT compared with other rapid methods.

Direct susceptibilities

Many of the commercially available molecular panels report genotypic resistance markers, but these have limited targets and do not provide a complete susceptibility profile for optimal patient treatment (current exception is Accelerate diagnostics assay). Laboratories that utilize these assays will still need to subculture positive bottles for full AST results, a process that can delay final reporting for up 48 h. To improve the TAT for AST results, several approaches have been studied, such as testing purified bacterial pellets on VITEK 2 (bioMérieux, Marcy l'Etolie, France) or BD Phoenix (BD Diagnostics, Sparks, MD) system or performing disk diffusion directly from positive blood cultures.

Disk diffusion from blood bottle

Use of Kirby-Bauer disk diffusion has been a standard method for AST in the clinical microbiology laboratory for many years. Protocols testing from positive blood culture require one to two drops of blood added to saline, and a "lawn" of bacteria is created from this dilution with concentrations varying between published protocols (85, 86). Results from these studies showed varied results ranging from combined error rates of 9 to 14.1% depending on drug-bug combination (85, 86). Gentamicin was particularly error prone for *Enterococcus* because very major errors were detected in 10.9% of specimens tested (86). Likely issues for these protocols may be the lack of inoculum standardization because the final CFU/ml can vary by organism. Despite these potential errors, the decrease in AST TAT can be beneficial. One study found a decreased time to administration of effective and targeted antibiotics in 9.3 and 14.3% of cases. However, laboratories still need to perform standardized AST from colonies to correct potential errors (86). The European Committee on Antimicrobial Susceptibility Testing (EUCAST) has released guidelines for performing and interpreting AST direct from blood cultures. To reduce misinterpretation of results, they suggest that all AST be repeated on pure colonies, results should not be reported if growth is visibly light, and results should be read after 16 to 20 h of incubation. However, reporting resistance prior to 16 to 20 h is likely valid. Finally, Etest can also be used instead of Kirby-Bauer disks with studies observing similar performance ranging from 83 to 100% correlation with standard Etests (87).

Automated AST systems

A few studies have evaluated the use of the VITEK 2 or the BD Phoenix for direct AST testing of blood cultures and/or phenotypic identification (88–91). One study compared both platforms using the same blood cultures. Results were comparable for either platform with performance concordant with product inserts (98.7% GN and 96.2% GP for the VITEK 2 and 99.0% GN and 99.5% GP for the BD Phoenix [91]). These data are supported by other studies demonstrating similar AST concordance ranging from 97.9 to 99.0% with GN organisms (88, 91). Differences between platform performance were noticed for identification functions, especially GP organisms where correct identifications were given in 43.7% (BD Phoenix) and 75% (VITEK 2) of isolates (91). Difficulties in GP identification directly from positive blood cultures have been previously recognized, because one study found that the BD Phoenix correctly identified 82% of 68 GP samples (89). In this study, detergents were used in the purification process, which may account for the increase in GP identification. However, it is possible that changes in the pelleting method could affect AST results, because 77% of the samples gave results concordant with the reference method with an error rate of 1.9% (89). These data suggest that direct testing of GN organisms with automated systems is reliable, but more data may be needed to optimize GP identification. The EUCAST guideline for direct AST of positive blood or urine cultures states that testing should not be performed by automated systems unless approved by the manufacturer.

Future Technology

Because blood culture is a critical value for the clinical laboratory, new methodologies that improve identification and reduce TAT will likely continue to be developed. Currently, there are several of these technologies in production that include the use of colorimetric arrays, DNA carrying particles, and sequence analysis. Some of these, such as sequence analysis, are already being used in a number of laboratories, but improvements such as simplifying workflow and reducing cost may be necessary before universal adaptation for use in blood culture. Other assays are currently under development and will likely be FDA cleared within the next few years.

Colorimetric Sensor Arrays

During growth and metabolism, various volatile chemicals are generated as by-products, the combination of which can be unique to certain bacterial and fungal species (92). Colorimetric sensor arrays (CSAs) are able to detect these chemical signatures including alcohols, amines, ethers, fatty acids, and other metabolites by using vapor-sensing metalloporphyrin dyes that respond to each chemical (93). These dyes are immobilized on the array allowing spot detection of various chemical by-products creating a volatile "fingerprint" of the recovered organisms. Identification is then performed by matching the pattern of colored dyes to a reference database of known organisms similar to MALDI-TOF MS identification (92). SpecID (Specific Technologies, Mountain View, CA) is one such assay currently in development using CSA to identify organisms growing directly from blood culture bottles. The system uses a CSA attached directly to the blood bottle, and a camera continuously monitors the CSA for colorimetric changes. This system can then be used to detect positive bottles and report an ID approximately 2 h after positivity, with the benefit of an identification, without the manipulation of the specimen by a technologist.

This technology is still early in development so literature on the performance of the system is limited. In two studies using the CSA from agar, one found 100% accuracy for detection of *Yersinia pestis* and *Bacillus anthracis* at low CFU/ml counts (n = 6), while the other using 1,894 plates and 15 bacterial species found the CSA to be 91.0% sensitive and 99.4% specific compared with reference testing (94, 95). One study used a blood bottle adapter to detect metabolites from blood cultures and observed 91.9% concordance using cultures spiked with known strains. When time to positivity was compared to conventional blood culture systems, the CSA detected growth approximately 2 h before the BacT/Alert 3D system (12.1 versus 14.9 h) (96). However, because this system is still in development, the performance of the assay along with the design of the system will likely be modified prior to commercial release.

Microcantilever

Cantilever sensors are highly sensitive detectors that measure mass through the change of deflection or resonant frequency shifts to detect a specific analyte (97). For use with microbial diagnostics, the system is able to measure the mass of individual cells and also determine the concentration of organisms in a specimen for identification. The technology has the ability to determine antimicrobial susceptibility by exposing organisms to a drug and detecting changes in organism load and cellular mass over time secondary to antimicrobial activity (98). The benefit of this technology is that it allows detection of low bacterial concentrations (as low as 200 bacterial cells or as low as 60 fungal spores) within a specimen (99, 100). In addition, AST TAT could be reduced to as few as 2 h by detecting changes to the mass of cells when exposed to antibiotics (101). The company Lifescale (Affinity Biosensors, Santa Barbara, CA) is currently in the process of developing assays using microcantilevers for AST.

Bioparticles and Microphage

A recent approach for microbial detection and AST has been the development of genus/species-specific delivery of DNA through the use of engineered particles or phages. Transfection of organisms with DNA carrying expressible reporter genes, such as luciferase or green-fluorescent protein, allows detection of the marker in viable organisms. AST can then be performed by adding antibiotics to the specimen and measuring the presence/absence of the marker as a proxy of growth (resistance) or no growth (susceptibility) to the antibiotic. One such system currently under development is the Smarticle technology (Roche Diagnostic, Indianapolis, IN) that specifically uses luciferase as a growth marker. Currently, there are no commercially available assays using the technology, but the potential for rapid ID and AST from positive blood cultures is obvious.

Optical Spectroscopy

Another approach for identification of organisms is to use intrinsic properties of organisms to differentiate based on spectroscopy. Technologies using these properties include Raman spectroscopy, Fourier transform infrared (FTIR) spectroscopy, and intrinsic fluorescence spectroscopy (IFS). Detection and identification rely on interpretation of the vibrational spectrum of the overall molecular composition of a specimen compared with a reference library of known spectra. Evaluation of Raman and FTIR spectroscopy on microcolonies from positive blood culture bottles found high accuracy for both Raman, 92.2%, and FTIR, 98.3%, compared with the laboratory standard of care (n=114) with results in 6 to 8 h after bottle positivity (102). IFS relies on fluorescence of naturally occurring substrates such as tryptophan and nicotinamide adenine dinucleotide + hydrogen (NADH), and identification is performed by comparing specimen fluorescent signatures to known databases. An evaluation using positive blood cultures following a short lysis, centrifugation, and detection found the assay to be 99.3% concordant at a genus level and 96.5% concordant at a species level of identification compared with a combination of VITEK 2 and MALDI-TOF MS identifications (n = 1,121) (103). These spectrometry technologies are an exciting new frontier in microbiology, but they do have their limitations because background interference from components of culture media is common, and so efficient purification is necessary for analysis.

Sequencing from Blood Culture

Sequence analysis of bacterial genomes is a widely accepted tool for the molecular identification of bacteria most often reserved for difficult to identify organisms that fail to be categorized by current technologies (104). However, the ability to quickly identify polymicrobial cultures using metagenomics sequence data and to provide (at the same time) genotypic resistance predictions from the contents of positive blood cultures is extremely exciting. Currently, several sequencing approaches have been evaluated ranging from broad-range 16S rRNA amplification to next-generation sequencing (NGS), each having their benefits and disadvantages (105, 106).

Similar to other diagnostic methods, sample preparation is key because inhibitors of amplification and human DNA will affect the quality results. Many published techniques follow protocols similar to those used for MALDI-TOF MS by performing differential centrifugation to remove matrix components followed by bacterial purification for either 16S sequencing or NGS. DNA/RNA is then extracted from bacterial pellets either through the use of detergents and heat to release nucleic acid or commercially available kits with standardized reagents (105, 106). Because NGS can detect small amounts of background nucleic acids, extraction controls should be processed with each run to determine background levels of extraneous DNA/RNA in reagents and contaminated platforms (107). After extraction, 16S PCR protocols use universal primers to amplify 16S rRNA followed by gel electrophoresis to confirm amplification prior to sequencing to reduce testing costs. Specimens with amplified product are then sequenced and analyzed using reference databanks such as GenBank or other curated genomic databases. NGS requires extended workflow (depending on the sequencing platform being used), i.e., the preparation of the NGS libraries, sequencing, annotation, and alignment of sequence reads and comparison of generated sequences with standardized databases for identification of organism and/or resistance markers. The American Academy of Microbiology convened a colloquium to define these issues to help improve the placement of NGS into the clinical microbiology laboratory. A review by Goldberg et al. highlights these concepts that were generated in the report (108).

Studies evaluating 16S rRNA demonstrate a reduction in TAT for identification compared with culture with some techniques such as pyrosequencing taking as little as 4 h from bottle positivity (109, 110). When comparing pyrosequencing targeting V1 and V3 regions of 16S rRNA to all positive blood bottles, one study found overall agreement with culture to be 84.3% (86/102) to a genus level and 64.7% (66/102) to a species level (109). It has been noted that the use of 16S rRNA can be limited in comparison with conventional methods because many organisms are not found within the comparators database, which can be a limitation to many studies (111). One study specifically using pyrosequencing targeting the 18S rRNA gene for yeast was able to correctly identify all 48 yeast isolates compared with the use of automated phenotypic systems (110). These data suggest that a targeted approach to quickly identifying yeast can be useful because speciation can aid in predicting antifungal susceptibility.

The use of NGS for positive blood cultures has not been reported, likely because of the overall cost and time to result at present. Data have been published using NGS directly from blood cultures (no incubation), which was discussed in chapter 7. If cost and time to result could be reduced, NGS from positive blood bottles could be beneficial for the clinical laboratories because both identification and genotypic resistance could be obtained for an expanded list of bug and drug combinations compared with current panel blood culture molecular assays.

Summary

Data suggest that identification of pathogens in blood culture specimens provides value for patient care, and that optimizing the time to results can improve outcomes. In a recent meta analysis of 31 articles, changing from a traditional method to a rapid diagnostics method for blood cultures had several benefits to patient care (112). Of the 5,920 patients reviewed, significant changes in mortality rate of bacteremia, but not candidemia, and significant decrease to length of stay and time to effective therapy. Impor-

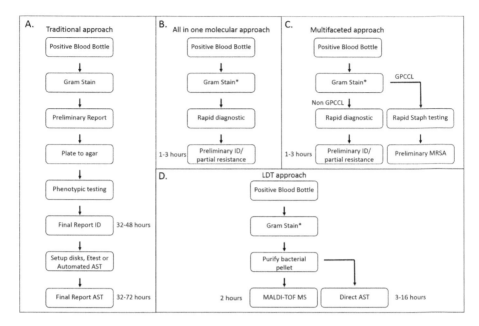

FIGURE 3 Various approaches to structuring laboratory policy of positive blood cultures. With the variety of assays available to identify organisms growing in blood cultures, laboratories can customize workflow to fit various criteria affecting turnaround time, cost, and complexity. Potential workflow approaches for laboratories are as follows. **(A)** The traditional method should not be used alone, because results are too delayed and several viable rapid options are available; however, plating should be applied to all rapid testing where the * is placed to confirm results and check for polymicrobial cultures. **(B)** For ease of workflow, a single molecular device can be used for all positive bottles. This is best done using a large panel that covers the most common blood pathogens. **(C)** To reduce cost or improve patient care, a multifaceted approach can be implemented where the rapid assay used changes based on the Gram stain result. For instance, using cheaper methicillin-resistant *S. aureus* (MRSA) assays for Gram-positive cocci in clusters (GPCCL) and a panel for all other testing. **(D)** Although it is labor intensive to bring on matrix-assisted laser desorption ionization–time of flight mass spectroscopy (MALDI-TOF MS) or use antimicrobial susceptibility testing (AST), panels of product that insert these assays likely have the shortest TAT for reporting susceptibilities. Combinations of these approaches can be used to fit the laboratories' needs and abilities.

tantly, significance was only found when rapid identification was combined with antimicrobial stewardship programs.

In the current clinical microbiology environment, there are numerous options for rapid identification of organisms in positive blood culture bottles. The simplest approach is a "sample to answer" assay (Fig. 3) where the laboratory runs all tests through a large panel such as Verigene, FilmArray, or ePlex that will detect several bacterial and genotypic targets. These systems are not only highly accurate, but the use of a single instrument reduces the initial investment cost and cost for validation that can vary based on the laboratories size. A multifaceted approach where different assays are run based on the Gram stain result has the potential to improve patient care and reduce laboratory costs. For instance, MRSA assays are both more rapid and less expensive than larger panels and so using these assays on blood cultures containing GPCCL may be beneficial for the laboratory. However, multifaceted approaches will increase policy complexity, training, and validation needed for testing blood cultures. MALDI-TOF MS is promising because it is able to identify a very large panel of microbes, and the consumable cost per assay is low. However, the lack of standardization of sample processing and FDA-approved test may limit the use of the technology to larger laboratories that have the funding and laboratory expertise to perform the extensive verification studies required. The use of MALDI-TOF MS for AST has added challenges for the laboratory because these assays do not have standardized reagents and laboratories will need to make solutions of antibiotics for testing, adding additional layers of complexity for performing quality control.

A question remaining in the field of blood culture is what is the clinical utility of a phenotypic susceptibility result compared with genotypic resistance determinant detection? Studies directly measuring this are needed, but the results are likely dependent on the organism/s being tested. Genotypic resistance is likely efficient for the treatment of common GP blood pathogens because knowledge of the presence of MRSA or VRE directly impacts the choice of optimal antimicrobial therapy. These resistant genotypes are easily detected by most molecular platforms, so rapid phenotypic testing may not be necessary for treating infections except for narrowing therapy. Treating GN infections may benefit more from phenotypic susceptibility reporting rather than just genotypic results because of the large variety of resistance mechanisms (ESBLs, AmpC, carbapenemases) and the genes involved. Couple this with the lack of predictive resistance among GN organisms, so genotypic resistance only informs the physician on what drugs will not be effective. Studies evaluating clinical impact will be essential in answering these questions.

Ultimately, the methodologies used by individual laboratories will vary with available laboratory resources, workforce, and budget, as well as the local epidemiology and patient population served. In time it is possible that these rapid assays will replace culture altogether as technology will continue to improve and the added value of culture fails to justify the cost and time of testing. Similar trends have been observed in virology, where culture of any type is obsolete compared with molecular counterparts and, more recently, molecular panels for stool testing have eliminated stool culture in some laboratories. All rapid methods available to date have limitations relative to conventional culture-based methods, and thus will not supplant conventional methods in the near term.

References

1. Levy MM, Rhodes A, Phillips GS, Townsend SR, Schorr CA, Beale R, Osborn T, Lemeshow S, Chiche JD, Artigas A, Dellinger RP. 2014. Surviving Sepsis Campaign: association between performance metrics and outcomes in a 7.5-year study. *Intensive Care Med* **40**:1623–1633.
2. Angus DC, Wax RS. 2001. Epidemiology of sepsis: an update. *Crit Care Med* **29** (Suppl):S109–S116.
3. Kumar A, Roberts D, Wood KE, Light B, Parrillo JE, Sharma S, Suppes R, Feinstein D, Zanotti S, Taiberg L, Gurka D, Kumar A, Cheang M. 2006. Duration of hypotension before initiation of effective antimicrobial therapy is the critical determinant of survival in human septic shock. *Crit Care Med* **34**:1589–1596.
4. Ibrahim EH, Sherman G, Ward S, Fraser VJ, Kollef MH. 2000. The influence of inadequate antimicrobial treatment of bloodstream infections on patient outcomes in the ICU setting. *Chest* **118**:146–155.
5. Shorr AF, Micek ST, Welch EC, Doherty JA, Reichley RM, Kollef MH. 2011. Inappropriate antibiotic therapy in Gram-negative sepsis increases hospital length of stay. *Crit Care Med* **39**:46–51.
6. Kerremans JJ, van der Bij AK, Goessens W, Verbrugh HA, Vos MC. 2009. Needle-to-incubator transport time: logistic factors influencing transport time for blood culture specimens. *J Clin Microbiol* **47**:819–822.
7. Sautter RL, Bills AR, Lang DL, Ruschell G, Heiter BJ, Bourbeau PP. 2006. Effects of delayed-entry conditions on the recovery and detection of microorganisms from BacT/ALERT and BACTEC blood culture bottles. *J Clin Microbiol* **44**:1245–1249.
8. Buetti N, Marschall J, Atkinson A, Kronenberg A, Swiss Centre for Antibiotic Resistance. 2016. National Bloodstream Infection Surveillance in Switzerland 2008-2014: different patterns and trends for university and community hospitals. *Infect Control Hosp Epidemiol* **37**:1060–1067. doi:10.1017/ice.2016.137.
9. Cockerill FR III, Reed GS, Hughes JG, Torgerson CA, Vetter EA, Harmsen WS, Dale JC, Roberts GD, Ilstrup DM, Henry NK. 1997. Clinical comparison of BACTEC 9240 plus aerobic/F resin bottles and the isolator aerobic culture system for detection of bloodstream infections. *J Clin Microbiol* **35**:1469–1472.
10. Karahan ZC, Mumcuoglu I, Guriz H, Tamer D, Balaban N, Aysev D, Akar N. 2006. PCR evaluation of false-positive signals from two automated blood-culture systems. *J Med Microbiol* **55**:53–57.
11. Ziegler R, Johnscher I, Martus P, Lenhardt D, Just HM. 1998. Controlled clinical laboratory comparison of two supplemented aerobic and anaerobic media used in

automated blood culture systems to detect bloodstream infections. *J Clin Microbiol* 36:657–661.

12. Durtschi JD, Erali M, Bromley LK, Herrmann MG, Petti CA, Smith RE, Voelkerding KV. 2005. Increased sensitivity of bacterial detection in cerebrospinal fluid by fluorescent staining on low-fluorescence membrane filters. *J Med Microbiol* 54:843–850.

13. Lauer BA, Reller LB, Mirrett S. 1981. Comparison of acridine orange and Gram stains for detection of microorganisms in cerebrospinal fluid and other clinical specimens. *J Clin Microbiol* 14:201–205.

14. Qian Q, Tang YW, Kolbert CP, Torgerson CA, Hughes JG, Vetter EA, Harmsen WS, Montgomery SO, Cockerill FR III, Persing DH. 2001. Direct identification of bacteria from positive blood cultures by amplification and sequencing of the 16S rRNA gene: evaluation of BACTEC 9240 instrument true-positive and false-positive results. *J Clin Microbiol* 39:3578–3582.

15. Winn WC, Koneman EW. 2006. *Koneman's Color Atlas and Textbook of Diagnostic Microbiology*, 6th ed. Lippincott Williams & Wilkins, Philadelphia, PA.

16. MacArthur RD, Miller M, Albertson T, Panacek E, Johnson D, Teoh L, Barchuk W. 2004. Adequacy of early empiric antibiotic treatment and survival in severe sepsis: experience from the MONARCS trial. *Clin Infect Dis* 38:284–288.

17. Miano TA, Powell E, Schweickert WD, Morgan S, Binkley S, Sarani B. 2012. Effect of an antibiotic algorithm on the adequacy of empiric antibiotic therapy given by a medical emergency team. *J Crit Care* 27:45–50.

18. Wang MC, Lin WH, Yan JJ, Fang HY, Kuo TH, Tseng CC, Wu JJ. 2015. Early identification of microorganisms in blood culture prior to the detection of a positive signal in the BACTEC FX system using matrix-assisted laser desorption/ionization-time of flight mass spectrometry. *J Microbiol Immunol Infect* 48:419–424.

19. Al-Soud WA, Rådström P. 2001. Purification and characterization of PCR inhibitory components in blood cells. *J Clin Microbiol* 39:485–493.

20. Clark AE, Kaleta EJ, Arora A, Wolk DM. 2013. Matrix-assisted laser desorption ionization-time of flight mass spectrometry: a fundamental shift in the routine practice of clinical microbiology. *Clin Microbiol Rev* 26:547–603.

21. Angeletti S. 2017. Matrix assisted laser desorption time of flight mass spectrometry (MALDI-TOF MS) in clinical microbiology. *J Microbiol Methods* 138:20–29. doi:10.1016/j.mimet.2016.09.003.

22. Ferreira L, Sánchez-Juanes F, González-Avila M, Cembrero-Fuciños D, Herrero-Hernández A, González-Buitrago JM, Muñoz-Bellido JL. 2010. Direct identification of urinary tract pathogens from urine samples by matrix-assisted laser desorption ionization-time of flight mass spectrometry. *J Clin Microbiol* 48:2110–2115.

23. Hsieh SY, Tseng CL, Lee YS, Kuo AJ, Sun CF, Lin YH, Chen JK. 2008. Highly efficient classification and identification of human pathogenic bacteria by MALDI-TOF MS. *Mol Cell Proteomics* 7:448–456.

24. La Scola B, Raoult D. 2009. Direct identification of bacteria in positive blood culture bottles by matrix-assisted laser desorption ionisation time-of-flight mass spectrometry. *PLoS One* 4:e8041.

25. Prod'hom G, Bizzini A, Durussel C, Bille J, Greub G. 2010. Matrix-assisted laser desorption ionization-time of flight mass spectrometry for direct bacterial identification from positive blood culture pellets. *J Clin Microbiol* 48:1481–1483.

26. Moussaoui W, Jaulhac B, Hoffmann AM, Ludes B, Kostrzewa M, Riegel P, Prévost G. 2010. Matrix-assisted laser desorption ionization time-of-flight mass spectrometry identifies 90% of bacteria directly from blood culture vials. *Clin Microbiol Infect* 16:1631–1638.

27. Bazzi AM, Rabaan AA, El Edaily Z, John S, Fawarah MM, Al-Tawfiq JA. 2017. Comparison among four proposed direct blood culture microbial identification methods using MALDI-TOF MS. *J Infect Public Health* 10:308–315. doi:10.1016/j.jiph.2016.05.011.

28. Verroken A, Defourny L, Lechgar L, Magnette A, Delmée M, Glupczynski Y. 2015. Reducing time to identification of positive blood cultures with MALDI-TOF MS analysis after a 5-h subculture. *Eur J Clin Microbiol Infect Dis* 34:405–413.

29. Gonzalez MD, Weber CJ, Burnham CA. 2016. Rapid identification of microorganisms from positive blood cultures by testing early growth on solid media using matrix-assisted laser desorption ionization-time of flight mass spectrometry. *Diagn Microbiol Infect Dis* 85:133–135.

30. Nonnemann B, Tvede M, Bjarnsholt T. 2013. Identification of pathogenic microorganisms directly from positive blood vials by matrix-assisted laser desorption/ionization time of flight mass spectrometry. *APMIS* 121:871–877.

31. Hazelton B, Thomas LC, Olma T, Kok J, O'Sullivan M, Chen SC, Iredell JR. 2014. Rapid and accurate direct antibiotic susceptibility testing of blood culture broths using MALDI Sepsityper combined with the BD Phoenix automated system. *J Med Microbiol* 63:1590–1594.

32. Morgenthaler NG, Kostrzewa M. 2015. Rapid identification of pathogens in positive blood culture of patients with sepsis: review and meta-analysis of the performance of the sepsityper kit. *Int J Microbiol* 2015:827416.

33. Yan Y, He Y, Maier T, Quinn C, Shi G, Li H, Stratton CW, Kostrzewa M, Tang YW. 2011. Improved identification of yeast species directly from positive blood culture media by combining Sepsityper specimen processing and Microflex analysis with the matrix-assisted laser desorption ionization Biotyper system. *J Clin Microbiol* 49:2528–2532.

34. Spanu T, Posteraro B, Fiori B, D'Inzeo T, Campoli S, Ruggeri A, Tumbarello M, Canu G, Trecarichi EM, Parisi G, Tronci M, Sanguinetti M, Fadda G. 2012. Direct MALDI-TOF mass spectrometry assay of blood culture broths for rapid identification of Candida species causing bloodstream infections: an observational study in two large microbiology laboratories. *J Clin Microbiol* 50:176–179.

35. Rychert J, Burnham CA, Bythrow M, Garner OB, Ginocchio CC, Jennemann R, Lewinski MA, Manji R, Mochon AB, Procop GW, Richter SS, Sercia L, Westblade LF, Ferraro MJ, Branda JA. 2013. Multicenter evaluation of the Vitek MS matrix-assisted laser desorption ionization-time of flight mass spectrometry system for identification of Gram-positive aerobic bacteria. *J Clin Microbiol* 51:2225–2231.

36. Wang XH, Zhang G, Fan YY, Yang X, Sui WJ, Lu XX. 2013. Direct identification of bacteria causing urinary tract infections by combining matrix-assisted laser desorption ionization-time of flight mass spectrometry with UF-1000i urine flow cytometry. *J Microbiol Methods* 92:231–235.

37. Loonen AJ, Jansz AR, Stalpers J, Wolffs PF, van den Brule AJ. 2012. An evaluation of three processing methods and the effect of reduced culture times for faster direct

identification of pathogens from BacT/ALERT blood cultures by MALDI-TOF MS. *Eur J Clin Microbiol Infect Dis* 31:1575–1583.

38. Meex C, Neuville F, Descy J, Huynen P, Hayette MP, De Mol P, Melin P. 2012. Direct identification of bacteria from BacT/ALERT anaerobic positive blood cultures by MALDI-TOF MS: MALDI Sepsityper kit versus an in-house saponin method for bacterial extraction. *J Med Microbiol* 61:1511–1516.

39. Almuhayawi M, Altun O, Abdulmajeed AD, Ullberg M, Özenci V. 2015. The performance of the four anaerobic blood culture bottles BacT/ALERT-FN, -FN Plus, BACTEC-Plus and -Lytic in detection of anaerobic bacteria and identification by direct MALDI-TOF MS. *PLoS One* 10:e0142398.

40. Schubert S, Weinert K, Wagner C, Gunzl B, Wieser A, Maier T, Kostrzewa M. 2011. Novel, improved sample preparation for rapid, direct identification from positive blood cultures using matrix-assisted laser desorption/ionization time-of-flight (MALDI-TOF) mass spectrometry. *J Mol Diagn* 13:701–706.

41. Buchan BW, Riebe KM, Ledeboer NA. 2012. Comparison of the MALDI Biotyper system using Sepsityper specimen processing to routine microbiological methods for identification of bacteria from positive blood culture bottles. *J Clin Microbiol* 50:346–352.

42. Randazzo A, Simon M, Goffinet P, Classen JF, Hougardy N, Pierre P, Kinzinger P, Mauel E, Goffinet JS. 2016. Optimal turnaround time for direct identification of microorganisms by mass spectrometry in blood culture. *J Microbiol Methods* 130:1–5.

43. Hrabák J, Chudáčková E, Walková R. 2013. Matrix-assisted laser desorption ionization-time of flight (MALDI-TOF) mass spectrometry for detection of antibiotic resistance mechanisms: from research to routine diagnosis. *Clin Microbiol Rev* 26:103–114.

44. Ghebremedhin B, Halstenbach A, Smiljanic M, Kaase M, Ahmad-Nejad P. 2016. MALDI-TOF MS based carbapenemase detection from culture isolates and from positive blood culture vials. *Ann Clin Microbiol Antimicrob* 15:5.

45. Kim JS, Kang GE, Kim HS, Kim HS, Song W, Lee KM. 2016. Evaluation of Verigene blood culture test systems for rapid identification of positive blood cultures. *BioMed Res Int* 2016:1081536.

46. Uno N, Suzuki H, Yamakawa H, Yamada M, Yaguchi Y, Notake S, Tamai K, Yanagisawa H, Misawa S, Yanagihara K. 2015. Multicenter evaluation of the Verigene Gram-negative blood culture nucleic acid test for rapid detection of bacteria and resistance determinants in positive blood cultures. *Diagn Microbiol Infect Dis* 83:344–348.

47. Ledeboer NA, Lopansri BK, Dhiman N, Cavagnolo R, Carroll KC, Granato P, Thomson R Jr, Butler-Wu SM, Berger H, Samuel L, Pancholi P, Swyers L, Hansen GT, Tran NK, Polage CR, Thomson KS, Hanson ND, Winegar R, Buchan BW. 2015. Identification of Gram-negative bacteria and genetic resistance determinants from positive blood culture broths by use of the Verigene Gram-negative blood culture multiplex microarray-based molecular assay. *J Clin Microbiol* 53:2460–2472.

48. Buchan BW, Ginocchio CC, Manii R, Cavagnolo R, Pancholi P, Swyers L, Thomson RB Jr, Anderson C, Kaul K, Ledeboer NA. 2013. Multiplex identification of gram-positive bacteria and resistance determinants directly from positive blood culture broths: evaluation of an automated microarray-based nucleic acid test. *PLoS Med* 10:e1001478.

49. Maatallah M, Vading M, Kabir MH, Bakhrouf A, Kalin M, Nauclér P, Brisse S, Giske CG. 2014. *Klebsiella variicola* is a frequent cause of bloodstream infection in the Stockholm area, and associated with higher mortality compared to *K. pneumoniae*. *PLoS One* 9:e113539.

50. Walker T, Dumadag S, Lee CJ, Lee SH, Bender JM, Cupo Abbott J, She RC. 2016. Clinical impact of laboratory implementation of Verigene BC-GN microarray-based assay for detection of Gram-negative bacteria in positive blood cultures. *J Clin Microbiol* 54:1789–1796.

51. Boom R, Sol CJ, Salimans MM, Jansen CL, Wertheim-van Dillen PM, van der Noordaa J. 1990. Rapid and simple method for purification of nucleic acids. *J Clin Microbiol* 28:495–503.

52. Altun O, Almuhayawi M, Ullberg M, Ozenci V. 2013. Clinical evaluation of the FilmArray blood culture identification panel in identification of bacteria and yeasts from positive blood culture bottles. *J Clin Microbiol* 51:4130–4136.

53. Salimnia H, Fairfax MR, Lephart PR, Schreckenberger P, DesJarlais SM, Johnson JK, Robinson G, Carroll KC, Greer A, Morgan M, Chan R, Loeffelholz M, Valencia-Shelton F, Jenkins S, Schuetz AN, Daly JA, Barney T, Hemmert A, Kanack KJ. 2016. Evaluation of the FilmArray blood culture identification panel: results of a multicenter controlled trial. *J Clin Microbiol* 54:687–698.

54. McCoy MH, Relich RF, Davis TE, Schmitt BH. 2016. Performance of the FilmArray® blood culture identification panel utilized by non-expert staff compared with conventional microbial identification and antimicrobial resistance gene detection from positive blood cultures. *J Med Microbiol* 65:619–625.

55. Southern TR, VanSchooneveld TC, Bannister DL, Brown TL, Crismon AS, Buss SN, Iwen PC, Fey PD. 2015. Implementation and performance of the BioFire FilmArray® Blood Culture Identification panel with antimicrobial treatment recommendations for bloodstream infections at a midwestern academic tertiary hospital. *Diagn Microbiol Infect Dis* 81:96–101.

56. Ward C, Stocker K, Begum J, Wade P, Ebrahimsa U, Goldenberg SD. 2015. Performance evaluation of the Verigene® (Nanosphere) and FilmArray® (BioFire®) molecular assays for identification of causative organisms in bacterial bloodstream infections. *Eur J Clin Microbiol Infect Dis* 34:487–496.

57. Messacar K, Hurst AL, Child J, Campbell K, Palmer C, Hamilton S, Dowell E, Robinson CC, Parker SK, Dominguez SR. 19 August 2016. Clinical impact and provider acceptability of real-time antimicrobial stewardship decision support for rapid diagnostics in children with positive blood culture results. *J Pediatric Infect Dis Soc* doi:10.1093/jpids/piw047.

58. Dodémont M, De Mendonça R, Nonhoff C, Roisin S, Denis O. 2015. Evaluation of Verigene Gram-Positive Blood Culture Assay performance for bacteremic patients. *Eur J Clin Microbiol Infect Dis* 34:473–477.

59. Buchan BW, Reymann GC, Granato PA, Alkins BR, Jim P, Young S. 2015. Preliminary evaluation of the research-use-only (RUO) iCubate iC-GPC assay for identification of select Gram-positive bacteria and their resistance determinants in blood culture broths. *J Clin Microbiol* 53:3931–3934.

60. Hensley DM, Tapia R, Encina Y. 2009. An evaluation of the advandx Staphylococcus aureus/CNS PNA FISH assay. *Clin Lab Sci* 22:30–33.

61. Chapin K, Musgnug M. 2003. Evaluation of three rapid methods for the direct identification of *Staphylococcus aureus* from positive blood cultures. *J Clin Microbiol* 41:4324–4327.

62. Aydemir G, Koç AN, Atalay MA. 2016. [Evaluation of peptide nucleic acid fluorescent in situ hybridization (PNA FISH) method in the identification of *Candida* species isolated from blood cultures]. *Mikrobiyol Bul* 50:293–299.

63. Faron ML CC, Buchan BW, Guralnik M, LaBombardi VJ, Ledeboer NA. 2016. Multicenter evaluation of the Miacom HemoFISH for bacterial identification from positive blood cultures. Poster presentation at American Society for Microbiology Microbe 2016.

64. Vincent JL, Guralnik M, Faron ML, Buchan BW, Ledeboer NA. 2016. Evaluation of the Miacom HemoFISH Assay for positive blood cultures. Poster presentation at European Congress of Clinical Microbiology and Infectious Diseases 2016.

65. Lob SH, Biedenbach DJ, Badal RE, Kazmierczak KM, Sahm DF. 2016. Discrepancy between genotypic and phenotypic extended-spectrum β-lactamase rates in *Escherichia coli* from intra-abdominal infections in the USA. *J Med Microbiol* 65:905–909.

66. Burnham CA, Frobel RA, Herrera ML, Wickes BL. 2014. Rapid ertapenem susceptibility testing and *Klebsiella pneumoniae* carbapenemase phenotype detection in *Klebsiella pneumoniae* isolates by use of automated microscopy of immobilized live bacterial cells. *J Clin Microbiol* 52:982–986.

67. Metzger S, Frobel RA, Dunne WM Jr. 2014. Rapid simultaneous identification and quantitation of *Staphylococcus aureus* and *Pseudomonas aeruginosa* directly from bronchoalveolar lavage specimens using automated microscopy. *Diagn Microbiol Infect Dis* 79:160–165.

68. Lisby GKS, Knudsen JD, Turng B, Metzger S, Littauer P. 2015. Performance of the new Accelerate ID/AAST System in highly resistant *Acinetobacter baumannii* bloodstream infection isolates, compared to routine laboratory testing. Poster presentation at European Congress of Clinical Microbiology and Infectious Diseases, 2015.

69. Price CDI, Tuttle E, Shorr A, Mensack M, Bessesen M, Miquirray S, Overdier K, Duarte N, Shamsheyeva A, Gamage D, Allers E, Hance K, Michel C, Turng B, Metzger S. 2015. Rapid identification and antimicrobial susceptibility testing of bacteria in bloodstream infections using the Accelerate ID/AST Technology. Poster presentation at European Congress of Clinical Microbiology and Infectious Diseases, 2015.

70. Diekema DJ, Beekmann SE, Chapin KC, Morel KA, Munson E, Doern GV. 2003. Epidemiology and outcome of nosocomial and community-onset bloodstream infection. *J Clin Microbiol* 41:3655–3660.

71. Bauer KA, West JE, Balada-Llasat JM, Pancholi P, Stevenson KB, Goff DA. 2010. An antimicrobial stewardship program's impact with rapid polymerase chain reaction methicillin-resistant *Staphylococcus aureus*/ *S. aureus* blood culture test in patients with *S. aureus* bacteremia. *Clin Infect Dis* 51:1074–1080.

72. Ruimy R, Dos-Santos M, Raskine L, Bert F, Masson R, Elbaz S, Bonnal C, Lucet JC, Lefort A, Fantin B, Wolff M, Hornstein M, Andremont A. 2008. Accuracy and potential usefulness of triplex real-time PCR for improving antibiotic treatment of patients with blood cultures showing clustered gram-positive cocci on direct smears. *J Clin Microbiol* 46:2045–2051.

73. Nguyen DT, Yeh E, Perry S, Luo RF, Pinsky BA, Lee BP, Sisodiya D, Baron EJ, Banaei N. 2010. Real-time PCR testing for mecA reduces vancomycin usage and length of hospitalization for patients infected with methicillin-sensitive staphylococci. *J Clin Microbiol* 48:785–790.

74. Snyder JW, Munier GK, Heckman SA, Camp P, Overman TL. 2009. Failure of the BD GeneOhm StaphSR assay for direct detection of methicillin-resistant and methicillin-susceptible *Staphylococcus aureus* isolates in positive blood cultures collected in the United States. *J Clin Microbiol* 47:3747–3748.

75. Stamper PD, Cai M, Howard T, Speser S, Carroll KC. 2007. Clinical validation of the molecular BD GeneOhm StaphSR assay for direct detection of *Staphylococcus aureus* and methicillin-resistant *Staphylococcus aureus* in positive blood cultures. *J Clin Microbiol* 45:2191–2196.

76. Wolk DM, Struelens MJ, Pancholi P, Davis T, Della-Latta P, Fuller D, Picton E, Dickenson R, Denis O, Johnson D, Chapin K. 2009. Rapid detection of *Staphylococcus aureus* and methicillin-resistant *S. aureus* (MRSA) in wound specimens and blood cultures: multicenter preclinical evaluation of the Cepheid Xpert MRSA/SA skin and soft tissue and blood culture assays. *J Clin Microbiol* 47:823–826.

77. Bartels MD, Boye K, Rohde SM, Larsen AR, Torfs H, Bouchy P, Skov R, Westh H. 2009. A common variant of staphylococcal cassette chromosome mec type IVa in isolates from Copenhagen, Denmark, is not detected by the BD GeneOhm methicillin-resistant *Staphylococcus aureus* assay. *J Clin Microbiol* 47:1524–1527.

78. Buchan BW, Allen S, Burnham CA, McElvania TeKippe E, Davis T, Levi M, Mayne D, Pancholi P, Relich RF, Thomson R, Ledeboer NA. 2015. Comparison of the next-generation Xpert MRSA/SA BC assay and the GeneOhm StaphSR assay to routine culture for identification of *Staphylococcus aureus* and methicillin-resistant *S. aureus* in positive-blood-culture broths. *J Clin Microbiol* 53:804–809.

79. Peacock SJ, Paterson GK. 2015. Mechanisms of methicillin resistance in *Staphylococcus aureus*. *Annu Rev Biochem* 84:577–601.

80. Heraud S, Freydiere AM, Doleans-Jordheim A, Bes M, Tristan A, Vandenesch F, Laurent F, Dauwalder O. 2015. Direct Identification of *Staphylococcus aureus* and determination of methicillin susceptibility from positive blood-culture bottles in a Bact/ALERT system using Binax Now *S. aureus* and PBP2a tests. *Ann Lab Med* 35:454–457.

81. Romero-Gómez MP, Quiles-Melero I, Navarro C, Paño-Pardo JR, Gómez-Gil R, Mingorance J. 2012. Evaluation of the BinaxNOW PBP2a assay for the direct detection of methicillin resistance in *Staphylococcus aureus* from positive blood culture bottles. *Diagn Microbiol Infect Dis* 72:282–284.

82. Yossepowitch O, Dan M, Kutchinsky A, Gottesman T, Schwartz-Harari O. 2014. A cost-saving algorithm for rapid diagnosis of *Staphylococcus aureus* and susceptibility to oxacillin directly from positive blood culture bottles by combined testing with BinaxNOW® *S. aureus* and Xpert MRSA/SA Assay. *Diagn Microbiol Infect Dis* 78:352–355.

83. Manickam K, Walkty A, Lagacé-Wiens PRS, Adam H, Swan B, McAdam B, Pieroni P, Alfa M, Karlowsky JA. 2013. Evaluation of MRSASelect (™) chromogenic medium for the early detection of methicillin-resistant *Staphylococcus aureus* from blood cultures. *Can J Infect Dis Med Microbiol* 24:e113–e116.

84. Harriau P, Ruffel F, Lardy JB. 2006. [Use of BioRad plating agar MRSASelect for the daily detection of methicillin resistant staphylococci isolated from samples taken from blood culture bottles]. *Pathol Biol (Paris)* **54**:506–509.

85. Menon V, Lahanas S, Janto C, Lee A. 2016. Utility of direct susceptibility testing on blood cultures: is it still worthwhile? *J Med Microbiol* **65**:501–509.

86. Stokkou S, Geginat G, Schlüter D, Tammer I. 2015. Direct disk diffusion test using European Clinical Antimicrobial Susceptibility Testing breakpoints provides reliable results compared with the standard method. *Eur J Microbiol Immunol (Bp)* **5**:103–111.

87. Hong T, Ndamukong J, Millett W, Kish A, Win KK, Choi YJ. 1996. Direct application of Etest to gram-positive cocci from blood cultures: quick and reliable minimum inhibitory concentration data. *Diagn Microbiol Infect Dis* **25**:21–25.

88. Funke G, Funke-Kissling P. 2004. Use of the BD PHOENIX automated identification and susceptibility testing positive blood cultures in a microbiology system for direct of gram-negative rods from three-phase trial. *J Clin Microbiol* **42**:1466–1470.

89. Lupetti A, Barnini S, Castagna B, Nibbering PH, Campa M. 2010. Rapid identification and antimicrobial susceptibility testing of Gram-positive cocci in blood cultures by direct inoculation into the BD Phoenix system. *Clin Microbiol Infect* **16**:986–991.

90. Hazelton B, Thomas LC, Olma T, Kok J, O'Sullivan M, Chen SCA, Iredell JR. 2014. Rapid and accurate direct antibiotic susceptibility testing of blood culture broths using MALDI Sepsityper combined with the BD Phoenix automated system. *J Med Microbiol* **63**:1590–1594.

91. Gherardi G, Angeletti S, Panitti M, Pompilio A, Di Bonaventura G, Crea F, Avola A, Fico L, Palazzo C, Sapia GF, Visaggio D, Dicuonzo G. 2012. Comparative evaluation of the Vitek-2 Compact and Phoenix systems for rapid identification and antibiotic susceptibility testing directly from blood cultures of Gram-negative and Gram-positive isolates. *Diagn Microbiol Infect Dis* **72**:20–31.

92. Carey JR, Suslick KS, Hulkower KI, Imlay JA, Imlay KR, Ingison CK, Ponder JB, Sen A, Wittrig AE. 2011. Rapid identification of bacteria with a disposable colorimetric sensing array. *J Am Chem Soc* **133**:7571–7576.

93. Rakow NA, Suslick KS. 2000. A colorimetric sensor array for odour visualization. *Nature* **406**:710–713.

94. Lonsdale CL, Taba B, Queralto N, Lukaszewski RA, Martino RA, Rhodes PA, Lim SH. 2013. The use of colorimetric sensor arrays to discriminate between pathogenic bacteria. *PLoS One* **8**:e62726.

95. Lim SH, Mix S, Anikst V, Budvytiene I, Eiden M, Churi Y, Queralto N, Berliner A, Martino RA, Rhodes PA, Banaei N. 2016. Bacterial culture detection and identification in blood agar plates with an optoelectronic nose. *Analyst (Lond)* **141**:918–925.

96. Lim SH, Mix S, Xu Z, Taba B, Budvytiene I, Berliner AN, Queralto N, Churi YS, Huang RS, Eiden M, Martino RA, Rhodes P, Banaei N, Land GA. 2014. Colorimetric sensor array allows fast detection and simultaneous identification of sepsis-causing bacteria in spiked blood culture. *J Clin Microbiol* **52**:592–598.

97. Lavrik NV, Sepaniak MJ, Datskos PG. 2004. Cantilever transducers as a platform for chemical and biological sensors. *Rev Sci Instrum* **75**:2229–2253.

98. Longo G, Alonso-Sarduy L, Rio LM, Bizzini A, Trampuz A, Notz J, Dietler G, Kasas S. 2013. Rapid detection of bacterial resistance to antibiotics using AFM cantilevers as nanomechanical sensors. *Nat Nanotechnol* **8**:522–526.

99. Gfeller KY, Nugaeva N, Hegner M. 2005. Micromechanical oscillators as rapid biosensor for the detection of active growth of *Escherichia coli*. *Biosens Bioelectron* 21:528–533.

100. Nugaeva N, Gfeller KY, Backmann N, Lang HP, Düggelin M, Hegner M. 2005. Micromechanical cantilever array sensors for selective fungal immobilization and fast growth detection. *Biosens Bioelectron* 21:849–856.

101. Gfeller KY, Nugaeva N, Hegner M. 2005. Rapid biosensor for detection of antibiotic-selective growth of *Escherichia coli*. *Appl Environ Microbiol* 71:2626–2631.

102. Maquelin K, Kirschner C, Choo-Smith LP, Ngo-Thi NA, van Vreeswijk T, Stämmler M, Endtz HP, Bruining HA, Naumann D, Puppels GJ. 2003. Prospective study of the performance of vibrational spectroscopies for rapid identification of bacterial and fungal pathogens recovered from blood cultures. *J Clin Microbiol* 41:324–329.

103. Walsh JD, Hyman JM, Borzhemskaya L, Bowen A, McKellar C, Ullery M, Mathias E, Ronsick C, Link J, Wilson M, Clay B, Robinson R, Thorpe T, van Belkum A, Dunne WM Jr. 2013. Rapid intrinsic fluorescence method for direct identification of pathogens in blood cultures. *MBio* 4:e00865-13.

104. Patel JB. 2001. 16S rRNA gene sequencing for bacterial pathogen identification in the clinical laboratory. *Mol Diagn* 6:313–321.

105. Hassan RM, El Enany MG, Rizk HH. 2014. Evaluation of broad-range 16S rRNA PCR for the diagnosis of bloodstream infections: two years of experience. *J Infect Dev Ctries* 8:1252–1258.

106. Grumaz S, Stevens P, Grumaz C, Decker SO, Weigand MA, Hofer S, Brenner T, von Haeseler A, Sohn K. 2016. Next-generation sequencing diagnostics of bacteremia in septic patients. *Genome Med* 8:73.

107. Salter SJ, Cox MJ, Turek EM, Calus ST, Cookson WO, Moffatt MF, Turner P, Parkhill J, Loman NJ, Walker AW. 2014. Reagent and laboratory contamination can critically impact sequence-based microbiome analyses. *BMC Biol* 12:87.

108. Goldberg B, Sichtig H, Geyer C, Ledeboer N, Weinstock GM. 2015. Making the leap from research laboratory to clinic: challenges and opportunities for next-generation sequencing in infectious disease diagnostics. *MBio* 6:e01888-15.

109. Motoshima M, Yanagihara K, Morinaga Y, Matsuda J, Hasegawa H, Kohno S, Kamihira S. 2012. Identification of bacteria directly from positive blood culture samples by DNA pyrosequencing of the 16S rRNA gene. *J Med Microbiol* 61:1556–1562.

110. Quiles-Melero I, García-Rodriguez J, Romero-Gómez MP, Gómez-Sánchez P, Mingorance J. 2011. Rapid identification of yeasts from positive blood culture bottles by pyrosequencing. *Eur J Clin Microbiol Infect Dis* 30:21–24.

111. Bosshard PP, Zbinden R, Abels S, Böddinghaus B, Altwegg M, Böttger EC. 2006. 16S rRNA gene sequencing versus the API 20 NE system and the VITEK 2 ID-GNB card for identification of nonfermenting Gram-negative bacteria in the clinical laboratory. *J Clin Microbiol* 44:1359–1366.

112. Timbrook TT, Morton JB, McConeghy KW, Caffrey AR, Mylonakis E, LaPlante KL. 2017. The Effect of molecular rapid diagnostic testing on clinical outcomes in bloodstream infections: a systematic review and meta-analysis. *Clin Infect Dis* 64:15–23.

The Dark Art of Blood Cultures
Edited by Wm. Michael Dunne, Jr. and Carey-Ann D. Burnham
© 2018 American Society for Microbiology, Washington, DC
doi:10.1128/9781555819811.ch12

Fungal and Mycobacterial Blood Cultures

12

Robert S. Liao[1] and William Lainhart[2]

Early and appropriate antimicrobial therapy of sepsis is associated with improved clinical outcomes, and the laboratory identification of the etiological agent of fungemia and/or mycobacteremia is very important for successful outcome. Fungi and some mycobacteria grow more slowly than many common pathogenic bacteria, and specialized broth culture media and methodologies are available for their isolation. Not surprisingly, there are reports of fungi, primarily yeast, being recovered more effectively using mycobacterial blood culture media compared with routine blood culture bottles intended for the detection of aerobic and anaerobic bacteria (1, 2). The laboratory diagnosis of mycobacteremia and fungemia often requires special consideration with the selection of blood culture testing and interpretation of results.

Fungal Blood Culture

The diagnosis of invasive fungal disease is often made via blood culture to detect the mold or yeast causing fungemia. Different filamentous fungi and *Candida* species have emerged over time as more common causes of infection with unique antifungal susceptibilities. The number of cases of sepsis in the United States caused by fungi increased 207% between 1979 and 2000, with 16,042 cases in 2000 (4.6% of cases) (3). The efforts to steadily improve fungal blood cultures have been driven by the need for more rapid and accurate fungal identification and susceptibility testing to help the medical

[1]PeaceHealth Laboratories, Springfield, OR 97477
[2]Washington University School of Medicine, St. Louis, MO 63110

management of patients with fungemia (4). Improvement in blood culture techniques for the detection of bacteria has also incrementally benefited the recovery of fungi in the laboratory, but these advances have been largely intended to optimize the detection of bacteremia, and diagnostic sensitivity remains an ongoing issue for the management of fungemia. Advances in instrumentation, blood bottles, and culture media over the past 40 years along with the adoption of best practice by clinical laboratories have resulted in the widespread adoption of continuous monitoring blood culture systems (CMBCSs), with some laboratories also opting to use a manual blood culture method with the lysis-centrifugation system. Ninety-three percent of laboratories licensed by the College of American Pathologists in 2015 routinely used either the Bactec (BD Diagnostics, Sparks, MD), BacT/Alert 3D (bioMérieux, Marcy-l'Étoile, France), or VersaTREK (Thermo Scientific Microbiology, Waltham, MA) (5). Specific mycological media bottles and lysis-centrifugation tubes remain a recommendation for the purpose of detecting fungemia (6).

Fungemia

Fungemia with yeast is commonly described with patients that have the following risk factors: immunosuppressive disease, intravenous access device, broad-spectrum antibiotics, hyperalimentation, and injury to the gastrointestinal mucosa. The most common pathogenic yeast isolated from blood culture include: *Candida albicans* (Fig. 1, top), *Candida glabrata* (Fig. 1, middle), *Candida parapsilosis*, *Candida tropicalis*, and *Cryptococcus neoformans*. Other *Candida* species, *Malassezia furfur*, *Trichosporon*, and *Rhodotorula* are less frequently recovered (7, 8). The term candidemia describes the presence of *Candida* species in the blood of which *C. albicans* is the most common species identified. The presence of *Candida* in a blood culture is never viewed as a contaminant initially, because dissemination from the primary source causing a bloodstream infection is common (4). Disseminated histoplasmosis caused by *Histoplasma capsulatum* has been recognized with increasing frequency in immunosuppressed patients (9) such as those with bone marrow and solid organ transplantation, AIDS, and hematologic malignancies. Other dimorphic fungi (*Blastomyces* and *Coccidioides*) are less frequently recovered (10–13). Once in the lung, these fungi can reach the bloodstream and continue to the central nervous system. Blood cultures may be positive for cryptococci in approximately two-thirds of AIDS-associated cases associated with meningoencephalitis (14). Of the filamentous fungi, species like *Fusarium* (Fig. 1, bottom) and *Scedosporium* appear to be more

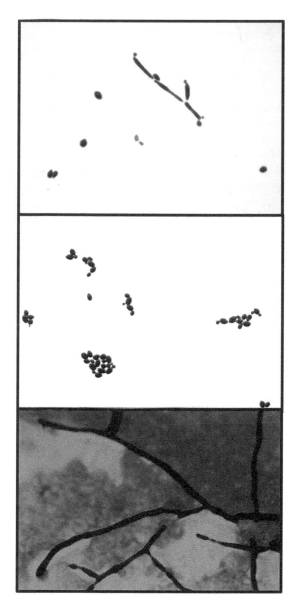

Figure 1 Gram stains of positive fungal blood cultures. **(Top)** *Candida albicans* (1000× magnification). (Middle) *Candida glabrata* (1000× magnification) **(Bottom)** *Fusarium* sp. (1000× magnification).

commonly isolated in blood culture, whereas isolates of *Aspergillus* or the *Zygomycetes* are infrequently detected in blood culture despite having a propensity for causing disseminated infections (15–17). Thus, blood cultures represent a limited diagnostic tool for invasive aspergillosis because

Aspergillus fungemia is rarely encountered, and its prognostic value in the setting of invasive disease is difficult to establish because of media contamination often yielding false-positive results (18). The basic differences observed in the microbiology between the yeast and filamentous fungi not surprisingly impact our capabilities to detect these fungi in blood culture.

Specialized Fungal-Specific Blood Culture Developed for CMBCSs

Specialized systems and blood culture bottles that promote the recovery of fungi from blood are available. Comparable performance has been demonstrated using aerobic broth culture media when CMBCSs from various vendors have been compared in the past for the detection of fungemia (19, 20). The BD Bactec MYCO/F Lytic and the bioMérieux BacT/Alert MB (currently not available) culture bottles that were designed for the selective culture of mycobacteria have also been demonstrated to preferentially support the growth of fungi, predominantly yeast-like fungi, better than traditional aerobic and anaerobic bacterial blood culture media (1, 2, 21). Cateau et al. (22) demonstrated that coincubation of *Candida* with faster-growing bacteria in standard blood culture media could prevent fungal detection in simulated blood cultures. Bactec MYCO/F Lytic bottles contain antibiotics intended to inhibit the growth of bacteria other than mycobacteria or fungi and are thus well suited to detect both mycobacteria and fungi. The BacT/Alert MB culture bottles did not contain antibiotics and were intended to detect mycobacteria only. A 2-year retrospective study of predominantly candidemic patients showed that the Bactec MYCO/F Lytic bottle allowed earlier *Candida* species detection by at least 1 day in 27.5% of cases compared with contemporaneously submitted routine blood culture bottles (Bactec Plus Aerobic/F and Anaerobic/F bottles) (23).

The only FDA-cleared blood culture bottle for the selective culture and recovery of fungi from blood is the BD Bactec Mycosis-IC/F blood culture bottle. The Bactec Mycosis-IC/F bottle contains fungal media, lysing reagent to cause hemolysis and release of phagocytized fungi, and antibiotics that prevent bacterial overgrowth (tobramycin and chloramphenicol) (24). The Bactec Mycosis-IC/F bottle has been optimized for the recovery of yeast but has not been proven effective for the recovery of dimorphic fungi as stated in the package insert (24). CMBCSs have a significant disadvantage with the detection of many clinically significant fungi other than *Candida* species which can be partially alleviated with the use of mycological broth bottles and blind subculture. The Bactec Mycosis-IC/F bottle has been shown to be more effective than the Bactec Plus Aerobic/F medium for the diagnosis of candidemia in terms of the positivity rate and the time to positivity (1). Meyer et al. (1) also demonstrated a significant advantage to patient testing using the Bactec Mycosis-IC/F bottle with a mean time savings of 8.8 h for *C. albicans* and 43.7 h for *C. glabrata*. Similarly, Fricker-Hidalgo et al. (25) observed a significant time savings of 9.5 h for *C. albicans* and 105.2 h for *C. glabrata* by using the Bactec Mycosis IC/F medium in comparison with the results seen with Bactec Plus Aerobic/F blood culture bottle.

Of the manual blood culture systems, the biphasic broth (Septi-Chek; Becton Dickinson Diagnostic Systems, Sparks, MD) and lysis-centrifugation systems (Wampole Isostat/Isolator Microbial System; Alere, Waltham, MA) have both been used to recover dimorphic and filamentous fungi. Poor performance of the biphasic culture system has been attributed to the need for continuous mixing of the bottles for the first 24 h of incubation and insufficient incubation time (26). With Isolator lysis-centrifugation, a blood specimen is inoculated into tubes containing a mixture of an anticoagulant, lysing agent, and fluorocarbon-cushioning agent (see also chapter 3). The lysed blood is centrifuged, and the sediment is used to inoculate mycology agar (27, 28). For optimal recovery of dimorphic and filamentous fungi using Isolator lysis-centrifugation, the concentrated blood sediment is inoculated onto multiple mycology agar-based media and incubated at 30°C ± 2°C in ambient air (27). Plates can be incubated for 3 weeks, with an extended incubation to 4 weeks if *Histoplasma* spp. are strongly suspected (29). The best evidence-based consensus that exists for the preferential use of the Isolator lysis-centrifugation system over other blood culture methods for fungal detection is with *Histoplasma capsulatum*. This advantage extends to both a higher sensitivity for detecting *H. capsulatum* (30–32) and a shorter time to positivity (33). With the exception of some isolates of *C. glabrata*, studies have shown that CMBCSs are equivalent to Isolator lysis-centrifugation blood culture for the recovery of *Candida* and *Cryptococcus* species from the blood (31). A significant and well-recognized drawback to the routine use of lysis-centrifugation tubes has been the high rate of contamination even when Isolator lysis-centrifugation tubes are processed by skilled laboratorians using class 2 biological safety cabinets (34, 35). In high-risk patients where fungal blood culture is more likely a consideration, the difficulty in distinguishing contamination from fungemia is likely to lead to unnecessary treatment. Additionally, the Isolator lysis-centrifugation method requires additional cost and labor, typically requiring an hour to process a specimen. A similar low utility of the Wampole Isolator 1.5-ml pediatric blood culture tube has been observed (36).

A consensus does not exist that specialized fungal culture microbiology is necessary (37, 38). In hospitalized patients with advanced HIV infection, Mess and Daar (37) observed that fungal-specific blood culture using Isolator lysis-centrifugation was of little diagnostic value, because *Candida* species and *C. neoformans* were effectively recovered using bacterial culture, and other diagnostic tests such as serology provided more rapid results. Inefficient use of specific fungal cultures using the Isolator lysis-centrifugation blood culture method has been observed when put into practice, as indicated by: (i) the poor recovery of fungi (39), or (ii) a recovery rate of clinically significant fungal isolates that are comparable to routine blood cultures (40). However, these authors do add a caveat and postulate that Isolator lysis-centrifugation blood cultures could be more helpful in geographic areas where dimorphic fungi such as *H. capsulatum* are more common and where delayed fungal growth is more typical (37–39).

Important Considerations for Fungal Culture: Yeast and Yeast-like Fungi

With the use of current CMBCSs, numerous studies have documented the improved recovery of yeasts in aerobic broth formulations, and, thus, it is generally regarded that special media formulated for the recovery of yeasts are thought to be unnecessary (31, 33). Agitation of broth-based systems increases aeration and was one of the important steps toward improving the recovery of yeasts (26). *Candida* species grow well in routine bacterial blood culture broth and will be detected even with low inoculum within a 5-day CMBCS protocol (2, 41). *C. albicans* will typically grow in an aerobic blood culture bottle in 1.9 days using either the Bactec or BacT/Alert 3D (20).

Exceptions to the ease of growing some species of yeast and yeast-like fungi in CMBCSs do exist. When using aerobic blood culture bottles to recover pathogenic yeast, the options that have been evaluated to assist in recovery include extended incubation and/or blind subculture. Blood containing *C. albicans* that has been previously treated with antifungal agents and other species such as *C. glabrata* may require extended incubation. The mean time to positivity using the Bactec MYCO/F Lytic (mycobacterial) bottle for *C. glabrata* fungemia was determined to be 56.5 h compared with 34.2 h for *C. albicans* (42). In a comparison using simulated growth in aerobic media, the time to positivity for 10 isolates of *C. glabrata* was 51.8 h (range, 39.3 to 64.8 h) using the BacT Alert 3D versus 106 h (range, 72.4 to

126.5 h) using the Bactec 9240 (2). By comparison, the time to positivity for *C. albicans* in aerobic blood culture using the BacT Alert 3D and Bactec 9240 was significantly shorter and less variable at 23.9 h and 23.5 h, respectively (2). Studies performed in the 1990s investigating the optimal length of incubation for CMBCSs did not always agree but did show that relevant *Candida* and *C. neoformans* species could be detected within a 5- to 6-day incubation protocol (43, 44). Terminal subcultures were shown to benefit the recovery of *C. glabrata* and *C. neoformans* when aerobic blood bottles were used in a small number of studies with patient specimens (20, 45) and a simulated candidemia model (2). Terminal blind subculture adds a significant cost to patient testing but may have value when selectively used as a potentially useful adjunctive step in high-risk patients (25). *Cryptococcus* may be recovered from CMBCSs with blind subcultures to fungal media at the end of a standard 5- or 7-day incubation (46). Cryptococcal antigen testing can guide the identification of cryptococcemia; however, blind subculturing from blood culture broth bottles to routine and mycological agar media has been recommended (47). *M. furfur* is a yeast that has a well-described requirement for supplementation of media with lipids to obtain optimal growth. *M. furfur* may be visible in blood culture smears as small monopolar budding yeasts that resemble bowling pins with a broad base at the point of attachment, and a collarette may be visible. However, *M. furfur* will not grow on routine fungal media without the addition of a thin film of sterile olive oil as a growth factor to the subculture agar (47). Growth is best supported by inoculation of Isolator lysis-centrifugation tube sediments onto mycological agar media (Sabouraud dextrose and brain heart infusion or potato flake agars) prepared before inoculation with a thin film of sterile olive oil (47).

Dimorphic fungi can grow in most commercially prepared aerobic blood culture broth media; however, detection with broth-based media is unreliable because CMBCSs may require an extended incubation of up to 2 to 4 weeks. Most data that exist to assess the performance of blood culture for growing dimorphic fungi pertain to *H. capsulatum*. Unlike most pathogenic yeasts, many *H. capsulatum* isolates are typically recovered after 2 weeks of incubation using Isolator lysis-centrifugation blood culture (31). On retrospective review of matched blood cultures, Lyon and Woods (32) observed that growth of 64 clinical isolates of *H. capsulatum* was detected in a mean of 11.8 days (range, 3 to 28 days) by using Isolator lysis-centrifugation blood culture; none of these were detected by using the BacT/Alert aerobic bottle. Fuller et al. (33) demonstrated that the Bactec MYCO/F Lytic (mycobacterial) bottle detected 18 of the 19 *H. capsulatum* isolates that grew by Isolator lysis-centrifugation blood culture. The mean time to detection in this study was 9.67 days (range, 4 to 23 days) using Isolator lysis-centrifugation and 18.4 days (range, 6 to 26 days) using the Bactec MYCO/F Lytic (mycobacterial) bottle (33). If infection with *H. capsulatum*, *Coccidioides immitis*, or *Blastomyces dermatitidis* is suspected, then blood should be processed with the lysis-centrifugation method and plated directly onto solid media for the fastest results (12, 48).

Important Considerations for Fungal Culture: Filamentous Fungi

The standard blood culture broths designed for CMBCSs have been optimized for bacteria and, although successful in recovering most yeast, will only rarely recover filamentous fungi. Filamentous fungi are best detected by using either a special mycological broth culture bottle (Bactec Mycosis-IC/F blood culture bottle) developed for use with the CMBC or by using the Isolator lysis-centrifugation system and plated onto fungal media (47). Some species of filamentous fungi like *Scedosporium* and *Fusarium* can grow within 3 to 5 days, but, if infection is suspected, they should be incubated for an extended time for a minimum of 4 weeks (6). In addition to the Isolator lysis-centrifugation system, the Bactec Mycosis-IC/F blood culture bottle may also be considered for recovery of filamentous fungi with subculture to mycological agar media (Sabouraud dextrose and brain heart infusion or potato flake agars) and incubation at $30°C \pm 2°C$ in ambient air for 4 weeks (33, 47, 49). Filamentous fungi can grow in the blood cultures of patients with invasive disease, but the culture growth will often not flag as positive by the CMBCS instrument (33, 50). The reasoning for this has not been clearly established, although there are large microbiological differences between filamentous fungal species. Rosa et al. (50) determined that subculture of *Aspergillus fumigatus* from inoculated Bactec Mycosis-IC/F blood culture bottles required vigorous agitation and a higher than expected sampling volume from presumptively positive flagged bottles to avoid false-negative results in the face of visible fungal balls in the bottle. So, although true *Aspergillus* fungemia appears to be a rare event in high-risk patients, optimal culture conditions and detection remain an issue. In contrast to aspergillosis, fusariosis has a high frequency of positive blood cultures in the context of disseminated disease, yielding positive blood cultures 41% of the time (51). It has been suggested that the difference may be due to the fact that *Fusarium* species produce yeast-like structures that enable dissemination and growth in blood (51).

Adoption of Specialized Fungal-Specific Blood Culture

Without a practice guideline, inefficient use of specific fungal culture by hospital clinicians has been observed with orders performed when facing diagnostic uncertainty and when managing patients who were sicker or had prior candidemia detected in routine blood cultures (38). It is difficult for clinicians to determine *a priori* if a septic patient has fungemia or bacteremia as was demonstrated in a study by McDonald et al. (28), where 82% of patients thought to be at risk for fungemia had only bacteria isolated from blood culture. Patients that have fungemia typically do not have a special request for fungal blood culture. Making an informed clinical decision about whether a result represents contamination and not fungemia when managing high-risk patients prone to opportunistic infection is complicated by the dependence on the laboratory result and need to initiate early antifungal treatment. The need for fungal-specific blood culture and how this testing is offered to clinicians should take into account the risk factors in the patient population and the prevalence of dimorphic fungi. The adoption of fungal-specific blood culture should be balanced with the excellent recovery of *Candida* from CMBCSs, the additional costs and resource requirements of the laboratory, and the conservation of blood. Blood drawn for fungal culture using the Bactec Mycosis IC/F bottle will not grow bacteria and thereby reduces the total blood volume available to detect bacteremia.

Enhanced Rapid Species Identification Technologies Used with Positive Blood Cultures and Direct Sample Testing

The diagnosis of fungemia could be improved by the development of adjunctive molecular and proteomic testing to identify fungal pathogens from a positive blood culture. Similarly, advances in the direct detection of fungi from a blood specimen, although not replacing the need for blood culture, would greatly enhance the management of patients with fungemia. To date, these advances in detecting fungemia have only applied to candidemia. The FDA-cleared products for direct detection of *Candida* species from a positive blood culture include: (i) peptide nucleic acid fluorescence *in situ* hybridization assay (PNA-FISH) and (ii) PCR-based multiplex panel testing. PNA-FISH is a mature technology that has been in use for the rapid identification of some *Candida* species in less than 2 h. AdvanDx (Woburn, MA) provides PNA-FISH kits that target specific fungal genomic regions of up to five *Candida* species depending of the probes in use (52). The bioMérieux/BioFire FilmArray blood culture identification (BCID) system is a two-stage, nested PCR test that is performed in a closed pouch that provides a sample-to-answer result in 1 h (53). The BCID system simultaneously identifies bacteria (and resistance genes) and five *Candida* species: *C. albicans*, *C. glabrata*, *C. krusei*, *C. parapsilosis*, and *C. tropicalis*. Potential sources of discordant results with routine fungal culture identification include: (i) polymicrobial infections with faster-growing bacteria that could inhibit the culture of *Candida*, (ii) detection of nonviable or very low levels of *Candida* by PCR, (iii) false positivity due to contamination with *Candida* DNA of supplies and reagents or at the point of blood collection and laboratory testing (54), and (iv) analytical limitations in discriminating between closely related species and multiple species of *Candida* growing together in a blood culture.

The T2 Biosystems (Lexington, MA) T2Candida Panel is a fully automated FDA-cleared test that detects *Candida* directly in whole blood without the need for culture using a magnetic resonance-based diagnostic approach to detect amplified nucleic acid (55). The assay rapidly detects candidemia caused by *C. albicans*, *C. glabrata*, *C. krusei*, *C. parapsilosis*, and *C. tropicalis* in 3 to 5 h with a sample-to-answer format. Prospective comparison studies that assess how the T2 Candida Panel works with large numbers of clinical specimens when used in comparison with traditional blood culture methodology are forthcoming. The application of this technology to filamentous and dimorphic fungi is keenly anticipated.

Mycobacterial Blood Culture

Epidemiology of Mycobacterial Infections Worldwide

Worldwide, the incidence of mycobacterial infections from all sources is decreasing, and reported *Mycobacterium tuberculosis* cases in the United States dropped by approximately 65% from 1992 to 2014 (56). However, in many resource-poor areas, these infections remain very prevalent, with 60% of the worldwide cases of *M. tuberculosis* occurring in six countries: China, India, Indonesia, Nigeria, Pakistan, and South Africa (57). Incidence of *Mycobacterium* spp. infection, especially with *Mycobacterium avium* complex (MAC), increased after the beginning of the worldwide HIV epidemic but decreased dramatically with the introduction of antiretroviral therapy (ART) and highly active antiretroviral therapy (HAART) in the mid-1990s in the United States (58), and began decreasing post-2000 in Africa (59).

Since the late 1980s, the relationship between HIV infection and disseminated *M. tuberculosis* infection has been well documented. Shafer et al. (60) sought to determine the prevalence of *M. tuberculosis* bacteremia in patients with a new diagnosis of tuberculosis: 59 patients (~46% HIV+) over a 4-month period. Of these patients, nine (seven HIV+, two intravenous drug users/HIV status unknown) had blood cultures positive for *M. tuberculosis*, with a mean time to positivity (TTP) of 43 days, suggesting that as many as 1/3 of HIV+ patients with a new diagnosis could have *M. tuberculosis* detected in their blood. A study by Oplustil et al. (61) prospectively analyzed blood cultures submitted from HIV+ patients with fever over a 19-month period at a university hospital in Brazil, and found that among the 254 HIV+ patients with fever and blood cultures, approximately 1/6 were positive for growth of mycobacteria (22 MAC, 15 *M. tuberculosis*, four with other *Mycobacterium* spp.). These studies illustrate the high prevalence of disseminated mycobacterial infection (both *M. tuberculosis* and MAC) in HIV+ patients. A more recent systematic review and meta-analysis, conducted by Pavlinac et al. (62), described the prevalence of disseminated tuberculosis in adults and children. While HIV infection increased the prevalence of mycobacteremia with *M. tuberculosis* in both populations, this presentation of the disease was much more common in adults (13.5% HIV– versus 15.5% HIV+) than in children (0.4% HIV– versus 0.8% HIV+) (62).

Over the past decade, the results of a number of studies have also underscored the importance of rapidly growing nontuberculous mycobacteria (RGM) with respect to catheter- and central line-associated bloodstream infections (63–69). A retrospective, single-center review (May 2004 to June 2005) identified six patients with long-term intravenous (IV) catheters that had RGM bloodstream infections (two *Mycobacterium mucogenicum*, two *Mycobacterium fortuitum*, and one each *Mycobacterium neoaurum* and *Mycobacterium septicum*). In all cases, the patients recovered with appropriate antibiotic therapy and removal of the catheter (63), a result confirmed by other studies of RGM-associated indwelling catheter infections (67, 68). Multiple studies have shown that risk factors for RGM bloodstream infections include comorbidities (on average, patients had three to four comorbidities), including malignancy or recent stem cell transplant, and indwelling catheters (68, 69). In Japan, an outbreak cluster of infections with nontuberculous mycobacteria (NTM) occurred on a hematology-oncology ward at a tertiary care center (October 2011 to February 2012) with five mycobacteremic patients (four with *M. mucogenicum* and one with *Mycobacterium canariasense*). All five patients had comorbidities (three with acute myeloid leukemia, one with acute lymphoblastic leukemia, and one with aplastic anemia) and were successfully treated with empiric therapy and removal of all central venous catheters (67). An outbreak investigation occurred, which implicated the water supply on the ward as the point source of infection; both pathogens were successfully cultured from the water, and 16S rRNA sequencing confirmed their match to patient isolates (67).

Risk Factors for Disseminated Mycobacterial Infection

Presently, most disseminated mycobacterial infections are caused by MAC (70), although bloodstream infections with *M. tuberculosis* and RGMs are also prevalent (64–66, 71–74). In a comparison between mycobacterial blood culture and bone marrow biopsy/culture to detect disseminated mycobacterial infection, Kilby et al. (75) found that culture of these specimens was equally sensitive, with bone marrow culture yielding positive cultures approximately 2 days earlier, on average, than blood culture (22 versus 24 days, respectively). Studies determining the prevalence of mycobacteremia in patients with suspected mycobacterial infection vary based on their patient population. In one study, approximately one-third of patients with unspecified HIV infection and suspect mycobacterial infection were mycobacteremic (16 patients with *M. tuberculosis*, seven with MAC) (76), whereas another study with 93 patients (~60% HIV+) found that one-sixth of patients with suspected tuberculosis were culture positive for *M. tuberculosis* in their blood cultures (77). When grouping these patients by HIV status, a third study found one-ninth of HIV– patients with suspected mycobacterial infection were mycobacteremic, whereas mycobacteremia was found in closer to one-third of HIV+ patients (78). In patients with laboratory-confirmed tuberculosis, nearly 50% (9/21) of HIV+ patients are mycobacteremic (77), underscoring the increased risk for disseminated infections in this population, although a separate study estimated a prevalence of ~39% in HIV+ patients (79). Despite this increased risk, use of antiretroviral therapy in HIV+ patients with tuberculosis (TB) has been shown to be protective against dissemination of infection (80).

In a 2012 prospective cohort study, 508 febrile patients were evaluated for disseminated *M. tuberculosis* infection by using blood culture to identify risk factors associated with *M. tuberculosis* mycobacteremia (71). In all, ~6% (29/508) cultures were positive with *M. tuberculosis*, and positivity of these cultures was statistically significantly associated with >1 month of coughing, >1 month of fever, >10% weight loss, lymphadenopathy, and HIV infection, and lower CD4+/total lymphocyte counts were associated with disseminated TB infection (71). Unfortunately, despite empiric treatment for *M. tuberculosis* infection and administration of antiretroviral therapy, 50% of patients with disseminated *M. tuberculosis* infection died within 36 days of enrollment in this study. Compared with those who survived, these patients exhibited lowered CD4+ ($P = 0.049$) and total lymphocyte cell counts ($P = 0.050$), suggesting that successful antiretroviral therapy and return of CD4+ cell counts to sufficient levels could be protective of death caused by disseminated *M. tuberculosis* infection (71). In a separate study, additional statistically significant risk factors for mycobacteremia were identified, including men who have sex with men, renal failure, and HIV viral loads >500,000 copies/ml (73). In a recent study, approximately 1/4 HIV+ patients (96/418) with smear-negative sputum specimens were found have *M. tuberculosis*-positive sputum and/or blood cultures (74). Statistically significant predictors for *M. tuberculosis* culture positivity in these patients included an abnormal chest X ray and a positive urine TB lipoarabinomannan (TB-LAM) test. In conjunction, these tests had 50% sensitivity and 86.1% specificity for predicting *M. tuberculosis* culture positivity among patients with CD4+ cell counts <100 cells/mm^3 (74). However, previous treatment for *M. tuberculosis* infection was associated with a statistically significant reduction in the likelihood of culture positivity (74).

Patients with mycobacteremia often present with fever and weight loss and have predisposing comorbid conditions, including HIV (46% of disseminated *M. tuberculosis* infections), immunosuppression (21%), alcoholism (12%), diabetes mellitus (12%), and hematologic disorders (8%) (81). A recent study found that in patients with advanced HIV (CD4 counts <200 cells/mm^3), *M. tuberculosis* infections are often atypical and likely to be disseminated (82). A study of HIV+ adults in Thailand showed that low CD4 cell count was associated with mycobacteremia ($P = 0.031$) (83). Additionally, HAART usage ($P = 0.017$) and focal (nondisseminated) mycobacterial infection ($P = 0.044$) were protective against mortality, while complications of infection (shock, for example; $P < 0.001$) significantly increased a patient's odds of succumbing to the infection (83).

Blood Culture for the Diagnosis of Disseminated Mycobacterial Infection

In multiple studies, blood culture has been shown to improve diagnostic yield in cases of suspected disseminated mycobacterial infection (72, 80). In fact, Nguyen et al. (72) found that all patients with prolonged fever who had positive mycobacterial blood cultures, in their study, were also HIV+, and that in ~65% of these positive patients, blood culture was the only positive specimen. In a 20-year descriptive, retrospective study of risk factors for and approaches to diagnose disseminated *M. tuberculosis* infection, mycobacterial blood culture was identified as an important diagnostic test, with a sensitivity comparable to bone marrow culture (58% versus 54%) (81). In 51 patients with advanced HIV disease, and *M. tuberculosis* isolated from both sputum and blood specimens, Ssengooba et al. (82) found that >50% of these patients were infected with more than one strain of *M. tuberculosis*. Through susceptibility testing (first-line drugs), spoligotyping, and 24 locus mycobacterial interspersed repeat units-variable number tandem repeat (MIRU-VNTR) testing, the authors showed that 26/51 patients had discordant *M. tuberculosis* strains in their sputum and blood and, in some cases, multiple infections in the same specimen (82). This study highlights the need to isolate mycobacteria from multiple specimens in patients where dissemination of infection is suspected.

Early methods of mycobacterial blood culture primarily included the Isolator system (Wampole Laboratories, Cranbury, NJ) and the Bactec 13A blood culture bottle (Becton Dickinson Microbiology Systems, Sparks, MD). Whereas the Isolator system is still commonly used in the mycobacteriology laboratory, the Bactec 13A culture bottle, for radiometric culture, is no longer produced, and other mycobacterial blood culture broths have been developed, including MYCO/F Lytic (Becton Dickinson Microbiology Systems, Sparks, MD), BacT/Alert MB Blood media (bioMérieux, Marcy-L'Étoile, France), and ESP II/VersaTREK Myco (Thermo Scientific, TREK Diagnostic Systems, Oakwood Village, OH) (Fig. 2). Septi-Chek AFB (Becton Dickinson Microbiology Systems) is a biphasic culture system with both broth (7H9) and solid agar (chocolate, egg-based, and 7H11) that allows for both culture types simultaneously (Fig. 2). These biphasic cultures are monitored intermittently to visualize growth of mycobacterial colonies or increased turbidity of the liquid medium (84). Typically, mycobacterial blood cultures are incubated for 6 to 8 weeks at 35°C. Because of their slow-growing nature (a combination of the growth characteristics of mycobacteria and the often low burden of organisms experienced during infection), two studies assessed the utility of late positive blood cultures (culture positive after the standard 6- to 8-week incubation period) for the diagnosis of disseminated mycobacterial infection. While it is true that some mycobacterial pathogens may require additional incubation time, including *Mycobacterium ulcerans* (generation time up to 36 hours) (70), both studies concluded that there was no benefit to extending the incubation time of mycobacterial blood cultures, because all clinically significant isolates were detected within the standard 6- to 8-week incubation window (85, 86).

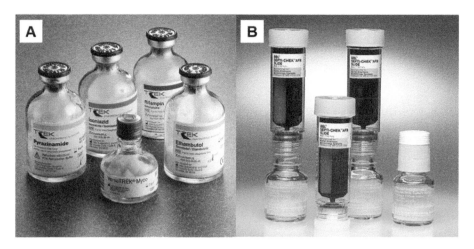

Figure 2 Exemplar images of mycobacterial blood culture media. (A) Thermo Scientific VersaTREK Myco blood culture bottle (front, center) and the Thermo Scientific VersaTREK Myco susceptibility kit (111). Photos courtesy of Thermo Fisher Scientific. Copying is prohibited. (B) BBL Septi-Chek AFB biphasic mycobacterial culture system (112).

Specimens for mycobacterial blood cultures can be processed and plated/ inoculated many different ways; each varies in percent recovery and time to positivity (studies of various mycobacteria, specimens, incubation systems, and mycobacterial blood culture media are summarized in Table 1). Many methods use either solid media, as in the Isolator 10 system, or liquid media with either manual, intermittent or automated, continuous detection of growth. Historically, mycobacterial blood culture in liquid media used manual, intermittent detection of growth in radiometric media (Bactec 13A), but, because of the burden of storing and discarding radioactive materials, current liquid media culture methods for mycobacterial blood cultures are nonradiometric and can be continuously monitored for growth using automated systems, including Bactec (460 TB, 9000, or 9240; Becton Dickinson, Sparks, MD), Difco ESP II/VersaTREK (Thermo Scientific, TREK Diagnostic Systems, Oakwood Village, OH), and MB/BacT/Alert (Classic or 3D; bioMérieux, Marcy-L'Étoile, France). However, a downside of liquid media culture is that isolated colonies are not available for quantitation of pathogen burden in the specimen and further workup (87), since growth on solid media is usually required prior to identification. Although the BD Mycobacterial Growth Indicator Tube (MGIT) system is often used in the mycobacteriology laboratory, its use is not recommended for

Table 1 Summary of studies comparing various media types and automated systems for the recovery and average time to positivity of mycobacterial blood cultures[a]

Source	Organism	# Pos. cultures	Specimen	Media	Unprocessed % Recovery	Unprocessed TTP	Lysis-centrifugation % Recovery	Lysis-centrifugation TTP	Liquid media observation (instrument)
Fojtasek and Kelly (93)	*M. chelonae*	17 (one patient)	Blood	Columbia blood agar	29.4%	>7 d	100%	2.5–2.7 d	Intermittent, radiometric
				Broth (unspecified)					
Kiehn et al. (94)	MAC	24	Blood	7H11 agar, LJ agar			2- to 5-fold increase	nd	Intermittent, radiometric
Salfinger et al. (89)[b]	MAC	47	Blood	7H11 agar			94.0%	9.6 d	Intermittent, radiometric
				7H12 broth			89.0%	6.6 d	Intermittent, radiometric
				7H13 broth	96.0%	11.5 d			
Wiebsky et al. (87)[b]	>4 species	72	Blood	Bactec 13A broth	94.4%	14.8 d			Intermittent, radiometric
				7H11 agar			93.1%	16.4 d	
	MAC	64	Blood	Bactec 13A broth	96.9%	nd			Intermittent, radiometric
				7H11 agar			nd		
	M. tuberculosis	4	Blood	Bactec 13A broth	100.0%	nd			Intermittent, radiometric
				7H11 agar			92.2%	nd	
	Other	4	Blood	Bactec 13A broth	50.0%	nd			Intermittent, radiometric
				7H11 agar			100.0%	nd	
Hanna et al. (113)[b]	MAC and *M. tuberculosis*	52	Blood	7H11 agar			100.0%	nd	Continuous (MGIT)
				MGIT			86.5%	21.0 d	
				LJ agar			78.8%	36.0 d	

Reference	Organism	No.	Specimen	Medium	Sensitivity	Time	System
van Griethuysen et al. (114)[b]	>7 species	131	Various	Biphasic culture[c]	80.2%	26.0 d	Intermittent (Septi-Chek AFB)
				MYCO/F-Lytic (7H9) broth	91.6%	17.6 d	Continuous (Bactec 9000 series)
		148	Various	LJ agar	79.9%	29.4 d	Continuous (Bactec 9000 series)
				MYCO/F-Lytic (7H9) broth	95.9%	17.6 d	
	M. tuberculosis	92	Various	Biphasic culture	81.5%	26.2 d	Intermittent (Septi-Chek AFB)
				MYCO/F-Lytic (7H9) broth	96.7%	18.0 d	Continuous (Bactec 9000 series)
		127	Various	LJ agar	83.5%	28.4 d	Continuous (Bactec 9000 series)
				MYCO/F-Lytic (7H9) broth	98.4%	18.0 d	
	Other	39	Various	Biphasic culture	76.9%	25.3 d	Intermittent (Septi-Chek AFB)
				MYCO/F-Lytic (7H9) broth	79.5%	15.9 d	Continuous (Bactec 9000 series)
		21	Various	LJ agar	57.0%	38.6 d	Continuous (Bactec 9000 series)
				MYCO/F-Lytic (7H9) broth	80.1%	15.9 d	

(continued on next page)

Table 1 (*continued*)

Source	Organism	# Pos. cultures	Specimen	Media	Unprocessed		Lysis-centrifugation		Liquid media observation (instrument)
					% Recovery	TTP	% Recovery	TTP	
Tholcken et al. (90)[b]	MAC and *M. tuberculosis*	73	Blood	ESP II vial			90.4%	15.6 d	Continuous (Difco ESP culture system II/VersaTREK)
				7H10/7H11 biplate			82.2%	19.0 d	
Woods et al. (115)	*M. tuberculosis*	53	Various	ESP II vial	88.7%	15.5 d			Continuous (Difco ESP culture system II/VersaTREK)
				Bactec 12B broth	92.5%	16.6 d			Continuous (Bactec 460)
	MAC	72	Various	ESP II vial	90.3%	nd			Continuous (Difco ESP culture system II/VersaTREK)
				Bactec 12B broth	73.6%	nd			Continuous (Bactec 460)
Manterola et al. (99)	5 species	106	Various	7H9 broth	94.3%	14.2 d			Continuous (MB BacT/Alert)
				LJ agar, Colestos agar	92.5%	26.1 d			

Study	Organism	No.	Specimen	Medium	% recovery	Mean time to detection (d)	Detection type
	M. tuberculosis	79	Various	7H12 broth	90.2%	11.7 d	Intermittent, radiometric
				7H9 broth	98.7%	20.2 d	Continuous (MB BacT/Alert)
				LJ/Colestos	93.7%	nd	
				7H12 broth	89.9%	22.5 d	Intermittent, radiometric
Archibald et al. (116)	MAC and *M. tuberculosis*	34	Blood	7H11 agar	41.2%	nd	
				MYCO/F-Lytic (7H9) broth	82.4%	nd	Continuous (Bactec 9000 series)
				Biphasic culture	76.5%	nd	Intermittent (Septi-Chek AFB)
Esteban et al. (117)	MAC	27	Blood	MYCO/F-Lytic (7H9) broth	nd	26.4 d	Continuous (Bactec 9000 series)
	M. tuberculosis			MYCO/F-Lytic (7H9) broth	nd	12.6 d	Continuous (Bactec 9000 series)
Martinez–Sanchez et al. (97)[b]	MAC and *M. tuberculosis*	23	Blood	Aerobic/F (7H9) broth, and LJ agar	47.8%	44.0 d	Continuous (Bactec 9000 series)
				MYCO/F-Lytic (7H9) broth	100.0%	17.0 d	Continuous (Bactec 9000 series)
Fuller et al. (33)	MAC	68	Blood	Bactec 13A broth	79.4%	nd	Intermittent, radiometric

(continued on next page)

Table 1 (*continued*)

Source	Organism	# Pos. cultures	Specimen	Media	Unprocessed		Lysis-centrifugation		Liquid media observation (instrument)
					% Recovery	TTP	% Recovery	TTP	
				MYCO/F-Lytic (7H9) broth	100.0%	nd			Continuous (Bactec 9000 series)
Vetter et al. (30)[b]	M. tuberculosis	3	Blood	MYCO/F-Lytic (7h9) broth	66.7%	23.5 d			Continuous (Bactec 9000 series)
				Agar[a] and Bactec 13a broth			33.3%	31.0 d	Intermittent, radiometric
Crump and Reller (81)	MAC	26	Blood	Bactec 13a broth	73.0%	12.6–15.3 d			Intermittent, radiometric
				MYCO/F-Lytic (7H9) broth	81.0%	12.8–13.2 d			Continuous (Bactec 9000 series)
				MB broth	85.0%	9.9–11.6 d			Continuous (MB BacT/Alert classic or 3d)
				7H10 agar			81.0%	19.0–20.4 d	

Study	Organism	No.	Specimen	Medium	% recovery	TTP	% recovery	TTP	System
Crump et al. (91)	M. tuberculosis	20	Blood	MB broth	60.0%	9.4–21.0 d			Continuous (MB BAcT/Alert 3d)
				MYCO/F-Lytic (7H9) broth	100.0%	14.9–27.0 d			Intermittent, fluorescence
				7H10 agar			45.0%	16.8–31.0 d	
Weighted average[e]	All			Solid media	79.9%	29.4 d	86.9%	20.0 d	
				Liquid media	95.6%	15.9 d	88.8%	14.8 d	

[a]TTP, time to positivity; d, days; MAC, M. avium complex; Other, mycobacterial species other than M. tuberculosis and MAC; Various, multiple specimen sources, including blood; nd, not determined.

[b]Studies included in these weighted averages.

[c]Biphasic culture–Septi-Chek AFB system uses modified Middlebrook 7H9 broth and a three-sided paddle containing chocolate, egg-based, and modified Middlebrook 7H11 solid agars.

[d]Solid agar: chocolate, brain heart infusion, and Sabouraud dextrose agar

[e]Weighted averages of % recovery and TTP, based on studies that had sufficient, discrete data.

mycobacterial blood cultures (88), because red blood cells can quench fluorescence of the MGIT tubes, resulting in false-negative cultures.

Various formulations of solid and liquid mycobacteriological media have been posited to affect sensitivity and TTP as well. Taken together, the studies looking at the ability of various media formulations for mycobacterial blood culture have found that the largest observed differences were between culture using solid media versus liquid media (Table 1). Overall, culture in liquid media (regardless of observation method, mycobacterial species, and specimen), on average, provides an advantage over solid media for both percent recovery of positive specimens and TTP in unprocessed and lysis-centrifuged specimens (Table 1). Use of lysis-centrifugation in conjunction with liquid media for culture does further improve TTP by approximately 1 day, on average, although a decrease in percent recovery of approximately 7% is also observed (Table 1). These overall observations are confirmed by multiple studies. One study compared mycobacterial blood culture on 7H11 agar with concentrated specimen, in 7H12 Bactec vials with concentrated specimen, and in 7H13 Bactec vials with nonconcentrated specimen (89). All three methods/media types performed similarly with respect to recovery of mycobacteria (94%, 89%, and 96%, respectively) (Table 1). However, concentrated specimen plated to solid media and unconcentrated specimen inoculated into liquid media had roughly the same TTP, although not concentrating the specimen increased the range of this metric (Table 1) (89). A separate study compared the Isolator system used in conjunction with 7H10/7H11 selective solid agar biplates to the Difco ESP II/ VersaTREK system, a continuously monitored, liquid media system (90). In this study, use of liquid media was shown to enhance recovery of mycobacteria from blood specimens and with shorter mean TTP for MAC and *M. tuberculosis* (Table 1) (90). Despite additionally finding that liquid mycobacterial blood culture provided reduced TTP, a third study found that the greatest predictor of TTP in patient samples was the burden of mycobacteria in blood ($r = -0.4920$) regardless of culture method (91).

The Isolator system of lysis-centrifugation for blood culture is different than other mycobacterial blood culture systems in that processing of the specimen concentrates any microorganisms, prior to plating, through lysis of blood cells followed by centrifugation, and plating on solid or inoculation into liquid media (92). This system has been shown to be an effective method to increase sensitivity and to decrease TTP of culture compared with direct plating of specimen to mycobacteriology media (Table 1) (93–95). In a paired comparison of directly plated specimen and the same specimen undergoing lysis-centrifugation, a 2- to 5-fold increase in isolated myco-bacteria was observed (94). Other groups have also observed increased sensitivity but also a decreased TTP of >4 days (Table 1) for specimens processed by lysis-centrifugation compared with conventional broth culture of specimen for the isolation of NTMs, such as *M. chelonae* (93).

Automated culture systems for mycobacterial blood culture have evolved over time from intermittent, radiometric detection to continuously moni-tored systems. The Bactec 460 TB system, a semiautomated radiometric system, remained a widely used mycobacterial culture instrument in the developing world through the early 2000s (96). However, because of issues with disposal of radioactive waste, MGITs have widely replaced these in-struments in these settings (97). Nonradiometric systems, including the Bactec 9000 series, and MB/BacT (does not agitate the specimens) and MB BacT/Alert (agitates the specimens) instruments are continuously monitored using fluorescent (Bactec 9000) or colorimetric indicators (MB BacT/Alert) that indicate growth in the culture (98–101). The VersaTREK blood culture system is also a nonradiometric, continuously monitored system, but unlike the Bactec 9000 series and MB BacT series instruments, this system detects and measures pressure differences associated with oxygen consumption as well as CO_2 or H_2 within the headspace of the culture bottle (102).

M. tuberculosis isolate susceptibility testing can be completed using the automated systems described above. In general, a suspension of the isolate (volume and concentration specified by the test manufacturer) is added to each of two culture bottles, one of which has a known concentration of the antimycobacterial drug of interest. An isolate is considered susceptible to the drug tested if the test culture (with drug) remains "no growth" for ≥ 3 days beyond the time it takes for the control culture (no drug) to flag as positive for growth. Growth in the test culture before this cutoff represents a resistant isolate (103, 104). Other susceptibility testing systems, such as that per-formed on the MGIT system, use an indicator system to quantify the amount of growth in a control tube to that seen in the various drug and drug concentration tubes.

Recently, an outbreak of *Mycobacterium chimaera* has been recognized in patients that underwent cardiac surgery in hospitals that use the Sorin 3T heater-cooler cardiopulmonary bypass device (105). These devices were implicated in this outbreak after atypical, extrapulmonary *M. chimaera* in-fections were observed in these patients in Europe (105, 106). It was found that *M. chimaera* was growing in the heated water bath used to maintain blood temperature in the instrument, which was shown to be contaminated with *M. chimaera* during the manufacturing process through epidemiological investigation. When this instrument is being used, the water is agitated, and the heater-cooler's exhaust fan can blow aerosolized *M. chimaera* into the operating room, where it can settle in the surgical field (106–108). In response to this outbreak, the manufacturer of the Sorin 3T instrument has released intensified cleaning and disinfection protocols to minimize the likelihood of transmission of this organism. Patients in this outbreak have presented with nonspecific symptoms, and it may take up to 4 years after the patient's surgery to identify this infection (105). Physicians caring for patients that may be included in this outbreak should be sure to collect and submit mycobacterial tissue or blood cultures.

Conclusion

Mycobacterial blood culture usage has declined in recent years for a number of reasons. In areas of the world with access to HAART, the incidence of mycobacterial blood infections in HIV+ patients has decreased. In general, specimens with high mycobacterial burden and those subjected to lysis-centrifugation have the shortest TTPs, although these times can be shortened further by inoculating the sediment from lysis-centrifugation into liquid media. Current blood culture systems automatically and continuously observe liquid media cultures for growth of mycobacteria. However, multiple studies have shown that concomitant plating of specimen, or lysis-centrifugation sediment, to solid media increases pathogen yield.

Production of mycobacterial blood culture media has become less profitable in the recent decade or so with decreasing incidence of disseminated mycobacterial infections in HIV+ patients, particularly in industrialized countries. In these areas, molecular diagnostics could enable clinical microbiology laboratories to quickly identify many species of mycobacteria. PCR assays, such as the Cepheid Xpert MTB/RIF assay (Sunnyvale, CA) and a multiplex MAC PCR (109) on primary specimens, or assays using DNA probe hybridization, mass spectrometry (MALDI TOF), 16S rRNA gene sequencing, and whole genome sequencing on cultured isolates could be very helpful in resource-poor settings, if manufactured cheaply enough to be affordable in these areas. However, if these methods are positive, there is no isolate available for further workup, including susceptibility testing, though current assays are able to determine resistance to certain antimycobacterial agents. Additionally, these tests need to be studied and verified for use in these settings, as research has shown that direct specimen testing can have poor sensitivity in some populations (110).

References

1. Meyer MH, Letscher-Bru V, Jaulhac B, Waller J, Candolfi E. 2004. Comparison of Mycosis IC/F and plus Aerobic/F media for diagnosis of fungemia by the bactec 9240 system. *J Clin Microbiol* **42**:773–777.

2. Horvath LL, George BJ, Murray CK, Harrison LS, Hospenthal DR. 2004. Direct comparison of the BACTEC 9240 and BacT/ALERT 3D automated blood culture systems for candida growth detection. *J Clin Microbiol* **42**:115–118.

3. Martin GS, Mannino DM, Eaton S, Moss M. 2003. The epidemiology of sepsis in the United States from 1979 through 2000. *N Engl J Med* **348**:1546–1554.

4. Fridkin SK. 2005. The changing face of fungal infections in health care settings. *Clin Infect Dis* **41**:1455–1460.

5. College of American Pathologists. 2015. *Blood culture participant summary-blood culture survey B (BCS-B)*. Northfield, IL.

6. CLSI. 2007. *Principles and Procedures for Blood Cultures. Approved guideline M47-A.* CLSI, Wayne, PA.

7. Geha DJ, Roberts GD. 1994. Laboratory detection of fungemia. *Clin Lab Med* **14**:83–97.

8. Guerra-Romero L, Edson RS, Cockerill FR III, Horstmeier CD, Roberts GD. 1987. Comparison of Du Pont Isolator and Roche Septi-Chek for detection of fungemia. *J Clin Microbiol* **25**:1623–1625.

9. Kauffman CA. 2007. Histoplasmosis: a clinical and laboratory update. *Clin Microbiol Rev* **20**:115–132.

10. Roberts GD, Washington JA II. 1975. Detection of fungi in blood cultures. *J Clin Microbiol* **1**:309–310.

11. Graybill JR. 1988. Histoplasmosis and AIDS. *J Infect Dis* **158**:623–626.

12. Paya CV, Roberts GD, Cockerill FR III. 1987. Laboratory methods for the diagnosis of disseminated histoplasmosis: clinical importance of the lysis-centrifugation blood culture technique. *Mayo Clin Proc* **62**:480–485.

13. Ampel NM, Ryan KJ, Carry PJ, Wieden MA, Schifman RB. 1986. Fungemia due to *Coccidioides immitis*. An analysis of 16 episodes in 15 patients and a review of the literature. *Medicine (Baltimore)* **65**:312–321.

14. Cox GM, Perfect JR. 1997. *Cryptococcus neoformans* var *neoformans* and *gattii* and *Trichosporon* species. *In* Edward LA (ed), *Topley and Wilson's Microbiology and Microbial Infections*, 9th ed. Arnold Press, London, UK.

15. Husain S, Muñoz P, Forrest G, Alexander BD, Somani J, Brennan K, Wagener MM, Singh N. 2005. Infections due to *Scedosporium apiospermum* and *Scedosporium prolificans* in transplant recipients: clinical characteristics and impact of antifungal agent therapy on outcome. *Clin Infect Dis* **40**:89–99.

16. Jensen TG, Gahrn-Hansen B, Arendrup M, Bruun B. 2004. *Fusarium fungaemia* in immunocompromised patients. *Clin Microbiol Infect* **10**:499–501.

17. Nucci M, Akiti T, Barreiros G, Silveira F, Revankar SG, Sutton DA, Patterson TF. 2001. Nosocomial fungemia due to *Exophiala jeanselmei* var. *jeanselmei* and a *Rhinocladiella* species: newly described causes of bloodstream infection. *J Clin Microbiol* **39**:514–518.

18. Denning DW. 1998. Invasive aspergillosis. *Clin Infect Dis* **26**:781–803; quiz 804-785.

19. Jorgensen JH, Mirrett S, McDonald LC, Murray PR, Weinstein MP, Fune J, Trippy CW, Masterson M, Reller LB. 1997. Controlled clinical laboratory comparison

of BACTEC plus aerobic/F resin medium with BacT/Alert aerobic FAN medium for detection of bacteremia and fungemia. *J Clin Microbiol* **35**:53–58.

20. Pohlman JK, Kirkley BA, Easley KA, Basille BA, Washington JA. 1995. Controlled clinical evaluation of BACTEC Plus Aerobic/F and BacT/Alert Aerobic FAN bottles for detection of bloodstream infections. *J Clin Microbiol* **33**:2856–2858.
21. Taniguchi T, Ogawa Y, Kasai D, Watanabe D, Yoshikawa K, Bando H, Yajima K, Tominari S, Shiiki S, Nishida Y, Uehira T, Shirasaka T. 2010. Three cases of fungemia in HIV-infected patients diagnosed through the use of mycobacterial blood culture bottles. *Intern Med* **49**:2179–2183.
22. Cateau E, Cognee AS, Tran TC, Vallade E, Garcia M, Belaz S, Kauffmann-Lacroix C, Rodier MH. 2012. Impact of yeast-bacteria coinfection on the detection of *Candida* sp. in an automated blood culture system. *Diagn Microbiol Infect Dis* **72**:328–331.
23. Zheng S, Ng TY, Li H, Tan AL, Tan TT, Tan BH. 2016. A dedicated fungal culture medium is useful in the diagnosis of fungemia: a retrospective cross-sectional study. *PLoS One* **11**:e0164668.
24. BD. 2016. BD BACTEC Mycosis-IC/F Culture Vial Package Insert. http://www.bd.com/ds/technicalCenter/inserts/PP113JAA(201002).pdf. Accessed December 1, 2016.
25. Fricker-Hidalgo H, Lebeau B, Pelloux H, Grillot R. 2004. Use of the BACTEC 9240 System with Mycosis-IC/F blood culture bottles for detection of fungemia. *J Clin Microbiol* **42**:1855–1856; author reply 1855–1856.
26. Murray PR. 1991. Comparison of the lysis-centrifugation and agitated biphasic blood culture systems for detection of fungemia. *J Clin Microbiol* **29**:96–98.
27. Procop GW, Cockerill FR III, Vetter EA, Harmsen WS, Hughes JG, Roberts GD. 2000. Performance of five agar media for recovery of fungi from isolator blood cultures. *J Clin Microbiol* **38**:3827–3829.
28. McDonald LC, Weinstein MP, Fune J, Mirrett S, Reimer LG, Reller LB. 2001. Controlled comparison of BacT/ALERT FAN aerobic medium and BATEC fungal blood culture medium for detection of fungemia. *J Clin Microbiol* **39**:622–624.
29. Hove MG, Woods GL. 1997. Duration of fungal culture incubation in an area endemic for *Histoplasma capsulatum*. *Diagn Microbiol Infect Dis* **28**:41–43.
30. Vetter E, Torgerson C, Feuker A, Hughes J, Harmsen S, Schleck C, Horstmeier C, Roberts G, Cockerill F III. 2001. Comparison of the BACTEC MYCO/F Lytic bottle to the isolator tube, BACTEC Plus Aerobic F/bottle, and BACTEC Anaerobic Lytic/10 bottle and comparison of the BACTEC Plus Aerobic F/bottle to the Isolator tube for recovery of bacteria, mycobacteria, and fungi from blood. *J Clin Microbiol* **39**:4380–4386.
31. Wilson ML, Davis TE, Mirrett S, Reynolds J, Fuller D, Allen SD, Flint KK, Koontz F, Reller LB. 1993. Controlled comparison of the BACTEC high-blood-volume fungal medium, BACTEC Plus 26 aerobic blood culture bottle, and 10-milliliter isolator blood culture system for detection of fungemia and bacteremia. *J Clin Microbiol* **31**:865–871.
32. Lyon R, Woods G. 1995. Comparison of the BacT/Alert and Isolator blood culture systems for recovery of fungi. *Am J Clin Pathol* **103**:660–662.
33. Fuller DD, Davis TE Jr, Denys GA, York MK. 2001. Evaluation of BACTEC MYCO/F Lytic medium for recovery of mycobacteria, fungi, and bacteria from blood. *J Clin Microbiol* **39**:2933–2936.

34. Henry NK, McLimans CA, Wright AJ, Thompson RL, Wilson WR, Washington JA II. 1983. Microbiological and clinical evaluation of the isolator lysis-centrifugation blood culture tube. *J Clin Microbiol* **17**:864–869.

35. Creger RJ, Weeman KE, Jacobs MR, Morrissey A, Parker P, Fox RM, Lazarus HM. 1998. Lack of utility of the lysis-centrifugation blood culture method for detection of fungemia in immunocompromised cancer patients. *J Clin Microbiol* **36**:290–293.

36. Campigotto A, Richardson SE, Sebert M, McElvania TeKippe E, Chakravarty A, Doern CD. 2016. Low utility of pediatric Isolator blood culture system for detection of fungemia in children: a 10-year review. *J Clin Microbiol* **54**:2284–2287.

37. Mess T, Daar ES. 1997. Utility of fungal blood cultures for patients with AIDS. *Clin Infect Dis* **25**:1350–1353.

38. Kosmin AR, Fekete T. 2008. Use of fungal blood cultures in an academic medical center. *J Clin Microbiol* **46**:3800–3801.

39. Morrell RM Jr, Wasilauskas BL, Steffee CH. 1996. Performance of fungal blood cultures by using the Isolator collection system: is it cost-effective? *J Clin Microbiol* **34**:3040–3043.

40. Kelly MT, Roberts FJ, Henry D, Geere I, Smith JA. 1990. Clinical comparison of isolator and BACTEC 660 resin media for blood culture. *J Clin Microbiol* **28**:1925–1927.

41. Horvath LL, George BJ, Hospenthal DR. 2007. Detection of fifteen species of *Candida* in an automated blood culture system. *J Clin Microbiol* **45**:3062–3064.

42. Lai CC, Wang CY, Liu WL, Huang YT, Hsueh PR. 2012. Time to positivity of blood cultures of different *Candida* species causing fungaemia. *J Med Microbiol* **61**:701–704.

43. Reisner BS, Woods GL. 1999. Times to detection of bacteria and yeasts in BACTEC 9240 blood culture bottles. *J Clin Microbiol* **37**:2024–2026.

44. Doern GV, Brueggemann AB, Dunne WM, Jenkins SG, Halstead DC, McLaughlin JC. 1997. Four-day incubation period for blood culture bottles processed with the Difco ESP blood culture system. *J Clin Microbiol* **35**:1290–1292.

45. Shigei JT, Shimabukuro JA, Pezzlo MT, de la Maza LM, Peterson EM. 1995. Value of terminal subcultures for blood cultures monitored by BACTEC 9240. *J Clin Microbiol* **33**:1385–1388.

46. Baron EJ, Weinstein MP, Dunne WM, Yagupsky P, Welch DF, Wilson DM. 2005. *Cumitech 1C, Blood Cultures IV*. ASM Press, Washington, DC.

47. Baron EJ, Scott JD, Tompkins LS. 2005. Prolonged incubation and extensive subculturing do not increase recovery of clinically significant microorganisms from standard automated blood cultures. *Clin Infect Dis* **41**:1677–1680.

48. Bille J, Stockman L, Roberts GD, Horstmeier CD, Ilstrup DM. 1983. Evaluation of a lysis-centrifugation system for recovery of yeasts and filamentous fungi from blood. *J Clin Microbiol* **18**:469–471.

49. Bianchi M, Robles AM, Vitale R, Helou S, Arechavala A, Negroni R. 2000. The usefulness of blood culture in diagnosing HIV-related systemic mycoses: evaluation of a manual lysis centrifugation method. *Med Mycol* **38**:77–80.

50. Rosa C, Araujo R, Rodrigues AG, Pinto-de-Sousa MI, Pina-Vaz C. 2011. Detection of *Aspergillus* species in BACTEC blood cultures. *J Med Microbiol* **60**:1467–1471.

51. Nucci M, Anaissie E. 2007. *Fusarium* infections in immunocompromised patients. *Clin Microbiol Rev* **20**:695–704.

52. Hall L, Le Febre KM, Deml SM, Wohlfiel SL, Wengenack NL. 2012. Evaluation of the Yeast Traffic Light PNA FISH probes for identification of *Candida* species from positive blood cultures. *J Clin Microbiol* 50:1446–1448.
53. Salimnia H, Fairfax MR, Lephart PR, Schreckenberger P, DesJarlais SM, Johnson JK, Robinson G, Carroll KC, Greer A, Morgan M, Chan R, Loeffelholz M, Valencia-Shelton F, Jenkins S, Schuetz AN, Daly JA, Barney T, Hemmert A, Kanack KJ. 2016. Evaluation of the FilmArray Blood Culture Identification Panel: results of a multicenter controlled trial. *J Clin Microbiol* 54:687–698.
54. Bonassoli LA, Bertoli M, Svidzinski TI. 2005. High frequency of *Candida parapsilosis* on the hands of healthy hosts. *J Hosp Infect* 59:159–162.
55. Pfaller MA, Wolk DM, Lowery TJ. 2016. T2MR and T2Candida: novel technology for the rapid diagnosis of candidemia and invasive candidiasis. *Future Microbiol* 11:103–117.
56. CDC. 2015. Tuberculosis in the United States: national tuberculosis surveillance system highlights from 2014. https://www.cdc.gov/tb/statistics/surv/surv2014/default.htm. Accessed January 10, 2017.
57. WHO. 2016. *Global Tuberculosis Report.* World Health Organization, Geneva, Switzerland.
58. Kirk O, Gatell JM, Mocroft A, Pedersen C, Proenca R, Brettle RP, Barton SE, Sudre P, Phillips AN, Lundgren JD. 2000. Infections with *Mycobacterium tuberculosis* and *Mycobacterium avium* among HIV-infected patients after the introduction of highly active antiretroviral therapy. EuroSIDA Study Group JD. *Am J Respir Crit Care Med* 162:865–872.
59. Lawn SD, Badri M, Wood R. 2005. Tuberculosis among HIV-infected patients receiving HAART: long term incidence and risk factors in a South African cohort. *AIDS* 19:2109–2116.
60. Shafer RW, Goldberg R, Sierra M, Glatt AE. 1989. Frequency of *Mycobacterium tuberculosis* bacteremia in patients with tuberculosis in an area endemic for AIDS. *Am Rev Respir Dis* 140:1611–1613.
61. Oplustil CP, Leite OH, Oliveira MS, Sinto SI, Uip DE, Boulos M, Mendes CF. 2001. Detection of mycobacteria in the bloodstream of patients with acquired immunodeficiency syndrome in a university hospital in Brazil. *Braz J Infect Dis* 5:252–259.
62. Pavlinac PB, Lokken EM, Walson JL, Richardson BA, Crump JA, John-Stewart GC. 2016. *Mycobacterium tuberculosis* bacteremia in adults and children: a systematic review and meta-analysis. *Int J Tuberc Lung Dis* 20:895–902.
63. Hawkins C, Qi C, Warren J, Stosor V. 2008. Catheter-related bloodstream infections caused by rapidly growing nontuberculous mycobacteria: a case series including rare species. *Diagn Microbiol Infect Dis* 61:187–191.
64. Yu F-L, Lee J-C, Wu T-H, Liang Y-L, Lin C-W, Chen T-T, Wang G-C. 2010. Isolation of *Mycobacterium fortuitum* from BACTEC 9240 blood culture system: a case report. *J Biomed Lab Sci* 22:70–72.
65. Su SH, Chen YH, Tsai TY, Huang SC, Lin CY, Chen TC, Lu PL. 2013. Catheter-related *Mycobacterium abscessus* bacteremia manifested with skin nodules, pneumonia, and mediastinal lymphadenopathy. *Kaohsiung J Med Sci* 29:50–54.
66. Takekoshi D, Al-Heeti O, Belvitch P, Schraufnagel DE. 2013. Native-valve endocarditis caused by *Mycobacterium chelonae*, misidentified as polymicrobial gram-positive bacillus infection. *J Infect Chemother* 19:754–756.

67. Tagashira Y, Kozai Y, Yamasa H, Sakurada M, Kashiyama T, Honda H. 2015. A cluster of central line-associated bloodstream infections due to rapidly growing nontuberculous mycobacteria in patients with hematologic disorders at a Japanese tertiary care center: an outbreak investigation and review of the literature. *Infect Control Hosp Epidemiol* **36**:76–80.

68. Abidi MZ, Ledeboer N, Banerjee A, Hari P. 2016. *Mycobacterium mucogenicum* bacteremia in immune-compromised patients, 2008-2013. *Diagn Microbiol Infect Dis* **85**:182–185.

69. Rodriguez-Coste MA, Chirca I, Steed LL, Salgado CD. 2016. Epidemiology of rapidly growing mycobacteria bloodstream infections. *Am J Med Sci* **351**:253–258.

70. Pfyffer GE. 2015. *Mycobacterium*: general characteristics, laboratory detection, and staining procedures. *In* Jorgensen JH, Pfaller MA (ed), *Manual of Clinical Microbiology*, 11th ed. ASM Press, Washington, DC.

71. Crump JA, Ramadhani HO, Morrissey AB, Saganda W, Mwako MS, Yang LY, Chow SC, Njau BN, Mushi GS, Maro VP, Reller LB, Bartlett JA. 2012. Bacteremic disseminated tuberculosis in sub-Saharan Africa: a prospective cohort study. *Clin Infect Dis* **55**:242–250.

72. Nguyen DN, Nguyen TV, Dao TT, Nguyen LT, Horby P, Nguyen KV, Wertheim HF. 2014. One year experience using mycobacterial blood cultures to diagnose tuberculosis in patients with prolonged fever in Vietnam. *J Infect Dev Ctries* **8**:1620–1624.

73. El Sahly HM, Teeter LD, Musser JM, Graviss EA. 2014. *Mycobacterium tuberculosis* bacteraemia: experience from a non-endemic urban centre. *Clin Microbiol Infect* **20**:263–268.

74. Nakiyingi L, Nonyane BA, Ssengooba W, Kirenga BJ, Nakanjako D, Lubega G, Byakika-Kibwika P, Joloba ML, Ellner JJ, Dorman SE, Mayanja-Kizza H, Manabe YC. 2015. Predictors for MTB culture-positivity among HIV-infected smear-negative presumptive tuberculosis patients in Uganda: application of new tuberculosis diagnostic technology. *PLoS One* **10**:e0133756.

75. Kilby JM, Marques MB, Jaye DL, Tabereaux PB, Reddy VB, Waites KB. 1998. The yield of bone marrow biopsy and culture compared with blood culture in the evaluation of HIV-infected patients for mycobacterial and fungal infections. *Am J Med* **104**:123–128.

76. von Gottberg A, Sacks L, Machala S, Blumberg L. 2001. Utility of blood cultures and incidence of mycobacteremia in patients with suspected tuberculosis in a South African infectious disease referral hospital. *Int J Tuberc Lung Dis* **5**:80–86.

77. David ST, Mukundan U, Brahmadathan KN, John TJ. 2004. Detecting mycobacteraemia for diagnosing tuberculosis. *Indian J Med Res* **119**:259–266.

78. Gopinath K, Kumar S, Singh S. 2008. Prevalence of mycobacteremia in Indian HIV-infected patients detected by the MB/BacT automated culture system. *Eur J Clin Microbiol Infect Dis* **27**:423–431.

79. Hanscheid T, Monteiro C, Cristino JM, Lito LM, Salgado MJ. 2005. Growth of *Mycobacterium tuberculosis* in conventional BacT/ALERT FA blood culture bottles allows reliable diagnosis of mycobacteremia. *J Clin Microbiol* **43**:890–891.

80. Heysell SK, Thomas TA, Gandhi NR, Moll AP, Eksteen FJ, Coovadia Y, Roux L, Babaria P, Lalloo U, Friedland G, Shah S. 2010. Blood cultures for the diagnosis of multidrug-resistant and extensively drug-resistant tuberculosis among HIV-infected patients from rural South Africa: a cross-sectional study. *BMC Infect Dis* **10**:344.

81. Crump JA, Reller LB. 2003. Two decades of disseminated tuberculosis at a university medical center: the expanding role of mycobacterial blood culture. *Clin Infect Dis* 37:1037–1043.
82. Ssengooba W, Cobelens FG, Nakiyingi L, Mboowa G, Armstrong DT, Manabe YC, Joloba ML, de Jong BC. 2015. High genotypic discordance of concurrent *Mycobacterium tuberculosis* isolates from sputum and blood of HIV-infected individuals. *PLoS One* 10:e0132581.
83. Kiertiburanakul S, Watcharatipagorn S, Chongtrakool P, Santanirand P. 2012. Epidemiology of bloodstream infections and predictive factors of mortality among HIV-infected adult patients in Thailand in the era of highly active antiretroviral therapy. *Jpn J Infect Dis* 65:28–32.
84. Sewell DL, Rashad AL, Rourke WJ Jr, Poor SL, McCarthy JA, Pfaller MA. 1993. Comparison of the Septi-Chek AFB and BACTEC systems and conventional culture for recovery of mycobacteria. *J Clin Microbiol* 31:2689–2691.
85. Dougherty MJ, Spach DH, Larson AM, Hooton TM, Coyle MB. 1996. Evaluation of an extended blood culture protocol to isolate fastidious organisms from patients with AIDS. *J Clin Microbiol* 34:2444–2447.
86. Greub G, Jaton K, Beer V, Prod'hom G, Bille J. 1998. The detection of mycobacteria in blood cultures using the Bactec system: 6 weeks versus 12 weeks of incubation? routine terminal Ziel-Neelsen? *Clin Microbiol Infect* 4:401–404.
87. Witebsky FG, Keiser JF, Conville PS, Bryan R, Park CH, Walker R, Siddiqi SH. 1988. Comparison of BACTEC 13A medium and Du Pont isolator for detection of mycobacteremia. *J Clin Microbiol* 26:1501–1505.
88. BD. 2017. BD BBL MGIT Package Insert. http://www.bd.com/ds/productCenter/245113.asp. Accessed January 30, 2017.
89. Salfinger M, Stool EW, Piot D, Heifets L. 1988. Comparison of three methods for recovery of *Mycobacterium avium* complex from blood specimens. *J Clin Microbiol* 26:1225–1226.
90. Tholcken CA, Huang S, Woods GL. 1997. Evaluation of the ESP Culture System II for recovery of mycobacteria from blood specimens collected in isolator tubes. *J Clin Microbiol* 35:2681–2682.
91. Crump JA, Morrissey AB, Ramadhani HO, Njau BN, Maro VP, Reller LB. 2011. Controlled comparison of BacT/Alert MB system, manual Myco/F lytic procedure, and isolator 10 system for diagnosis of *Mycobacterium tuberculosis* bacteremia. *J Clin Microbiol* 49:3054–3057.
92. Esteban J, Molleja A, Fernández-Roblas R, Soriano F. 1998. Number of days required for recovery of mycobacteria from blood and other samples. *J Clin Microbiol* 36:1456–1457.
93. Fojtasek MF, Kelly MT. 1982. Isolation of *Mycobacterium chelonei* with the lysis-centrifugation blood culture technique. *J Clin Microbiol* 16:403–405.
94. Kiehn TE, Edwards FF, Brannon P, Tsang AY, Maio M, Gold JW, Whimbey E, Wong B, McClatchy JK, Armstrong D. 1985. Infections caused by *Mycobacterium avium* complex in immunocompromised patients: diagnosis by blood culture and fecal examination, antimicrobial susceptibility tests, and morphological and seroagglutination characteristics. *J Clin Microbiol* 21:168–173.
95. Kiehn TE, Cammarata R. 1986. Laboratory diagnosis of mycobacterial infections in patients with acquired immunodeficiency syndrome. *J Clin Microbiol* 24:708–711.

96. Rodrigues CS, Shenai SV, Almeida D, Sadani MA, Goyal N, Vadher C, Mehta AP. 2007. Use of bactec 460 TB system in the diagnosis of tuberculosis. *Indian J Med Microbiol* **25**:32–36.

97. Martínez-Sánchez L, Ruiz-Serrano J, Bouza E, Torres L, Díaz M, Alcalá L, Rodríguez-Créixems M. 2000. Utility of the BACTEC Myco/F lytic medium for the detection of mycobacteria in blood. *Diagn Microbiol Infect Dis* **38**:223–226.

98. Benjamin WH Jr, Waites KB, Beverly A, Gibbs L, Waller M, Nix S, Moser SA, Willert M. 1998. Comparison of the MB/BacT system with a revised antibiotic supplement kit to the BACTEC 460 system for detection of mycobacteria in clinical specimens. *J Clin Microbiol* **36**:3234–3238.

99. Manterola JM, Gamboa F, Padilla E, Lonca J, Matas L, Hernández A, Giménez M, Cardona PJ, Viñado B, Ausina V. 1998. Comparison of a nonradiometric system with Bactec 12B and culture on egg-based media for recovery of mycobacteria from clinical specimens. *Eur J Clin Microbiol Infect Dis* **17**:773–777.

100. Piersimoni C, Scarparo C, Callegaro A, Tosi CP, Nista D, Bornigia S, Scagnelli M, Rigon A, Ruggiero G, Goglio A. 2001. Comparison of MB/Bact alert 3D system with radiometric BACTEC system and Löwenstein-Jensen medium for recovery and identification of mycobacteria from clinical specimens: a multicenter study. *J Clin Microbiol* **39**:651–657.

101. BD. 2017. *BD BACTEC 9000 Series Product Information.* http://www.bd.com/ds/productCenter/BC-Bactec.asp. Accessed January 30, 2017.

102. Thermo Scientific. 2017. *VersaTREK Instrumentation.* http://www.trekds.com/products/versatrek/instrumentation.asp. Accessed January 30, 2017.

103. Gravet A, Souillard N, Habermacher J, Moser A, Lohmann C, Schmitt F, Delarbre JM. 2011. [Culture and susceptibility testing of mycobacteria with VersaTREK]. *Pathol Biol (Paris)* **59**:32–38.

104. Espasa M, Salvadó M, Vicente E, Tudó G, Alcaide F, Coll P, Martin-Casabona N, Torra M, Fontanals D, González-Martín J. 2012. Evaluation of the VersaTREK system compared to the Bactec MGIT 960 system for first-line drug susceptibility testing of *Mycobacterium tuberculosis*. *J Clin Microbiol* **50**:488–491.

105. Kohler P, Kuster SP, Bloemberg G, Schulthess B, Frank M, Tanner FC, Rössle M, Böni C, Falk V, Wilhelm MJ, Sommerstein R, Achermann Y, Ten Oever J, Debast SB, Wolfhagen MJ, Brandon Bravo Bruinsma GJ, Vos MC, Bogers A, Serr A, Beyersdorf F, Sax H, Böttger EC, Weber R, van Ingen J, Wagner D, Hasse B. 2015. Healthcare-associated prosthetic heart valve, aortic vascular graft, and disseminated *Mycobacterium chimaera* infections subsequent to open heart surgery. *Eur Heart J* **36**:2745–2753.

106. Sax H, Bloemberg G, Hasse B, Sommerstein R, Kohler P, Achermann Y, Rössle M, Falk V, Kuster SP, Böttger EC, Weber R. 2015. Prolonged outbreak of *Mycobacterium chimaera* infection after open-chest heart surgery. *Clin Infect Dis* **61**:67–75.

107. Sommerstein R, Rüegg C, Kohler P, Bloemberg G, Kuster SP, Sax H. 2016. Transmission of *Mycobacterium chimaera* from heater-cooler units during cardiac surgery despite an ultraclean air ventilation system. *Emerg Infect Dis* **22**:1008–1013.

108. Sommerstein R, Schreiber PW, Diekema DJ, Edmond MB, Hasse B, Marschall J, Sax H. 2017. *Mycobacterium chimaera* outbreak associated with heater-cooler devices: piecing the puzzle together. *Infect Control Hosp Epidemiol* **38**:103–108.

109. Kulski JK, Khinsoe C, Pryce T, Christiansen K. 1995. Use of a multiplex PCR to detect and identify *Mycobacterium avium* and *M. intracellulare* in blood culture fluids of AIDS patients. *J Clin Microbiol* **33**:668–674.

110. Pohl C, Rutaihwa LK, Haraka F, Nsubuga M, Aloi F, Ntinginya NE, Mapamba D, Heinrich N, Hoelscher M, Marais BJ, Jugheli L, Reither K. 2016. Limited value of whole blood Xpert(®) MTB/RIF for diagnosing tuberculosis in children. *J Infect* **73**:326–335.

111. ThermoFisher Scientific. 2017. VersaTrek(TM) Myco susceptibility kit. http://www.thermofisher.com/order/catalog/product/7115-60. Accessed February 20, 2017.

112. BD. 2017. Septi-Chek(TM) AFB culture bottle. http://www.bd.com/ds/productCenter/243558.asp. Accessed February 20, 2017.

113. Hanna BA, Walters SB, Bonk SJ, Tick LJ. 1995. Recovery of mycobacteria from blood in mycobacteria growth indicator tube and Lowenstein-Jensen slant after lysis-centrifugation. *J Clin Microbiol* **33**:3315–3316.

114. van Griethuysen AJ, Jansz AR, Buiting AG. 1996. Comparison of fluorescent BACTEC 9000 MB system, Septi-Chek AFB system, and Lowenstein-Jensen medium for detection of mycobacteria. *J Clin Microbiol* **34**:2391–2394.

115. Woods GL, Fish G, Plaunt M, Murphy T. 1997. Clinical evaluation of difco ESP culture system II for growth and detection of mycobacteria. *J Clin Microbiol* **35**:121–124.

116. Archibald LK, McDonald LC, Addison RM, McKnight C, Byrne T, Dobbie H, Nwanyanwu O, Kazembe P, Reller LB, Jarvis WR. 2000. Comparison of BACTEC MYCO/F LYTIC and WAMPOLE ISOLATOR 10 (lysis-centrifugation) systems for detection of bacteremia, mycobacteremia, and fungemia in a developing country. *J Clin Microbiol* **38**:2994–2997.

117. Esteban J, Fernández-Roblas R, Cabria F, Soriano F. 2000. Usefulness of the BACTEC MYCO/F lytic system for detection of mycobacteremia in a clinical microbiology laboratory. *J Microbiol Methods* **40**:63–66.

The Dark Art of Blood Cultures
Edited by Wm. Michael Dunne, Jr. and Carey-Ann D. Burnham
© 2018 American Society for Microbiology, Washington, DC
doi:10.1128/9781555819811.ch13

The Bacterial Blood Microbiota/Microbiome

13

Eileen M. Burd[1] and Lars F. Westblade[2]

Introduction

Many surfaces on the human body are continually exposed to microorganisms in the external environment and become colonized before or shortly after birth with a normal resident microbiota, the collection of microorganisms in a particular environment, which matures over time and persists throughout life. These nonsterile surfaces include the skin, mucous membranes, lower gastrointestinal tract, upper respiratory system, and anterior urethra. The community of microorganisms harbored in or on these sites is a highly complex mixture that varies in composition depending on nutrient availability, moisture, temperature, pH, and other environmental conditions. The composition of the normal microbiota can also be affected by host factors such as age, nutrition, and immune status.

In 2007, the National Institutes of Health launched the Human Microbiome Project to survey the human microbiome, the collective genome of microorganisms associated with the human body, using culture-independent technologies. Researchers from approximately 80 academic and scientific institutions reported their findings after 5 years of work. Polymerase chain reaction (PCR) amplification of the bacterial 16S rRNA gene coupled with characterization by high-throughput DNA sequencing has revealed that more than 10,000 bacterial species comprise the human microbiome of

[1]Department of Pathology and Laboratory Medicine, Department of Medicine, Division of Infectious Diseases, Emory Antibiotic Resistance Center, Emory University School of Medicine, Atlanta, GA
[2]Department of Pathology and Laboratory Medicine, Department of Medicine, Division of Infectious Diseases, Weill Cornell Medicine, New York, NY

healthy adults and contribute about 8 million unique protein-coding genes (1–3). It is presumed that there are continuous dynamic interactions among the organisms that comprise the normal microbiota as well as between the organisms and the host. These organisms derive from their host a steady supply of nutrients, a stable environment, protection, and transport. At the same time, they provide direct benefits to the host by protecting against colonization and infection by pathogenic microorganisms, producing substances such as vitamin K and enzymes that aid in nutrition and digestion, and stimulating the development and activity of the immune system.

There is a growing body of evidence that indicates the composition of the microbiome in healthy individuals is different from those who are ill (4, 5). Alterations in the microbiome are thought to contribute to the pathogenesis of disorders such as Crohn's disease, inflammatory bowel disease, ulcerative colitis, obesity, esophageal cancer, psoriasis, atopic dermatitis, rheumatoid arthritis, bacterial vaginosis, preterm delivery, and many others (4–10). Furthermore, many of the microorganisms that comprise the normal microbiota are opportunistic pathogens and can cause illness if there is a breach in host resistance. Disruption of resistance barriers allows microorganisms to overpopulate their normal habitat or enter areas of the body where they are not normally found.

The ability to detect and sequence bacterial DNA has dramatically changed our understanding of sterility. In the absence of disease, areas of the body that are typically considered to be sterile include bone and bone marrow, tissues and organs of the body cavity, lower respiratory tract, upper urogenital regions, central nervous system, inner and middle ear, aqueous and vitreous humor, amniotic fluid, and the small amounts of fluid that are found in joints and in the pleural, pericardial, and peritoneal cavities. Specimens from these sites are negative by standard culture techniques, but the presence of bacteria has been inferred using 16S rRNA gene sequencing methodologies in the bladder and urine, breast, brain, fetal side of the placenta, and other sites (11–13), and some of these organisms can be cultured using techniques that inoculate a larger volume of specimen. These organisms do not induce infection, although at least some of them naturally have the capacity to do so. This raises many questions about the nature of their presence and their role in health and disease.

Nature of the Blood Microbiota/Microbiome

In addition to the aforementioned anatomical sites, it is generally assumed that the bloodstream of healthy humans is sterile. When bacteremia is suspected, standard practice is to culture blood by inoculating two sets of blood culture bottles (aerobic and anaerobic) with each set obtained from a separate venipuncture (see chapter 10, Best Practices in Blood Culture). Blood culture bottles are incubated on continuously monitored systems for 5 days or in standard incubators with visual inspection for 7 days. It is normally expected that even fastidious microorganisms will grow within the 5- or 7-day timeframe, and, if there is no growth, the probability that a person has a blood infection caused by bacteria or yeast is low. If an organism grows in a blood culture, it is considered to be associated with true bloodstream infection. The exception is when skin contaminants are introduced into the culture in the process of drawing blood into the bottle.

Intracellular pathogens such as *Brucella* species, *Bartonella* species, fungi, and *Mycobacterium* species are best cultured using lysis-centrifugation (see chapter 3). Some organisms such as *Legionella* species, *Mycoplasma* species, *Leptospira* species, *Tropheryma whipplei*, and *Coxiella burnetii* do not grow in traditional blood culture systems because they require specialized media or culture conditions. Serology tests demonstrating IgM or high or rising IgG titers or PCR amplification of the bacterial 16S rRNA gene with subsequent sequencing of the amplicon can successfully identify these pathogens in some cases.

The majority (68%) of bloodstream pathogens are recovered within the first 24 h of incubation of blood culture bottles (14). Recovery increases to 88.3% within 48 h and to 96% within 72 h (14). Prolonged incubation can allow recovery of the organism in standard blood culture for some cases of infection with *Brucella* species and *Cardiobacterium* species, but, otherwise, extended incubation is not recommended (15–17), and, in general, does not recover organisms associated with true bloodstream infections but rather indicates the presence of small numbers of organisms either in circulation, as can occur after tooth brushing, or on the skin at the time of sample collection.

Evidence for and Origin of the Human Blood Microbiota/Microbiome

Evidence, albeit scarce, of a blood microbiota and/or microbiome is derived from studies describing the detection of microorganisms, or their components (e.g., lipopolysaccharide [LPS]), in blood, or various fractions post-collection for donation, using culture and immunologic methods (18, 19). Furthermore, culture-positive bacteremia after use of oral irrigation devices or tooth brushing is well appreciated (20, 21), and supports the notion that bacteria can circulate in the bloodstream of well-appearing individuals, even if transiently. Observation of pleomorphic bacterial-like structures in the blood of healthy individuals seemed to confirm the existence of a blood microbiota (22), although these structures have since been identified as microparticles derived from red blood cells (Fig. 1) (23). Because of their culture-independent nature, which permits detection of dormant or (seemingly) uncultivable organisms, DNA sequencing and other nucleic acid-based methods have played a central role in investigating the abundance and composition of bacterial species in the blood of humans. However, as with any specimen probed for the presence of microbes using molecular methods, these data only reflect the presence of DNA sequences derived from microorganisms in the specimen and not the microorganisms themselves. Thus, microbial DNA sequences in blood could correspond to freely circulating bacteria, bacteria associated with specific blood components, or DNA resulting from immune degradation or translocation from other anatomic sites (24), and could easily be confounded by contaminating DNA introduced during phlebotomy and subsequent manipulation, and/or associated with reagents and enzyme preparations commonly utilized in molecular biology. The issue of contamination is especially pronounced when specimens contain low microbial biomass (and therefore provide little

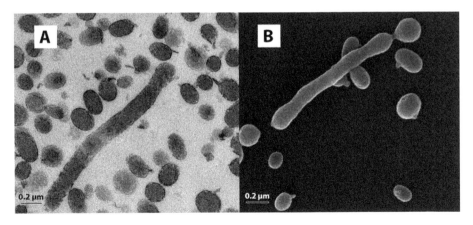

Figure 1 (**A**) Thin-section transmission electron microscopy image showing rod-shaped and ellipsoid red blood cell-derived microparticles (average diameter, 0.190 to 0.288 μm [23]) recovered from the supernatant of donor red blood cell storage units. (**B**) Scanning electron microscopy image of the red blood cell microparticles. Images courtesy of Charles D. Searles, Division of Cardiology, Department of Medicine, Emory University, Atlanta, and section of Cardiology, Atlanta VA Medical Center.

template DNA to compete with that potentially in the reagents) (25), as may be encountered in blood specimens, and DNA sequencing and nucleic acid-based data should be interpreted with caution and only in the setting of stringent controls.

One of the first studies designed to determine if circulating blood of healthy individuals harbored microbial DNA employed a broad-range, semiquantitative bacterial 16S rRNA gene PCR assay to interrogate venous whole-blood specimens collected from four individuals without clinical signs or symptoms of infection (26). More 16S rRNA gene DNA was observed in blood specimens compared with matched reagent controls, prompting the authors to suggest that blood specimens do contain bacterial DNA. Amplified 16S rRNA gene PCR products from a blood specimen obtained from a single individual and a matched control (sterile water drawn into an identical EDTA-containing tube and processed in an identical manner) were cloned and sequenced to determine the identity of blood-associated bacterial DNA sequences. Compared with reagent-associated DNA sequences, human blood contained DNA sequences closely corresponding to *Bacillus globisporus* (renamed *Sporosarcina globispora*), *Pseudomonas putida*, *Riemerella anatipestifer*, and *Stenotrophomonas maltophilia*. In contrast, DNA sequences closely related to *Acidovorax defluvii*, *Propionibacterium acnes* (renamed *Cutibacterium acnes*), and *Pseudomonas fluorescens* were detected in control and blood specimens; while DNA related to *Microbacterium schleiferi* was exclusively associated with the control, indicating these sequences were experimental contaminants perhaps derived from DNA polymerase preparations, other reagents, or during collection. Ultimately, the authors could not determine if the source of the DNA solely associated with blood specimens was blood, skin (because of contamination during blood collection), or a combination of both.

Work focused on detecting and annotating bacterial DNA sequences in blood drawn from donors to inform the safety of the blood supply has greatly contributed to our understanding of the microbiome in the circulatory system. In one of the most extensive studies of its kind, the bacterial microbiome present in whole blood and different fractions (buffy coat, plasma, and red blood cell pellet) collected from 30 healthy blood donors (21 women and nine men; age range, 18 to 53 years) was determined using a combination of quantitative 16S rRNA gene PCR and high-throughput 16S rRNA gene sequencing platforms optimized to decrease contaminating DNA (24). One of the key findings of the work revealed that most bacterial DNA present in blood is associated with the buffy coat (93.74% on average), and red blood cells contain much more bacterial DNA than plasma (6.23% versus 0.03%). Furthermore, either on average or per individual donor, the quantity of 16S rRNA gene copies in 1 ml of whole blood was equivalent to the sum of quantities measured in the three different fractions. Finally, the distribution of 16S rRNA gene copies was spread over a relatively broad range among donors; e.g., for whole blood, 1.8×10^7 to 7.6×10^7 16S rRNA gene copies/ml (mean, 4.2×10^7; standard deviation, 1.3×10^7). The quantity of 16S rRNA gene copies in the buffy coat correlated among donors with the white blood cell concentration but did not correlate with the red blood cell concentration. The authors concluded that this implied that the average amount of bacterial DNA per white blood cell is constant among donors, while the quantity associated with red blood cells is more variable. There was no significant difference in 16S rRNA gene concentration between male and female subjects.

After review and analysis of the 16S rRNA gene high-throughput DNA sequencing data, bacterial diversity, as determined using the Shannon diversity index (which reflects the richness and evenness of organisms present in a specimen), was more pronounced in the red blood cell fraction compared to buffy coat or plasma fractions, and the variability in diversity between subjects was relatively high in all fractions with no distinct differences between male and female donors. At the phyla level, DNA from the *Proteobacteria* phylum was predominant (>80%) followed by *Actinobacteria* (between 6.7 and 10.0% depending on the fraction), with a lower proportion of *Firmicutes* (between 3.0 and 6.4% depending on the fraction), and *Bacteroidetes* (between 2.5 and 3.4% depending on the fraction). Organisms significantly more associated with red blood cells compared with other fractions included members of the genera *Acinetobacter*, *Escherichia/Shigella*, *Corynebacterium*, *Pseudomonas*, *Staphylococcus*, *Stenotrophomonas*, and *Shewanella*, and further analysis allowed accurate identification of sequences due to *Acinetobacter baumannii* and *S. maltophilia*. Several bacterial organisms causing overt disease can invade red blood cells, e.g., *Bartonella quintana*, *Francisella tularensis*, and *Streptococcus pneumoniae*, to name a few (27), suggesting that red blood cells may provide a sanctuary for both pathogens and a resident microbiota. In contrast, the *Sphingobacteriia* class was primarily found in the buffy coat and plasma, yet poorly represented in red blood cells, and clostridia were more prevalent in plasma and red blood cells.

The origin of the blood microbiota/microbiome is postulated to be the gut (27), although it is not inconceivable that other anatomic sites (e.g., oral cavity and lungs) contribute. The translocation of bacteria from the gut into blood could occur via various mechanisms, including injury/inflammation to the epithelium or directly through cellular uptake by human cells associated with the immune system, e.g., M cells overlaying the Peyer's patches (27). The concentration of organisms, or their components (e.g., LPS), translocated could vary depending on meal composition and fasting status (24, 28). Consequently, the blood microbiota/microbiome is likely to be highly dynamic in terms of both composition and concentration. Interestingly, the gut microbiome is dominated by the *Firmicutes* and *Bacteroidetes* (29), while the blood microbiome is significantly enriched for *Proteobacteria* and *Actinobacteria* (24). A possible explanation for this difference, as suggested by Païssé and colleagues, could be selective filtering of the gut microbiome by intestinal or immune cells. Additionally, members of the phyla *Proteobacteria* and *Actinobacteria* may be equipped with traits that permit their relocation to the blood from the gut, or various anatomic sites.

Despite evidence suggestive of a blood microbiome, it is important to be mindful that data are extremely sparse and may suffer from artifacts. For instance, some organisms (e.g., members of the genera *Acinetobacter*, *Pseudomonas*, and *Stenotrophomonas*) detected in the blood of subjects using DNA sequencing-based methodologies have been associated with contamination due to reagents used in DNA extraction and PCR kits (25). Therefore, studies that employ a multidisciplinary approach and are designed to reduce contaminants, be they DNA, other biomolecules, or microorganisms themselves, are desperately needed to validate existing evidence.

Function of the Blood Microbiota/Microbiome
Noncommunicable Diseases
The finding of bacterial DNA sequences and components of bacterial organisms in human blood compels us to rethink the concept of infection. Emerging scientific evidence suggests that dormant bacteria in blood may play a role in chronic noncommunicable diseases such as diabetes mellitus, arthritis, Alzheimer's disease, Parkinson's disease, and others. Although many factors contribute to these disorders, research has provided substantial insight into the dysfunction of a broad range of processes that could potentially be attributed to dormant bacteria in the host blood.

Alzheimer's disease is the most extensively studied of the diseases with a possible connection to a blood microbiota/microbiome. Alzheimer's disease is a slowly progressive dementia with early symptoms of difficulty remembering newly learned information and gradual development of more serious memory loss, personality changes, and difficulty speaking, swallowing,

walking, and performing everyday activities. As a result of improved lon-
gevity, higher proportions of people have Alzheimer's disease in industrialized regions than in developing areas of the world. Alzheimer's disease is
most common in Western Europe, closely followed by East Asia, South
Asia, and North America (30). Specifically in the United States, it is estimated that one in nine people 65 years of age or older has Alzheimer's
disease (31). Aging, family history, environmental factors, and several genes
(APOE-e4, TREM2, CD33) have been implicated in placing older individuals at higher risk for developing Alzheimer's disease (32–34).

Microscopic changes in the brain that are associated with Alzheimer's
disease develop well before clinical symptoms appear. Two abnormal
structures, plaques and tangles, are microscopic hallmarks of the disease
(Fig. 2). Plaques are a result of a progressive abnormal accumulation of the
protein fragment beta-amyloid that builds up between neurons. Tangles
are formed inside neurons when the microtubule protein, tau, becomes
hyperphosphorylated and the proteins bind together and form twisted
strands. Most people develop some plaques and tangles as they age, but
individuals with Alzheimer's disease have much more. In Alzheimer's
disease, plaques and tangles initially develop in areas of the brain that are
central for memory functions and then spread through the cortex as the
disease progresses.

Figure 2 Alzheimer's disease pathology is characterized by the cerebral cortical accumulation
of neurofibrillary tangles (red arrow) that are formed within pyramidal neurons and the
development of neuritic plaques (green arrow) with beta-amyloid cores (original magnification, 400×, Bielschowsky stain). Image courtesy of Daniel J. Brat, MD, PhD, Department of
Pathology and Laboratory Medicine, Emory University School of Medicine.

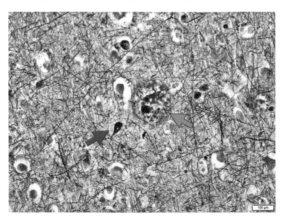

In addition to the morphologic changes in the brain, Alzheimer's disease is characterized by a prominent inflammatory component that includes neuroinflammation (triggered by activated astrocytes and microglia), systemic inflammation, oxidative stress, and excessive clotting (35, 36). The eventual result is that nerve cells are damaged and destroyed and there are fewer synapses than in a healthy brain. It is the reduction in nerve cells and synapses that causes the memory failure and other symptoms of Alzheimer's disease.

The cause of Alzheimer's disease is still unknown and there are likely several pathways (37). The deposition of tau tangles and beta-amyloid plaques has traditionally been considered to be the trigger for the inflammation and degeneration of neurons in the brain, and it is thought that somehow these structures block communication among nerve cells and disrupt processes that cells need to survive, but a mechanistic link has not been established (38, 39). Traumatic head injury, stroke, irradiation, and chemicals such as heavy metals, pesticides, and others have long been considered as potential initiators of Alzheimer's disease (37). An additional view has recently emerged that advocates that, in at least some cases of Alzheimer's disease, the beta-amyloid plaques are a response to an etiologic agent rather than causative of an innate immune response in the central nervous system (37, 38).

Since Alzheimer's disease has a strong inflammatory component suggestive of infection and beta-amyloid is known to have antibacterial, antiviral, and antifungal properties, researchers have sought a virus or other infectious agent as the cause of Alzheimer's disease for many years (40, 41). An increasing number of studies are generating evidence that support this theory. Notably, it has been suggested that herpes simplex virus type 1, *Chlamydophila pneumoniae*, bacteria associated with periodontal disease, and some other common pathogens find a niche in the brains of some individuals during primary infection where they remain latent and reactivate during aging and plausibly produce the clinical and pathologic changes associated with Alzheimer's disease (33, 40). A latent tissue microbiota has also been implicated in some other conditions such as sarcoidosis and preeclampsia (42, 43).

Other theories are that a chronic imbalance in either gut or oral microbiota provides a continual source of bacteria that may promote the development of Alzheimer's disease, either directly as a result of bacteria entering the bloodstream or indirectly by transit of inflammatory mediators that reach distant sites and produce tissue-specific damage (44–46). Oral bacteria from chronically infected periodontal pockets can enter the bloodstream and produce recurrent episodes of symptomless transient bacteremia (45, 47). Similarly, intestinal microbiota imbalance, particularly overgrowth of *Escherichia coli* but also of members of the genera *Streptococcus*, *Lactobacillus*, *Bacteroides*, and *Enterococcus*, may be a consequence of a variety of disorders and practices (e.g., illness, altered intestinal motility, diverticula, use of proton pump inhibitors, etc.) (44, 48). The excessive numbers of bacteria can subsequently disrupt the intestinal barrier function and allow for translocation of any number of foreign substances to gradually enter the bloodstream. Among those foreign substances are bacteria and/or bacterial antigens such as LPS.

Elevated fecal calprotectin levels found in many diagnosed Alzheimer's patients indicate intestinal permeability (33). In addition, plasma LPS levels in patients with Alzheimer's disease have been found to be three times higher than healthy controls (49) and could indicate a Gram-negative bacterial source originating in the gut (33). Some researchers suggest that bacteria themselves can pass from the gut or other colonized areas of the body into the blood where they are nondetectable by culture but exist in a nonproliferating state (27).

Although the identification of these organisms is not known, further work has been done to establish that blood microbiota could be the stimulus responsible for the inflammation, hypercoagulation, and beta-amyloid protein deposits seen in Alzheimer's disease. Of particular interest is the altered systemic iron profile with low transferrin and high ferritin seen in the serum of Alzheimer's disease patients (36). It has been suggested that when high levels of iron are introduced in blood, the dormant bacteria are revived and Gram-negative bacteria are stimulated to release LPS (50).

LPS is a powerful immunostimulant, and there is mounting evidence that recurrent low-grade LPS-induced inflammation can lead to the pathologic processes associated with Alzheimer's disease (45, 50):

- **LPS in the brain leads to oxidative stress.** Recent research has shown that, in individuals with a genetic predisposition to Alzheimer's disease, there is evidence of activated glial cells as early as 7 years before the expected onset of dementia (34). Although the stimulus for this activation has not been directly defined, it is known that LPS can reach the brain where it binds primarily to glial cells (45). Stimulated glial cells initiate phagocytosis and produce proinflammatory cytokines, oxygen free radicals, and nitric oxide (45). Because the brain lacks antioxidants to counteract oxidative stress, it is highly vulnerable to the cellular damage caused by reactive oxygen and nitrogen molecules and constant production of cytotoxic mediators by activated glial cells can result in damage and death of neurons (51, 52). The finding that LPS is neurotoxic only in the presence of microglia provides further support for the role of activated glial cells in LPS-induced inflammation in the brain (52).

- **LPS in the brain causes beta-amyloid formation.** In addition to causing neuroinflammation, LPS can also cause beta-amyloid deposition. LPS and bacterial peptidoglycan have been successfully used for many years as the stimulus in experimental models of inflammation and amyloidosis. In recent studies, beta-amyloid accumulation in the brain has been initiated experimentally by intraperitoneal injection of LPS in mice (53) or intracranial injection of LPS in monkeys (54). Other researchers have found that microorganisms themselves can cause beta-amyloid deposition. Direct challenge with *Salmonella* or *Candida albicans* in cell culture, nematode, and mouse models has been shown to prompt formation of amyloid plaques with the microorganisms trapped in the amyloid fibrils (55). Furthermore, a connection of gut microbiota to the development of beta-amyloid plaques has been demonstrated in mouse models of Alzheimer's disease (56, 57).

- **LPS and tau tangles:** Previous evidence indicated that beta-amyloid deposition drives tau pathology, but recent studies have shown that LPS-induced inflammatory stimuli in the absence of beta-amyloid increases phosphorylation of tau in neuronal and nonneuronal cells (58). The relationship between activated glial cells, amyloid plaques, neurons damaged by tau tangles, and the immune system is complex, and dichotomous effects have been noted in different experimental models, which makes the linkage of influences difficult to establish. It is interesting that peptides containing the microtubule binding sites on tau proteins have also been shown to have antimicrobial properties *in vitro* (59).

- **LPS-mediated hypercoagulation.** The hypercoagulability seen in Alzheimer's disease may also be triggered by LPS. When thrombin is added to platelet-poor plasma from Alzheimer's disease patients *in vitro*, the fibrin networks produced are composed of thicker fibers than seen with plasma from healthy individuals (36). To show that LPS could be responsible for this, further *in vitro* studies have shown that, when fibrinogen and very tiny amounts of LPS are mixed with platelet-poor plasma, aberrant clots with a matted net of thicker heterogeneous fibrin fibers are rapidly produced (50).

Chronic inflammation involving beta-amyloid, hyperphosphorylated tau, and other inflammatory proteins, overactive clotting, and excess levels of iron in the blood have been implicated in other neurodegenerative and chronic inflammatory diseases such as Parkinson's disease, multiple sclerosis, type 2 diabetes mellitus, atherosclerosis, rheumatoid arthritis, and others (27, 60–66). Many findings and observations support the theory of an infectious cause, with one possibility being that a dormant blood microbiota plays a role. While these diseases have underlying mechanisms in common, they manifest in fundamentally different tissue types. A general explanation offered for the variety of presentations is that the nature of the causative microorganisms might be different in different tissue locations (67). Furthermore, relatively little is known about LPS and the complex effects of different inflammatory molecules that may vary depending on the genetic background of the host (67).

Communicable Diseases

Bacterial contamination of donor blood and its separated components is an infrequent but important cause of transfusion-associated morbidity and mortality. Bacterial contamination occurs at the time of blood collection and could be a result of asymptomatic donor bacteremia due to a circulating blood microbiota or microorganisms on the surface of the skin that enter the blood during venipuncture.

Platelet products have a higher risk of developing significant bacterial contamination than red blood cell concentrates or plasma because they are stored at room temperature (20 to 24°C) for more than 5 days, and this provides the opportunity for any contaminating microorganisms to survive and multiply (68, 69). Most microorganisms in reported cases of transfusion-related bacterial infections are Gram-positive aerobic bacteria that are natural microbiota of the skin (68, 70), while Gram-negative organisms, primarily *Enterobacteriaceae*, cause the highest mortality associated with transfusion of infected blood products (59.7%). Platelet concentrates in the United States are screened using conventional blood culture systems such as BacT/Alert (bioMérieux Inc., Durham, NC), but other blood fractions are not routinely subject to screening.

However, when samples from red blood cell and plasma fractions from donors over 50 years of age were cultured on Trypticase soy blood agar and blue lactose plates under both aerobic and anaerobic conditions in one study, a surprisingly high proportion of blood units (62%) were found to contain viable bacteria (19). The organisms found included *Staphylococcus epidermidis* (38%), *Propionibacterium acnes* (renamed *Cutibacterium acnes*) (23%), *Staphylococcus caprae* species (8%), *Micrococcus luteus* (5%), and *Acinetobacter lwoffi* (3%) (19). The finding of viable bacteria in this study and others, as well as detection of microbial DNA sequences in blood of healthy donors, suggests that donor units contain an unrecognized reservoir of bacteria (19, 24). Larger studies to identify viable bacteria in blood components and assess the impact on risk associated with blood transfusion are needed to strengthen these findings and inform potential changes in screening programs (19, 24).

Therapeutic Potential and Areas of Future Research

Although available evidence indicates an infection-mediated pathologic mechanism and a positive association between a blood microbiota and some chronic inflammatory diseases, many questions remain and carefully controlled studies are required. An initial approach may involve culture to isolate microorganisms to determine their identity and for further characterization (27). Additional research, including longitudinal studies, is needed to discriminate cause and effect (27). As questions are resolved, new approaches for treating some chronic diseases could emerge.

The potential efficacy of metal chelators to restore metal ion homeostasis in the treatment of Alzheimer's disease and other neurodegenerative disorders has been shown in transgenic mice as well as in diagnosed patients, but clinical trials are needed (39, 71–77). Most attempted treatments have involved the use of immunosuppressive drugs because these are generally considered to be inflammatory diseases rather than caused by an infectious agent(s). Nonsteroidal anti-inflammatory drugs and other immune-system-modulating agents have not been shown to have any significant overall benefits for Alzheimer's disease patients, but the effectiveness may be based on timing (78). Small preclinical studies seem to suggest that activation of immune responses may be beneficial at some stages of the disease, and inhibiting the immune system may be beneficial at other times (78). Several novel immune-system-enhancing and -suppressing agents are currently in development and are intended to target the inflammatory component of Alzheimer's disease. These include microglial modulators, peroxisome proliferator-activated receptor, and retinoid X receptor agonists, agents that enhance systemic immunity, agents that suppress proinflammatory pathways, and antioxidation agents (78).

If it is verified that infectious agents are the etiologic drivers of Alzheimer's disease and other disorders, potential therapies might involve the use of antimicrobials or some other means of removing the causative microorganisms (79, 80). Probiotics or dietary modifications may potentially be effective in manipulating the gut microbiota and altering the development of the resultant inflammatory disorders (81). The complexity of the pathobiology of these processes and the gaps in our understanding make it difficult to know what treatment approach(es) might work best. Rigorous studies are needed to provide sound evidence for the existence of a blood microbiota/microbiome and clarify its role in health and disease. Therapies will continue to be refined as the field matures in the years to come.

Acknowledgments

The authors are grateful to Dr. Benjamin Lelouvier for expert review and to Donna Martin for assistance in preparation of the figures.

References

1. **Human Microbiome Project Consortium.** 2012. Structure, function and diversity of the healthy human microbiome. *Nature* **486:**207–214.
2. **Jumpstart Consortium Human Microbiome Project Data Generation Working Group.** 2012. Evaluation of 16S rDNA-based community profiling for human microbiome research. *PLoS One* **7:**e39315. doi:10.1371/journal.pone.0039315.
3. **Wylie KM, Truty RM, Sharpton TJ, Mihindukulasuriya KA, Zhou Y, Gao H, Sodergren E, Weinstock GM, Pollard KS.** 2012. Novel bacterial taxa in the human microbiome. *PLoS One* **7:**e35294. doi:10.1371/journal.pone.0035294.
4. **Cho I, Blaser MJ.** 2012. The human microbiome: at the interface of health and disease. *Nat Rev Genet* **13:**260–270.
5. **McDonald D, Ackermann G, Khailova L, Baird C, Heyland D, Kozar R, Lemieux M, Derenski K, King J, Vis-Kampen C, Knight R, Wischmeyer PE.** 2016. Extreme dysbiosis of the microbiome in critical illness. *mSphere.* e00199-16. doi:10.1128/mSphere.00199-16.
6. **Sartor RB.** 2008. Microbial influences in inflammatory bowel diseases. *Gastroenterology* **134:**577–594.
7. **Turnbaugh PJ, Hamady M, Yatsunenko T, Cantarel BL, Duncan A, Ley RE, Sogin ML, Jones WJ, Roe BA, Affourtit JP, Egholm M, Henrissat B, Heath AC, Knight R, Gordon JI.** 2009. A core gut microbiome in obese and lean twins. *Nature* **457:**480–484.
8. **Huffnagle GB.** 2010. The microbiota and allergies/asthma. *PLoS Pathog* **6:**e1000549. doi:10.1371/journal.ppat.1000549.
9. **Han YW, Fardini Y, Chen C, Iacampo KG, Peraino VA, Shamonki JM, Redline RW.** 2010. Term stillbirth caused by oral *Fusobacterium nucleatum.Obstet Gynecol* **115** (Supplement):442–445.
10. **Ravel J, Gajer P, Abdo Z, Schneider GM, Koenig SS, McCulle SL, Karlebach S, Gorle R, Russell J, Tacket CO, Brotman RM, Davis CC, Ault K, Peralta L, Forney**

LJ. 2011. Vaginal microbiome of reproductive-age women. *Proc Natl Acad Sci USA* **108** (Suppl 1):4680–4687.

11. Branton WG, Ellestad KK, Maingat F, Wheatley BM, Rud E, Warren RL, Holt RA, Surette MG, Power C. 2013. Brain microbial populations in HIV/AIDS: α-proteobacteria predominate independent of host immune status. *PLoS One* **8:**e54673. doi:10.1371/journal.pone.0054673.

12. Urbaniak C, Gloor GB, Brackstone M, Scott L, Tangney M, Reid G. 2016. The microbiota of breast tissue and its association with breast cancer. *Appl Environ Microbiol* **82:**5039–5048.

13. Hilt EE, McKinley K, Pearce MM, Rosenfeld AB, Zilliox MJ, Mueller ER, Brubaker L, Gai X, Wolfe AJ, Schreckenberger PC. 2014. Urine is not sterile: use of enhanced urine culture techniques to detect resident bacterial flora in the adult female bladder. *J Clin Microbiol* **52:**871–876.

14. Pardo J, Klinker KP, Borgert SJ, Trikha G, Rand KH, Ramphal R. 2014. Time to positivity of blood cultures supports antibiotic de-escalation at 48 hours. *Ann Pharmacother* **48:**33–40.

15. Durmaz G, Us T, Aydinli A, Kiremitci A, Kiraz N, Akgün Y. 2003. Optimum detection times for bacteria and yeast species with the BACTEC 9120 aerobic blood culture system: evaluation for a 5-year period in a Turkish university hospital. *J Clin Microbiol* **41:**819–821.

16. Baron EJ, Scott JD, Tompkins LS. 2005. Prolonged incubation and extensive subculturing do not increase recovery of clinically significant microorganisms from standard automated blood cultures. *Clin Infect Dis* **41:**1677–1680.

17. Forward KR. 2006. An evaluation of extended incubation time with blind subculture of blood cultures in patients with suspected endocarditis. *Can J Infect Dis Med Microbiol* **17:**186–188.

18. Granfors K, Merilahti-Palo R, Luukkainen R, Möttönen T, Lahesmaa R, Probst P, Märker-Hermann E, Toivanen P. 1998. Persistence of Yersinia antigens in peripheral blood cells from patients with *Yersinia enterocolitica* O:3 infection with or without reactive arthritis. *Arthritis Rheum* **41:**855–862.

19. Damgaard C, Magnussen K, Enevold C, Nilsson M, Tolker-Nielsen T, Holmstrup P, Nielsen CH. 2015. Viable bacteria associated with red blood cells and plasma in freshly drawn blood donations. *PLoS One* **10:**e0120826. doi:10.1371/journal.pone.0120826.

20. Berger SA, Weitzman S, Edberg SC, Casey JI. 1974. Bacteremia after the use of an oral irrigation device. A controlled study in subjects with normal-appearing gingiva: comparison with use of toothbrush. *Ann Intern Med* **80:**510–511.

21. Maharaj B, Coovadia Y, Vayej AC. 2012. An investigation of the frequency of bacteraemia following dental extraction, tooth brushing and chewing. *Cardiovasc J Afr* **23:**340–344.

22. McLaughlin RW, Vali H, Lau PC, Palfree RG, De Ciccio A, Sirois M, Ahmad D, Villemur R, Desrosiers M, Chan EC. 2002. Are there naturally occurring pleomorphic bacteria in the blood of healthy humans? *J Clin Microbiol* **40:**4771–4775.

23. Mitchell AJ, Gray WD, Schroeder M, Yi H, Taylor JV, Dillard RS, Ke Z, Wright ER, Stephens D, Roback JD, Searles CD. 2016. Pleomorphic structures in human blood are red blood cell-derived microparticles, not bacteria. *PLoS One* **11:**e0163582. doi:10.1371/journal.pone.0163582.

24. Païssé S, Valle C, Servant F, Courtney M, Burcelin R, Amar J, Lelouvier B. 2016. Comprehensive description of blood microbiome from healthy donors assessed by 16S targeted metagenomic sequencing. *Transfusion* 56:1138–1147.
25. Salter SJ, Cox MJ, Turek EM, Calus ST, Cookson WO, Moffatt MF, Turner P, Parkhill J, Loman NJ, Walker AW. 2014. Reagent and laboratory contamination can critically impact sequence-based microbiome analyses. *BMC Biol* 12:87. doi:10.1186/s12915-014-0087-z.
26. Nikkari S, McLaughlin IJ, Bi W, Dodge DE, Relman DA. 2001. Does blood of healthy subjects contain bacterial ribosomal DNA? *J Clin Microbiol* 39:1956–1959.
27. Potgieter M, Bester J, Kell DB, Pretorius E. 2015. The dormant blood microbiome in chronic, inflammatory diseases. *FEMS Microbiol Rev* 39:567–591.
28. Kelly CJ, Colgan SP, Frank DN. 2012. Of microbes and meals: the health consequences of dietary endotoxemia. *Nutr Clin Pract* 27:215–225.
29. Turnbaugh PJ, Ley RE, Mahowald MA, Magrini V, Mardis ER, Gordon JI. 2006. An obesity-associated gut microbiome with increased capacity for energy harvest. *Nature* 444:1027–1031.
30. Prince M, Comas-Herrera A, Knapp M, Guerchet M, Karagiannidou M. *World Alzheimer Report 2016*. https://www.alz.co.uk. Accessed December 2016.
31. Alzheimer's Association. 2016. 2016 Alzheimer's disease facts and figures. *Alzheimers Dement* 12:459–509.
32. Naj AC, *et al.*, Alzheimer Disease Genetics Consortium. 2014. Effects of multiple genetic loci on age at onset in late-onset Alzheimer disease: a genome-wide association study. *JAMA Neurol* 71:1394–1404.
33. Hu X, Wang T, Jin F. 2016. Alzheimer's disease and gut microbiota. *Sci China Life Sci* 59:1006–1023.
34. Suárez-Calvet M, Kleinberger G, Araque Caballero MÁ, Brendel M, Rominger A, Alcolea D, Fortea J, Lleó A, Blesa R, Gispert JD, Sánchez-Valle R, Antonell A, Rami L, Molinuevo JL, Brosseron F, Traschütz A, Heneka MT, Struyfs H, Engelborghs S, Sleegers K, Van Broeckhoven C, Zetterberg H, Nellgård B, Blennow K, Crispin A, Ewers M, Haass C. 2016. sTREM2 cerebrospinal fluid levels are a potential biomarker for microglia activity in early-stage Alzheimer's disease and associate with neuronal injury markers. *EMBO Mol Med* 8:466–476.
35. Lyman M, Lloyd DG, Ji X, Vizcaychipi MP, Ma D. 2014. Neuroinflammation: the role and consequences. *Neurosci Res* 79:1–12.
36. Bester J, Soma P, Kell DB, Pretorius E. 2015. Viscoelastic and ultrastructural characteristics of whole blood and plasma in Alzheimer-type dementia, and the possible role of bacterial lipopolysaccharides (LPS). *Oncotarget* 6:35284–35303.
37. Li CQ, Zheng Q, Wang Q, Zeng QP. 2016. Biotic/abiotic stress-driven Alzheimer's disease. *Front Cell Neurosci* 10:269. doi:10.3389/fncel.2016.00269.
38. Agostini M, Fasolato C. 2016. When, where and how? Focus on neuronal calcium dysfunctions in Alzheimer's disease. *Cell Calcium* 60:289–298.
39. Wang P, Wang Z-Y. 2017. Metal ions influx is a double edged sword for the pathogenesis of Alzheimer's disease. *Ageing Res Rev* 35:265–290.
40. Itzhaki RF, Lathe R, Balin BJ, Ball MJ, Bearer EL, Braak H, Bullido MJ, Carter C, Clerici M, Cosby SL, Del Tredici K, Field H, Fulop T, Grassi C, Griffin WS,

Haas J, Hudson AP, Kamer AR, Kell DB, Licastro F, Letenneur L, Lövheim H, Mancuso R, Miklossy J, Otth C, Palamara AT, Perry G, Preston C, Pretorius E, Strandberg T, Tabet N, Taylor-Robinson SD, Whittum-Hudson JA. 2016. Microbes and Alzheimer's disease. *J Alzheimers Dis* **51**:979–984.

41. Soscia SJ, Kirby JE, Washicosky KJ, Tucker SM, Ingelsson M, Hyman B, Burton MA, Goldstein LE, Duong S, Tanzi RE, Moir RD. 2010. The Alzheimer's disease-associated amyloid beta-protein is an antimicrobial peptide. *PLoS One* **5**:e9505. doi:10.1371/journal.pone.0009505.

42. Dubaniewicz A, Kalinowski L, Dudziak M, Kalinowska A, Singh M. 2015. Peroxynitrite in sarcoidosis: relation to *Mycobacterium* stationary phase. *Adv Exp Med Biol* **866**:41–49.

43. Kell DB, Kenny LC. 2016. A dormant microbial component in the development of preeclampsia. *Front Med (Lausanne)* **3**:60. doi:10.3389/fmed.2016.00060.

44. Bouhnik Y, Alain S, Attar A, Flourié B, Raskine L, Sanson-Le Pors MJ, Rambaud JC. 1999. Bacterial populations contaminating the upper gut in patients with small intestinal bacterial overgrowth syndrome. *Am J Gastroenterol* **94**:1327–1331.

45. Poole S, Singhrao SK, Kesavalu L, Curtis MA, Crean S. 2013. Determining the presence of periodontopathic virulence factors in short-term postmortem Alzheimer's disease brain tissue. *J Alzheimers Dis* **36**:665–677.

46. Scannapieco FA, Cantos A. 2016. Oral inflammation and infection, and chronic medical diseases: implications for the elderly. *Periodontol 2000* **72**:153–175.

47. Lockhart PB, Brennan MT, Sasser HC, Fox PC, Paster BJ, Bahrani-Mougeot FK. 2008. Bacteremia associated with toothbrushing and dental extraction. *Circulation* **117**:3118–3125.

48. Lynch SV, Pedersen O. 2016. The human intestinal microbiome in health and disease. *N Engl J Med* **375**:2369–2379.

49. Zhang R, Miller RG, Gascon R, Champion S, Katz J, Lancero M, Narvaez A, Honrada R, Ruvalcaba D, McGrath MS. 2009. Circulating endotoxin and systemic immune activation in sporadic amyotrophic lateral sclerosis (sALS). *J Neuroimmunol* **206**:121–124.

50. Pretorius E, Mbotwe S, Bester J, Robinson CJ, Kell DB. 2016. Acute induction of anomalous and amyloidogenic blood clotting by molecular amplification of highly substoichiometric levels of bacterial lipopolysaccharide. *J R Soc Interface* **13**:20160539.

51. Park J, Min JS, Kim B, Chae UB, Yun JW, Choi MS, Kong IK, Chang KT, Lee DS. 2015. Mitochondrial ROS govern the LPS-induced pro-inflammatory response in microglia cells by regulating MAPK and NF-κB pathways. *Neurosci Lett* **584**:191–196.

52. Block ML, Zecca L, Hong JS. 2007. Microglia-mediated neurotoxicity: uncovering the molecular mechanisms. *Nat Rev Neurosci* **8**:57–69.

53. Lee JW, Lee YK, Yuk DY, Choi DY, Ban SB, Oh KW, Hong JT. 2008. Neuro-inflammation induced by lipopolysaccharide causes cognitive impairment through enhancement of beta-amyloid generation. *J Neuroinflammation* **5**:37. doi:10.1186/1742-2094-5-37.

54. Philippens IH, Ormel PR, Baarends G, Johansson M, Remarque EJ, Doverskog M. 2017. Acceleration of amyloidosis by inflammation in the amyloid-beta marmoset monkey model of Alzheimer's disease. *J Alzheimers Dis* **55**:101–113.

55. Kumar DK, Choi SH, Washicosky KJ, Eimer WA, Tucker S, Ghofrani J, Lefkowitz A, McColl G, Goldstein LE, Tanzi RE, Moir RD. 2016. Amyloid-β peptide protects

against microbial infection in mouse and worm models of Alzheimer's disease. *Sci Transl Med* **8**:340ra72. doi:10.1126/scitranslmed.aaf1059.

56. Harach T, Marungruang N, Dutilleul N, Cheatham V, Mc Coy KD, Neher JJ, Jucker M, Fåk F, Lasser T, Bolmont T. 2015. *Reduction of Alzheimer's disease beta-amyloid pathology in the absence of gut microbiota.* arXiv:1509.02273v2 [q-bio.MN].

57. Minter MR, Zhang C, Leone V, Ringus DL, Zhang X, Oyler-Castrillo P, Musch MW, Liao F, Ward JF, Holtzman DM, Chang EB, Tanzi RE, Sisodia SS. 2016. Antibiotic-induced perturbations in gut microbial diversity influences neuro-inflammation and amyloidosis in a murine model of Alzheimer's disease. *Sci Rep* **6**:30028. doi:10.1038/srep30028.

58. Lee DC, Rizer J, Selenica LB, Reid P, Kraft C, Johnson A, Blair L, Gordon MN, Dickey CA, Morgan D. 2010. LPS-induced inflammation exacerbates phospho-tau pathology in rTg4510 mice. *J Neuroinflammation* **7**:56. doi:10.1186/1742-2094-7-56.

59. Kobayashi N, Masuda J, Kudoh J, Shimizu N, Yoshida T. 2008. Binding sites on tau proteins as components for antimicrobial peptides. *Biocontrol Sci* **13**:49–56.

60. He Q, Yu W, Wu J, Chen C, Lou Z, Zhang Q, Zhao J, Wang J, Xiao B. 2013. Intranasal LPS-mediated Parkinson's model challenges the pathogenesis of nasal cavity and environmental toxins. *PLoS One* **8**:e78418. doi:10.1371/journal.pone.0078418.

61. Chukkapalli SS, Rivera-Kweh MF, Velsko IM, Chen H, Zheng D, Bhattacharyya I, Gangula PR, Lucas AR, Kesavalu L. 2015. Chronic oral infection with major perio-dontal bacteria *Tannerella forsythia* modulates systemic atherosclerosis risk factors and inflammatory markers. *Pathog Dis* **73**:ftv009. doi:10.1093/femspd/ftv009.

62. Felice VD, Quigley EM, Sullivan AM, O'Keeffe GW, O'Mahony SM. 2016. Microbiota-gut-brain signalling in Parkinson's disease: implications for non-motor symptoms. *Parkinsonism Relat Disord* **27**:1–8.

63. Miklossy J, McGeer PL. 2016. Common mechanisms involved in Alzheimer's disease and type 2 diabetes: a key role of chronic bacterial infection and inflammation. *Aging (Albany NY)* **8**:575–588.

64. Marietta EV, Murray JA, Luckey DH, Jeraldo PR, Lamba A, Patel R, Luthra HS, Mangalam A, Taneja V. 2016. Human gut-derived *Prevotella histicola* suppresses inflammatory arthritis in humanized mice. *Arthritis Rheumatol* **68**:2878–2888.

65. Chen J, Wright K, Davis JM, Jeraldo P, Marietta EV, Murray J, Nelson H, Matteson EL, Taneja V. 2016. An expansion of rare lineage intestinal microbes characterizes rheumatoid arthritis. *Genome Med* **8**:43. doi:10.1186/s13073-016-0299-7.

66. Colpitts SL, Kasper LH. 2017. Influence of the gut microbiome on autoimmunity in the central nervous system. *J Immunol* **198**:596–604.

67. Kell DB, Pretorius E. 2015. On the translocation of bacteria and their lipopolysac-charides between blood and peripheral locations in chronic, inflammatory diseases: the central roles of LPS and LPS-induced cell death. *Integr Biol* **7**:1339–1377.

68. Brecher ME, Hay SN. 2005. Bacterial contamination of blood components. *Clin Microbiol Rev* **18**:195–204.

69. Bihl F, Castelli D, Marincola F, Dodd RY, Brander C. 2007. Transfusion-transmitted infections. *J Transl Med* **5**:25. doi:10.1186/1479-5876-5-25.

70. Hillyer CD, Josephson CD, Blajchman MA, Vostal JG, Epstein JS, Goodman JL. 2003. Bacterial contamination of blood components: risks, strategies, and regulation:

joint ASH and AABB educational session in transfusion medicine. *Hematology (Am Soc Hematol Educ Program)* **2003**:575–589.

71. Savory J, Huang Y, Wills MR, Herman MM. 1998. Reversal by desferrioxamine of tau protein aggregates following two days of treatment in aluminum-induced neuro-fibrillary degeneration in rabbit: implications for clinical trials in Alzheimer's disease. *Neurotoxicology* **19**:209–214.

72. Cherny RA, Atwood CS, Xilinas ME, Gray DN, Jones WD, McLean CA, Barnham KJ, Volitakis I, Fraser FW, Kim Y, Huang X, Goldstein LE, Moir RD, Lim JT, Beyreuther K, Zheng H, Tanzi RE, Masters CL, Bush AI. 2001. Treatment with a copper-zinc chelator markedly and rapidly inhibits beta-amyloid accumulation in Alzheimer's disease transgenic mice. *Neuron* **30**:665–676.

73. Opazo C, Barría MI, Ruiz FH, Inestrosa NC. 2003. Copper reduction by copper binding proteins and its relation to neurodegenerative diseases. *Biometals* **16**:91–98.

74. Ibach B, Haen E, Marienhagen J, Hajak G. 2005. Clioquinol treatment in familiar early onset of Alzheimer's disease: a case report. *Pharmacopsychiatry* **38**:178–179.

75. Adlard PA, Cherny RA, Finkelstein DI, Gautier E, Robb E, Cortes M, Volitakis I, Liu X, Smith JP, Perez K, Laughton K, Li QX, Charman SA, Nicolazzo JA, Wilkins S, Deleva K, Lynch T, Kok G, Ritchie CW, Tanzi RE, Cappai R, Masters CL, Barnham KJ, Bush AI. 2008. Rapid restoration of cognition in Alzheimer's transgenic mice with 8-hydroxy quinoline analogs is associated with decreased interstitial Abeta. *Neuron* **59**:43–55.

76. Squitti R. 2012. Metals in Alzheimer's disease: a systemic perspective. *Front Biosci (Landmark Ed)* **17**:451–472.

77. Robert A, Liu Y, Nguyen M, Meunier B. 2015. Regulation of copper and iron homeostasis by metal chelators: a possible chemotherapy for Alzheimer's disease. *Acc Chem Res* **48**:1332–1339.

78. Deardorff WJ, Grossberg GT. 2017. Targeting neuroinflammation in Alzheimer's disease: evidence for NSAIDs and novel therapeutics. *Expert Rev Neurother* **17**:17–32.

79. El-Shimy IA, Heikal OA, Hamdi N. 2015. Minocycline attenuates Aβ oligomers-induced pro-inflammatory phenotype in primary microglia while enhancing Aβ fibrils phagocytosis. *Neurosci Lett* **609**:36–41.

80. Budni J, Garcez ML, de Medeiros J, Cassaro E, Bellettini-Santos T, Mina F, Quevedo J. 2016. The anti-inflammatory role of minocycline in Alzheimer's disease. *Curr Alzheimer Res* **13**:1319–1329.

81. Winek K, Dirnagl U, Meisel A. 2016. The gut microbiome as therapeutic target in central nervous system diseases: implications for stroke. *Neurotherapeutics* **13**:762–774.

The Dark Art of Blood Cultures
Edited by Wm. Michael Dunne, Jr. and Carey-Ann D. Burnham
© 2018 American Society for Microbiology, Washington, DC
doi:10.1128/9781555819811.ch14

Postmortem Blood Culture 14

Robin R. Chamberland[1] and Carl O. Deetz[2]

Background

Autopsy has historically played a critical role in our understanding of normal anatomy, disease and treatment efficacies, or adverse effects of medications. Despite the importance of autopsy as a teaching tool, it is now limited to an ancillary role in modern medical education (1). This effect may continue to be amplified as physicians who did not observe autopsies during their training are less likely to request an autopsy later on in the course of their careers (2). In the 1970s, the Joint Commission on Accreditation of Healthcare Organizations (JCAHO) eliminated the requirement for a minimum autopsy rate from its accreditation process, and Medicare stopped reimbursing for autopsies in 1986 (3). Reasons physicians do not request an autopsy have reportedly included trepidation regarding the lack of training on how to seek autopsy permission, fear of offending the family, and fear of malpractice litigation. In addition, confidence in contemporary diagnostic technology and the ever present desire to reduce health care spending have also been cited as reasons (2, 4–9). Given the forces aligned against this procedure, autopsy rates have declined in the United States and other Western countries over the past 3 decades (4). Unfortunately, the sequelae of this decline include the loss of an established teaching tool along with the inability to identify and correct clinical errors and missed diagnoses (4).

A previously used classification scheme for medical errors discovered at autopsy divides these into class I, II, and III type errors, where class I errors

[1]Saint Louis University School of Medicine, Saint Louis, MO 63104
[2]Analytical Pathology Services, Saint Louis, MO 63136

result from a missed diagnosis that affects clinical outcome and class II and III type errors have, respectively, declining impacts on expected prognosis (3, 10). One study reported class I errors in 10% of autopsies over the course of 30 years at a Boston teaching hospital (11), while class I and II errors combined were found in 35% of autopsies in another study (10). These numbers might be subject to a selection bias, although it is interesting to note that further studies have shown that physicians are generally unable to predict which cases will show a major discrepancy at autopsy (12). This observation alone suggests the importance of autopsy in education and in revealing missed clinical diagnosis. It has been observed that the three most common missed diagnoses identified at autopsy include aortic dissection (AD), pulmonary embolism (PE), and active tuberculosis (TB). Calculating the expected prevalence of missed cases among patients not autopsied reduced the rate of detection from 93% to 82% for aortic dissection, 97% to 91% for pulmonary embolism, and 96% to 83% for active tuberculosis (3).

Since the report of Shojania and Burton (3) was derived from hospital-based autopsies where active tuberculosis was one of the most overlooked diagnoses, clinical microbiology testing may be a more important component of hospital autopsies than generally appreciated. The continued risk of a rapidly spreading influenza or other pandemic and the threat of a potential bioterrorism attack taken together with the fact that active tuberculosis is one of the most commonly missed diagnoses in autopsy studies makes clinical microbiology, in general, and blood culture, specifically, critically important postmortem diagnostic tools. In addition, the high prevalence of immunodeficiency in the setting of HIV, transplant, oncology, or aging not only emphasizes the relevance of an infectious disease-based argument for reversing the trend of declining postmortem examinations but also underscores the importance of blood culture in this setting. Currently, clinical microbiology might play less of a role in hospital autopsy than in forensic autopsy since hospital-directed autopsies are usually performed on patients with premortem cultures from a variety of sites already in progress and on individuals who might have received antimicrobial therapy prior to death. Still, the clinical microbiology laboratory frequently receives specimens for culture collected at autopsy when an autopsy is performed. The results generated from these culture requests can variably provide valuable information or produce confusion, and this depends in large part on variables including the selection of sites to sample, collection technique, and interpretation of results in the context of data available from patient history and other pathology-based evaluations.

Skepticism surrounds the role of microbiology at autopsy given discrepancies in findings between organisms isolated from living patients and those subsequently recovered from postmortem sampling (13, 14). We suggest that there is a useful, if limited, role for autopsy microbiology, in particular, blood culture. Appropriate subject selection, a high index of suspicion for an infectious agent as a cause or cofactor of death, attention to collection technique, and interpretation of findings are absolutely critical.

The Decision to Collect Cultures at Autopsy

The samples yielding the most useful information from postmortem microbiological testing have historically been blood, cerebrospinal fluid (CSF), and lung tissue (15). Growth in cultures from normally sterile sites such as blood can result from several possible scenarios. (i) The organism may have been present prior to death, either transiently or causing infection. The presence of signs and symptoms of infection or inflammation can aid in distinguishing these two options. (ii) Agonal spread of organisms to normally sterile sites is thought to result from physical trauma associated with resuscitation attempts or loss of integrity of mucosal surfaces due to ischemia at the time of death. (iii) Translocation of normal gastrointestinal and oropharyngeal flora after death, which is less likely with appropriate storage. (iv) Growth in cultures may result from contamination introduced at the time of autopsy specimen collection.

The European Society of Clinical Microbiology and Infectious Diseases Study Group for Forensic and Postmortem Microbiology (ESGFOR) conducted a survey to determine pathologist practice regarding microbiology at autopsy, demonstrating three primary indications for which it was used: clinical suspicion of infection not diagnosed antemortem, signs of infection at autopsy, and standard practice in fetal, perinatal, and pediatric deaths (16). The samples collected most frequently were blood from the heart or femoral artery (66% and 49%, respectively) followed by tissue from spleen or lung.

Morris et al. (17) conducted an extensive literature review on postmortem culture from blood and CSF, revealing that careful attention to sterile collection technique resulted in negative blood cultures two-thirds of the time, while two-thirds of positive autopsy blood cultures are monomicrobic and the remainder are polymicrobic. In a large study of 2,033 autopsies of infants through adults, only 7% yielded more than one organism (18), a rate that is not markedly higher than blood culture contamination rates from living patients in some settings. These findings suggest that agonal spread or postmortem translocation of normal flora across mucosal surfaces is unlikely to be common, given that mixed blood cultures make up a minority of positive results. In addition, the time to culture collection after death does not change these findings within the first 48 h if the body is stored appropriately at 4°C (15, 19).

Other studies have demonstrated far higher positive postmortem blood culture rates (13, 19), along with a greater preponderance of mixed cultures rather than a single organism, even with appropriate storage. These findings suggest that samples are often contaminated during the collection process, rather than supporting the notion that translocation of polymicrobial flora occurs in the setting of some studies and not others, and emphasize the attention that must be paid to sterile collection technique to obtain meaningful results. As might be expected, sterilization of the collection site before specimen collection and use of sterile instruments yield a lower rate of positive cultures than does collection with nonsterile instruments (20–22). While this point would seem obvious, careful attention to sterile technique at autopsy could potentially alleviate much of the poor reputation that autopsy microbiology has attained. Details of techniques for avoiding contamination in sample collection and handling are beyond the scope of this work, and have been described elsewhere (23, 24).

The best data supporting the use of postmortem blood culture is in the setting of sudden unexpected deaths in infants and young people. A British study evaluating the contribution of microbiology testing in the evaluation of sudden unexpected death in infancy (SUDI) demonstrated that 16% of blood cultures collected at autopsy revealed a potential pathogen, defined as an organism that would be considered a pathogen if recovered from blood of a living patient, or if recovered from multiple sites, with 90% of autopsies performed during the study period including blood culture (25). This was in a setting in which guidelines were in place for blood, CSF, and nasopharyngeal aspirate culture collection in all unexplained infant deaths, along with cultures from any site with findings that raised concern for infection, such as inner ear exudate. A potential pathogen was revealed in 49% of cases when all culture sites were considered, allowing cases to be classified as infectious rather than sudden infant death syndrome (SIDS).

A similar survey was conducted in the United States evaluating the use of infectious disease testing in cases of sudden unexpected infant deaths (SUIDs) (26). Aerobic and anaerobic blood cultures were routinely performed in SUIDs cases by 77.8% of respondents. Substantially fewer pathologists reported routine collection of samples to evaluate for viral etiologies, or bacterial cultures from other anatomic sites. Studies have demonstrated that routine collection of microbiological and histologic data at autopsy allows determination of definitive cause of death in 20 to 30% of SUID investigations, preventing overclassification of SIDS (26). These findings have led to defined autopsy protocols in many European countries, but such protocols do not yet exist in the United States. A 2006 study reported that one in eight infant deaths in the United States meets criteria for unexplained deaths due to possible infectious causes (UDPIC), noting infants' increased risk for infectious-disease-related death (27). These findings suggest that a defined protocol for infectious disease testing in unexplained infant death in the United States, along with guidelines for interpretation of the resulting data, could lead to more accurate classification of these deaths.

A study conducted in Spain revealed that 16% of sudden deaths in young people (age ≤34 years) were classified as sudden unexpected death from infectious diseases (SUDID), with that number rising to 32% in children aged 1 to 14 years (28). An infectious agent was identified in 74% of SUDID cases in which microbiological studies were performed. Toxicology studies demonstrated that 48% of subjects between ages 25 and 34 with death attributed to infectious causes had recently used illicit drugs. An association was observed between methadone use, often along with benzodiazepines, and deaths due to pneumonia, presumably due to respiratory aspiration during periods of decreased consciousness. Trends in use of opiates could drive numbers of infectious disease deaths related to these practices upward. While the incidence of sudden death due to undiagnosed infectious disease is low, microbiological studies can help to elucidate an etiologic agent when suspected.

Specific recommendations for sample collection in instances of sudden death were proposed by Fernández-Rodríguez et al. and grouped into the following categories: (i) infants through age 16 years without accompanying clinical syndrome, (ii) young people age 17 to 35 without clinical syndrome, (iii) any age with clinical syndrome, and (iv) traumatic or iatrogenic death (29). Recommendations for each group included blood culture for bacterial pathogens, as well as sample collection from other sites to evaluate for the presence of both bacterial and viral infectious etiologies, with breadth of testing dependent on group classification. Those recommendations were the result of studies indicating the usefulness of postmortem microbiology, especially in sudden death because little histologic evidence of inflammation may be observed (16).

Blood Culture Collection

Suspicion of undiagnosed infectious disease is the principal driving force for postmortem blood culture. Patients who die under medical care may already have positive blood culture in which case it is not necessary to attempt to recapitulate these findings at autopsy (30). However, more meaningful results may be obtained in the person who dies outside the hospital setting with signs and symptoms of sepsis.

The lack of standardization of postmortem microbiology testing practices led to the development by a group of European forensic pathologists, microbiologists, and physicians of a consensus proposed sampling protocol for the most commonly encountered scenarios (29). General recommendations include storage of the body at 4°C with autopsy within 24 h of death, skin disinfection with water-based antiseptic, collection of blood at the beginning of autopsy, and timely sample transport to the laboratory. Preference in site of blood collection in decreasing order is peripheral femoral, subclavian, carotid, jugular, and then left ventricle. Reznicek and Koontz recommend collection of heart blood and spleen, because identical isolates from both sites support a diagnosis of sepsis (24).

Diagnosis of bacteremia in living patients is typically accomplished through the collection of more than one set of blood cultures, which permits increased sensitivity by collecting optimal blood volumes, while also aiding in differentiating contamination from true-positive cultures. A similar approach was tested by evaluating pairs of postmortem blood cultures collected from both cardiac ventricles or the aorta and vena cava following decontamination of the vessel surfaces with 70% alcohol and 10% povidone iodine (31). This approach allowed collection of adequate blood volumes, along with mitigating risk of contamination that may be introduced when samples are collected by puncturing the skin. Findings from this study are described below.

Interpretation of Culture Results

Determining the significance of a positive blood culture is not always straightforward, and must be approached with care. The organism identified is an independent correlate of true bacteremia in living patients (32), with certain organisms nearly always (>90%) indicative of a "true positive," including *Enterobacteriaceae*, *Staphylococcus aureus*, *Streptococcus pneumoniae*, *Pseudomonas aeruginosa*, and *Candida albicans* (33, 34). Other organisms that usually represent true infection include *Streptococcus pyogenes*, *Streptococcus agalactiae*, *Listeria monocytogenes*, *Neisseria meningitidis*, *Neisseria gonorrhoeae*, *Haemophilus influenzae*, *Bacteroides fragilis* group organisms, *Cryptococcus neoformans*, and *Candida* spp. other than *albicans*, while organisms such as *Corynebacterium* spp., *Bacillus* spp. other than *anthracis*, and

Propionibacterium acnes are frequent contaminants (33, 34). Findings that are difficult to interpret include growth of coagulase-negative *Staphylococcus* spp. and viridans group streptococci, which can represent contamination or infection, highlighting the importance of corroborating clinical and histologic information (33, 34).

Interpretation of positive results should take into account the identification of the organism (likely pathogen versus likely contaminant), whether it is a pure or mixed culture, whether it was isolated from other sites as well, and whether the result is consistent with the patient's clinical course (24).

Sunagawa and Sugitani evaluated the use of paired blood cultures collected at autopsy. Recommended criteria for determination of bacteremia were defined as recovery of a single bacterial species that is a likely cause of bacteremia, recovery of a single species that is aerobic or facultatively anaerobic, and growth of the single organism in both sets of cultures (31). These parameters were based on assumptions that most cases of bacteremia are monomicrobial and that anaerobic organisms may be the result of compromised mucosal surfaces which could occur postmortem. Paired blood cultures were collected from 31 autopsy cases, 18 of which yielded growth, with a single bacterial species recovered in 12 cases. In five cases demonstrating growth of the single organism in both cultures of the pair, all three recommended criteria for bacteremia were met. An additional three cases met two of the three criteria, single species that is associated with bacteremia and aerobic or facultatively anaerobic, and were classified as likely bacteremia. Two additional isolates obtained from single cultures were excluded as the organisms were anaerobes and part of normal intestinal flora. The remaining six culture sets yielded multiple organisms and five were considered unlikely to be the cause of antemortem bacteremia. The sixth mixed culture, from which *Staphylococcus epidermidis* and *H. influenzae* were recovered, was classified as likely bacteremia because the two organisms did not represent likely intestinal flora, and *H. influenzae* in blood culture is among the organisms that nearly always represent a true positive finding antemortem (34). This study demonstrates that there may be a role for paired blood culture samples, collected from separate sites, in postmortem diagnosis of bacteremia, but that the data obtained must be interpreted carefully along with clinical and pathological findings.

The case for postmortem bacteriology studies in adults is more nebulous than in infants and young people with sudden unexpected deaths. Palmiere et al. conducted a study examining the role of microbiology in adult autopsy, specifically examining the effects of sampling contamination and postmortem bacterial translocation in interpretation of culture findings (35). The study included 100 medicolegal autopsies, with death having occurred outside the hospital setting, and microbiology testing performed when infection or sepsis was suspected. All cases included aerobic and anaerobic culture of blood aspirated from the right atrium after searing with a heated scalpel blade, along with collection from a second site, which included spleen, liver, and/or lungs. In addition, serum biochemical analysis for markers of infection included procalcitonin, C-reactive protein, interleukin-6, lipopolysaccharide binding protein, and others. Using a combination of parameters, including histopathology, increases in biochemical markers of inflammation/infection, and number and type of bacterial species identified, findings were classified as undetermined (5%), infection (35%), death unrelated to infection (19%), contamination (22%), or translocation (19%). Organisms isolated most commonly from true infections included *Enterobacteriaceae*, *P. aeruginosa*, *S. pneumoniae*, and *S. aureus*. Cases designated contamination most commonly revealed coagulase-negative staphylococci, sometimes along with *Micrococcus*, *Corynebacterium*, or *Propionibacterium*. Cases defined as translocation were characterized by findings of organisms of likely gastrointestinal origin (*Enterobacteriaceae*, enterococci, or lactobacilli), along with normal biochemical markers. While culture was useful in revealing the causative agent in 35% of cases in this study, 41% of positive results were related to contamination or bacterial translocation. Given that the biochemical markers used to determine the classification of results in these cases are not routinely used, it remains necessary to carefully evaluate and interpret microbiological findings from autopsy.

Molecular Testing for Blood Pathogens

The development of molecular testing has advanced the diagnosis of infectious diseases beyond many of the limitations of culture-, microscopy-, or serology-based detection of organisms, and has been applied to research, clinical diagnostics, and modern autopsy. Molecular technology encompasses methods used to detect or characterize genetic material (RNA or DNA) via probe, amplification, or sequencing. These techniques allow for the rapid detection and, in some cases, quantification of a variety of pathogens. These techniques are used in the clinical laboratory for applications such as diagnosis of respiratory tract, central nervous system, gastrointestinal, and sexually transmitted infections, in nasopharyngeal, cerebrospinal fluid, feces, urine, and genital samples (36). Molecular testing is also used for infection control and prevention purposes such as screening for patient colonization with methicillin-resistant *Staphylococcus aureus* or vancomycin-resistant *Enterococcus*, or maternal carriage of group B streptococci. Sequencing of the 16S rRNA gene following amplification from tissue or body fluid samples has proven helpful in the identification of bacterial causes of infection that cannot be recovered by conventional culture-based methods following antimicrobial therapy, or in infections with organisms that are not amenable to routine culture techniques (37). While this testing has bolstered the diagnostic capability of clinical laboratories, a notable limitation is in bacterial detection directly from blood, with most molecular testing on blood serving to identify or quantify viral pathogens. Several assays have been developed commercially for bacterial detection from whole blood (38), but have not proven sufficiently sensitive or specific to replace culture, and have not been approved by the Food and Drug Administration (FDA) or marketed in the United States. Instead, identification of bacterial organisms from blood is primarily conducted by multiplex PCR from positive blood culture supernatant, in which bacterial nucleic acids have been amplified through organism growth. Nucleic acid amplification tests have been developed for detection from whole blood or plasma of some bacterial organisms that do not readily grow in blood culture, such as *Coxiella burnetii*, *Tropheryma whipplei*, *Ehrlichia chaffeensis*, *Anaplasma phagocytophilum*, *Mycoplasma pneumoniae*, and *Bartonella* spp. (39).

Select Agents and Autopsy

The U.S. Department of Health and Human Services has deemed a number of organisms select agents based upon their potential to pose a severe threat to public health and safety. A subset of these organisms is further classified as tier 1 select agents based on their potential for malevolent misuse for purposes of bioterrorism. These agents are chosen based on criteria laid out in the Public Health Security and Bioterrorism Preparedness and Response Act of 2002 which include effect on human health, degree and method of contagiousness, and availability of treatments and immunizations. It should be noted that while these pathogens have the potential to be used in acts of bioterrorism, they may also be encountered when there is no suspicion of such an event, as many also cause naturally occurring infection. Bacterial pathogens categorized as tier 1 select agents are *Bacillus anthracis*, *Francisella tularensis*, *Yersinia pestis*, *Burkholderia mallei*, *Burkholderia pseudomallei*, and *Clostridium* species producing botulinum neurotoxin (https://www.selectagents.gov/faq-general.html). If there is any suspicion that a select agent may be recovered at autopsy, it is critical to take proper precautions while performing the procedure, to notify the laboratory that will be handling samples as to the suspected agents, and to follow all regulatory requirements for notification and waste disposal.

Summary: Autopsy and the Relevance of Microbiology Testing

Hill and Anderson (40) have reiterated what might be assumed from our historical understanding of the development of medicine that physiological discovery at autopsy provides the foundation upon which modern medicine rests, and, as outlined in this chapter, that blood culture can play a critical ancillary role in this continued process of discovery. Despite much debate as to the relevance of an autopsy in current medicine, and even more debate on the usefulness that microbiology plays in this setting, fears that agonal spread or postmortem translocation of normal flora across mucosal surfaces might limit interpretation of cultures are somewhat negated by a number of independent studies. When autopsies are used in a targeted approach, such as investigating the sudden death of infants or presumed previously healthy young people, or for obtaining timely information in an outbreak, be it natural or man-made, the value increases dramatically (41). In an environment of emerging and reemerging pathogens, and bioterrorism, the use of postmortem blood culture provides an additional layer of vigilance. In the context of protocols for the careful selection and collection of samples and interpretation of results, postmortem culture can add valuable diagnostic information to the autopsy report.

REFERENCES

1. Horowitz RE, Naritoku WY. 2007. The autopsy as a performance measure and teaching tool. *Hum Pathol* **38**:688–695.
2. Stolman CJ, Castello F, Yorio M, Mautone S. 1994. Attitudes of pediatricians and pediatric residents toward obtaining permission for autopsy. *Arch Pediatr Adolesc Med* **148**:843–847.
3. Shojania KG, Burton EC. 2008. The vanishing nonforensic autopsy. *N Engl J Med* **358**:873–875.
4. Xiao J, Krueger GR, Buja LM, Covinsky M. 2009. The impact of declining clinical autopsy: need for revised healthcare policy. *Am J Med Sci* **337**:41–46.
5. Peacock SJ, Machin D, Duboulay CE, Kirkham N. 1988. The autopsy: a useful tool or an old relic? *J Pathol* **156**:9–14.
6. Cottreau C, McIntyre L, Favara BE. 1989. Professional attitudes toward the autopsy. A survey of clinicians and pathologists. *Am J Clin Pathol* **92**:673–676.

7. Karunaratne S, Benbow EW. 1997. A survey of general practitioners' views on autopsy reports. *J Clin Pathol* **50**:548–552.
8. Start RD, McCulloch TA, Silcocks PB, Cotton WK. 1994. Attitudes of senior pathologists towards the autopsy. *J Pathol* **172**:81–84.
9. Grunberg SM, Sherrod A, Muellenbach R, Renshaw M, Zaretsky S, Levine AM. 1994. Analysis of physician attitudes concerning requests for autopsy. *Cancer Invest* **12**:463–468.
10. Gibson TN, Shirley SE, Escoffery CT, Reid M. 2004. Discrepancies between clinical and postmortem diagnoses in Jamaica: a study from the University Hospital of the West Indies. *J Clin Pathol* **57**:980–985.
11. Goldman L, Sayson R, Robbins S, Cohn LH, Bettmann M, Weisberg M. 1983. The value of the autopsy in three medical eras. *N Engl J Med* **308**:1000–1005.
12. Shojania KG, Burton EC, McDonald KM, Goldman L. 2003. Changes in rates of autopsy-detected diagnostic errors over time: a systematic review. *JAMA* **289**:2849–2856.
13. Wilson SJ, Wilson ML, Reller LB. 1993. Diagnostic utility of postmortem blood cultures. *Arch Pathol Lab Med* **117**:986–988.
14. Koneman EW, Davis MA. 1974. Postmortem bacteriology. 3. Clinical significance of microorganisms recovered at autopsy. *Am J Clin Pathol* **61**:28–40.
15. Lobmaier IV, Vege A, Gaustad P, Rognum TO. 2009. Bacteriological investigation—significance of time lapse after death. *Eur J Clin Microbiol Infect Dis* **28**:1191–1198.
16. Saegeman V, Cohen MC, Alberola J, Ziyade N, Farina C, ESCMID Study Group for Forensic and Postmortem Microbiology, Cornaglia G, Fernandez-Rodríguez A. 24 February 2017. How is post-mortem microbiology appraised by pathologists? Results from a practice survey conducted by ESGFOR. *Eur J Clin Microbiol Infect Dis* doi:10.1007/s10096-017-2943-6.
17. Morris JA, Harrison LM, Partridge SM. 2007. Practical and theoretical aspects of postmortem bacteriology. *Curr Diagn Pathol* **13**:65–74.
18. Carpenter HM, Wilkins RM. 1964. Autopsy bacteriology: review of 2,033 cases. *Arch Pathol* **77**:73–81.
19. Weber MA, Hartley JC, Brooke I, Lock PE, Klein NJ, Malone M, Sebire NJ. 2010. Post-mortem interval and bacteriological culture yield in sudden unexpected death in infancy (SUDI). *Forensic Sci Int* **198**:121–125.
20. Dolan CT, Brown AL Jr, Ritts RE Jr. 1971. Microbiological examination of post-mortem tissues. *Arch Pathol* **92**:206–211.
21. Wise R. 1976. The 'septic spleen'—a critical evaluation. *J Clin Pathol* **29**:228–230.
22. Morris JA, Harrison LM, Partridge SM. 2006. Postmortem bacteriology: a re-evaluation. *J Clin Pathol* **59**:1–9.
23. de Jongh DS, Loftis JW, Green GS, Shively JA, Minckler TM. 1968. Postmortem bacteriology: a practical method for routine use. *Am J Clin Pathol* **49**:424–428.
24. Reznicek MJ, Koontz FP. 2002. Autopsy microbiology, p 1256–1265. *In* McClatchey KD (ed), *Clinical Laboratory Medicine*, 2nd ed. Lippincott Williams & Wilkins, Philadelphia, PA.
25. Prtak L, Al-Adnani M, Fenton P, Kudesia G, Cohen MC. 2010. Contribution of bacteriology and virology in sudden unexpected death in infancy. *Arch Dis Child* **95**:371–376.

26. Brooks EG, Gill JR, Buchsbaum R, Utley S, Sathyavagiswaran L, Peterson DC, National Association of Medical Examiners NAME Ad Hoc Committee for Bioterrorism and Infectious Disease. 2015. Testing for infectious diseases in sudden unexpected infant death: a survey of medical examiner and coroner offices in the United States. *J Pediatr* **167**:178–82.e1.

27. Taylor CA, Holman RC, Callinan LS, Zaki SR, Blau DM. 2013. Unexplained death due to possible infectious diseases in infants-United States, 2006. *J Pediatr* **162**:195–201.e3.

28. Morentin B, Suárez-Mier MP, Aguilera B, Arrieta J, Audicana C, Fernández-Rodríguez A. 2012. Clinicopathological features of sudden unexpected infectious death: population-based study in children and young adults. *Forensic Sci Int* **220**:80–84.

29. Fernández-Rodríguez A, Cohen MC, Lucena J, Van de Voorde W, Angelini A, Ziyade N, Saegeman V. 2015. How to optimise the yield of forensic and clinical postmortem microbiology with an adequate sampling: a proposal for standardisation. *Eur J Clin Microbiol Infect Dis* **34**:1045–1057.

30. Waters BL. 2009. *Handbook of Autopsy Practice*, 4th ed. Humana Press, Totowa, NJ.

31. Sunagawa K, Sugitani M. 2017. Post-mortem detection of bacteremia using pairs of blood culture samples. *Leg Med (Tokyo)* **24**:92–97.

32. Bates DW, Lee TH. 1992. Rapid classification of positive blood cultures. Prospective validation of a multivariate algorithm. *JAMA* **267**:1962–1966.

33. Weinstein MP, Towns ML, Quartey SM, Mirrett S, Reimer LG, Parmigiani G, Reller LB. 1997. The clinical significance of positive blood cultures in the 1990s: a prospective comprehensive evaluation of the microbiology, epidemiology, and outcome of bacteremia and fungemia in adults. *Clin Infect Dis* **24**:584–602.

34. Weinstein MP. 2003. Blood culture contamination: persisting problems and partial progress. *J Clin Microbiol* **41**:2275–2278.

35. Palmiere C, Egger C, Prod'Hom G, Greub G. 2016. Bacterial translocation and sample contamination in postmortem microbiological analyses. *J Forensic Sci* **61**:367–374.

36. Emmadi R, Boonyaratanakornkit JB, Selvarangan R, Shyamala V, Zimmer BL, Williams L, Bryant B, Schutzbank T, Schoonmaker MM, Amos Wilson JA, Hall L, Pancholi P, Bernard K. 2011. Molecular methods and platforms for infectious diseases testing a review of FDA-approved and cleared assays. *J Mol Diagn* **13**:583–604.

37. Sontakke S, Cadenas MB, Maggi RG, Diniz PP, Breitschwerdt EB. 2009. Use of broad range 16S rDNA PCR in clinical microbiology. *J Microbiol Methods* **76**:217–225.

38. Skvarc M, Stubljar D, Rogina P, Kaasch AJ. 2013. Non-culture-based methods to diagnose bloodstream infection: does it work? *Eur J Microbiol Immunol (Bp)* **3**:97–104.

39. Baron EJ, Miller JM, Weinstein MP, Richter SS, Gilligan PH, Thomson RB Jr, Bourbeau P, Carroll KC, Kehl SC, Dunne WM, Robinson-Dunn B, Schwartzman JD, Chapin KC, Snyder JW, Forbes BA, Patel R, Rosenblatt JE, Pritt BS. 2013. A guide to utilization of the microbiology laboratory for diagnosis of infectious diseases: 2013 recommendations by the Infectious Diseases Society of America (IDSA) and the American Society for Microbiology (ASM)(a). *Clin Infect Dis* **57**:e22–e121.

40. Hill RB, Anderson RE. 1988. *The Autopsy: Medical Practice and Public Policy*. Butterworths, Boston, MA.

41. Mazuchowski EL II, Meier PA. 2005. The modern autopsy: what to do if infection is suspected. *Arch Med Res* **36**:713–723.

Index

Difco ESP blood culture system, 15–16, 16,
115–120
BacT/Alert *vs.* DifcoTREK ESP/
VersaTREK, 103–104
challenging incubation time, 119–120
comparison to BacT/Alert system,
117–118, 119
comparison to Isolator system, 118
media types, 116
mycobacterial culture, 259
performance of, 117
photograph, 115
workflow, 116–117
see also TREK blood culture systems
Difco Laboratories, 113, 115
DiGuiseppi, James, 16, 85, 87, 89, 91, 91,
92, 94, 95
DNA sequencing from blood culture,
232–233
Dorn, Gordon, 13, 14, 39
Driscoll, Richard, 88

E

Ehrlichia chaffeensis, 305
E. I. de Pont de Nemours & Co., 41
Emory University, 65
Enterobacter spp., 163, 164
Enterobacteriaceae, 27, 28, 34
Bactec 9000 series, 70–71
blood culture media, 157
extended-spectrum β-lactamases, 166
isolation, 45
mortality, 288
PNA-FISH, 223
postmortem blood culture, 302, 304
recovery of, 68
system comparisons, 102–104
Enterococcus spp., 286
Bactec 9000 series, 71
bloodstream infection, 163, 164
Difco ESP system, 119
pediatric bloodstream infection, 167
postmortem blood culture, 305
recovery from blood culture, 173, 174
recovery with Isolator, 118
vancomycin-resistant, 187
VersaTREK system, 126
Enterococcus avium, detection assay, 217
Enterococcus faecalis, 73, 166, 217
Enterococcus faecium, 166, 217

EpiCenter Microbiology Data Management
System, 62, 78, 79, 80
Epicoccum spp., recovery from blood culture,
173, 174
Escherichia, 282
Escherichia coli, 9, 34
BacT/Alert *vs.* Bactec, 102
Bactec 225 studies, 64
Bactec FX studies, 72–73
bloodstream infection, 163, 164
intestinal microbiota, 286
pediatric bacteremia, 152–153
pediatric bloodstream infection, 167
PNA-FISH, 223
recovery from blood culture, 173, 174
recovery with Isolator, 118
European Committee on Antimicrobial
Susceptibility Testing (EUCAST),
229
European Congress of Clinical Microbiology
and Infectious Diseases
(ECCMID), 224
European Society of Clinical Microbiology
and Infectious Diseases Study
Group for Forensic and
Postmortem Microbiology
(ESGFOR), 299
Exserohilum sp., 49
Extended spectrum β-lactamases (ESBL)
Enterobacteriaceae, 166

F

Federal regulation
role of FDA, 190–191
verification and validation of blood
culture systems, 188–190
Finegoldia magna
anaerobe, 164
recovery from Isolator microbial tube,
45–46, 52
Firmicutes, 282, 283
Flagella, 2
Food, Drug, and Cosmetic Act, 188
Food and Drug Administration (FDA),
190–191, 305
Fourier transform infrared spectroscopy
(FTIR), 231–232
Francisella tularensis, 208, 282, 305
Fungal blood culture, 245–254
adoption of specialized fungal-specific, 253